Palliative Care and End of Life Care

Guest Editor

MARGARET M. MAHON, PhD, RN, FAAN

NURSING CLINICS
OF NORTH AMERICA

www.nursing.theclinics.com

Consulting Editor
SUZANNE S. PREVOST, RN, PhD, COI

September 2010 • Volume 45 • Number 3

SAUNDERS an imprint of ELSEVIER, Inc.

W.B. SAUNDERS COMPANY

A Division of Elsevier Inc.

1600 John F. Kennedy Blvd., Suite 1800 • Philadelphia, PA 19103-2899

http://www.theclinics.com

NURSING CLINICS OF NORTH AMERICA Volume 45, Number 3
September 2010 ISSN 0029-6465, ISBN-13: 978-1-4377-1842-3

Editor: Katie Hartner
Developmental Editor: Donald Mumford

Nursing Clinics of North America (ISSN 0029-6465) is published quarterly by Elsevier Inc., 360 Park Avenue South, New York, NY 10010-1710. Months of issue are March, June, September, and December. Periodicals postage paid at New York, NY and additional mailing offices. Subscription price per year is, $133.00 (US individuals), $306.00 (US institutions), $228.00 (international individuals), $374.00 (international institutions), $184.00 (Canadian individuals), $374.00 (Canadian institutions), $70.00 (US students), and $115.00 (international students). To receive student/resident rate, orders must be accompanied by name of affiliated institution, date of term, and the signature of program/residency coordinator on institution letterhead. Orders will be billed at individual rate until proof of status is received. Foreign air speed delivery is included in all *Clinics* subscription prices. All prices are subject to change without notice. **POSTMASTER:** Send address changes to *Nursing Clinics*, Elsevier Health Sciences Division, Subscription Customer Service, 3251 Riverport Lane, Maryland Heights, MO 63043. **Customer Service: Telephone: 1-800-654-2452** (U.S. and Canada); **1-314-447-8871 (outside U.S. and Canada). Fax: 1-314-447-8029. E-mail: journalscustomerservice-usa@elsevier.com** (for print support) and **journalsonlinesupport-usa@elsevier.com** (for online support).

Nursing Clinics of North America is covered in *EMBASE/Excerpta Medica, MEDLINE/PubMed (Index Medicus), Social Sciences Citation Index, Current Contents, ASCA, Cumulative Index to Nursing, RNdex Top 100,* and Allied Health Literature and International Nursing Index (INI).

Printed and bound by CPI Group (UK) Ltd, Croydon, CR0 4YY

Transferred to Digital Print 2011

Contributors

CONSULTING EDITOR

SUZANNE S. PREVOST, RN, PhD, COI
Associate Dean, Practice and Community Engagement, University of Kentucky, Lexington, Kentucky

GUEST EDITOR

MARGARET M. MAHON, PhD, RN, FAAN
Advanced Practice Nurse, Palliative Care and Ethics; Associate Professor, School of Nursing, George Mason University, Fairfax, Virginia

AUTHORS

JEAN BELLO BELASCO, MD
Clinical Professor of Pediatrics, Division of Oncology, Children's Hospital of Philadelphia, Philadelphia, Pennsylvania

MYRA BLUEBOND-LANGNER, PhD, FPNC
Distinguished Professor of Anthropology, Department of Sociology, Anthropology and Criminal Justice, Rutgers University, Camden, New Jersey; True Colours Chair in Palliative Care for Children and Young People, Louis Dundas Centre for Children's Palliative Care, UCL Institute of Child Health - Great Ormond Street Hospital, London, England

MARILYN BOOKBINDER, RN, PhD, FPCN
Director of Nursing and Quality, Department of Pain Medicine and Palliative Care, Beth Israel Medical Center, New York, New York

†KAREN BUHLER-WILKERSON, PhD, RN, FAAN
Professor Emerita of Community Health Nursing and Director Emerita, Barbara Bates Center for the Study of the History of Nursing, University of Pennsylvania School of Nursing, Philadelphia, Pennsylvania

MARGARET L. CAMPBELL, PhD, RN, FAAN
Assistant Professor, Research, Center for Health Research, College of Nursing, Wayne State University; Administrative Director, Nursing Research, Nursing Administration, Detroit Receiving Hospital, Detroit, Michigan

PATRICK J. COYNE, MSN, APRN, FAAN
Clinical Director, Palliative Care Services, Massey Cancer Center, Medical College of Virginia Hospitals, Virginia Commonwealth University, Richmond, Virginia

---

† Deceased.

JULIE J. EXLINE, PhD
Associate Professor, Department of Psychology, Case Western Reserve University, Cleveland, Ohio

LISSI HANSEN, PhD, RN
Associate Professor, School of Nursing, Oregon Health and Science University, Portland, Oregon

PAMELA S. HINDS, PhD, RN, FAAN
Director, Department of Nursing Research and Quality Outcomes, Children's National Medical Center; Professor of Pediatrics, The George Washington University, Washington, DC

BONNYE JOHNSON, MS, RN
Community Health Education and Outreach Coordinator, Department of Medicine, College of Medicine and Comprehensive Sickle Cell Center, Chicago, Illinois

KATHERINE PATTERSON KELLY, PhD, RN
Pediatric Clinical Nurse Specialist, Department of Nursing Research and Quality Outcomes, Children's National Medical Center; Clinical Assistant Professor, The George Washington University, Washington, DC

KATHLEEN O. KREUTZER, MEd
Assistant Professor, Curriculum, Virginia Commonwealth University School of Medicine, Richmond, Virginia

RICHARD LABOTKA, MD
Professor, College of Medicine and Comprehensive Sickle Cell Center, Chicago, Illinois

LAURIE J. LYCKHOLM, MD
Professor of Medicine, Division of Hematology/Oncology and Palliative Care, Massey Cancer Center, Virginia Commonwealth University School of Medicine, Richmond, Virginia

A. KYLE MACK, MD
Assistant Professor of Pediatrics, Division of Pediatric Hematology/Oncology/Stem Cell Transplantation, Children's Memorial Hospital, Northwestern University-Feinberg School of Medicine, Chicago, Illinois

MARGARET M. MAHON, PhD, RN, FAAN
Advanced Practice Nurse, Palliative Care and Ethics; Associate Professor, School of Nursing, George Mason University, Fairfax, Virginia

MARLENE E. MCHUGH, DNP, FNP-BC, RN
Associate Director, Palliative Care Service, Montefiore Medical Center, Bronx; Assistant Professor, Clinical Nursing, Columbia University School of Nursing, New York, New York

ROBERT E. MOLOKIE, MD
Assistant Professor, Department of Medicine, College of Medicine, Department of Biopharmaceutical Sciences, College of Pharmacy and Comprehensive Sickle Cell Center; Jesse Brown Veterans Affairs Medical Center, Chicago, Illinois

LAURA PETRI, RN, PhD
Director of Faculty Programs, American Association of Colleges of Nursing (AACN), Washington, DC

MARYJO PRINCE-PAUL, PhD, APRN, ACHPN
Assistant Professor, Frances Payne Bolton School of Nursing, Case Western Reserve University; Research Associate and Advanced Practice Palliative Care Nurse, Hospice of the Western Reserve, Inc, Cleveland, Ohio

VISWANATHAN RAMAKRISHNAN, PhD
Associate Professor, Department of Biostatistics, Massey Cancer Center, Virginia Commonwealth University School of Medicine, Richmond, Virginia

ANNA SASAKI, MD, PhD
Medical Director of Hepatology and Liver Transplantation, Portland Veterans Affairs Medical Center; Associate Professor, Oregon Health and Science University, Portland, Oregon

DENICE K. SHEEHAN, PhD, RN
Assistant Professor of Nursing, Department of Nursing, Kent State University, Kent, Ohio

THOMAS J. SMITH, MD
Professor of Medicine, Division of Hematology/Oncology and Palliative Care, Massey Cancer Center, Virginia Commonwealth University School of Medicine, Richmond, Virginia

NEVILLE E. STRUMPF, PhD, RN, FAAN
Edith Clemmer Steinbright Professor Emerita, Associate Director, Hartford Center of Geriatric Nursing Excellence, University of Pennsylvania School of Nursing, Philadelphia, Pennsylvania

MARLA DEMESQUITA WANDER, MS
Graduate Student, Department of Childhood Studies, Rutgers University, Camden, New Jersey

DEBRA L. WIEGAND, RN, PhD, CCRN, FAAN
Assistant Professor, University of Maryland School of Nursing, Baltimore, Maryland

DIANA J. WILKIE, PhD, RN, FAAN
Professor and Harriet H. Werley Endowed Chair for Nursing Research, Director, Department of Biobehavioral Health Science, Center for End of Life Transition Research; Member, Comprehensive Sickle Cell Center, University of Illinois at Chicago, Chicago, Illinois

BETSY ZUCKER, MSN, FNP
Liver Clinic/DHSM, Portland Veterans Affairs Medical Center, Portland, Oregon

Contents

There is a need for generalist- and specialist-level palliative care clinicians proficient in symptom management and care coordination. Major factors contributing to this need include changed disease processes and trajectories, improved medical techniques and diagnostic testing, successful screening for chronic conditions, and drugs that often prolong life. The rapid progressive illnesses and deaths that plagued the first half of the twentieth century have been replaced in the twenty-first century by increased survival rates. Conditions that require ongoing medical care beyond a year define the current chronic illness population. Long years of survival are often accompanied by a reduced quality of life that requires more medical and nursing care and longer home care. This article reviews the management of selected symptoms in palliative and end of life care.

Pediatric societies in North America and in the United Kingdom and Europe take the position that children should be part of the decision-making process. Less clear, however, is how that should be accomplished. This article outlines what needs to be considered when taking on the challenge of involving children with life-threatening and life-limiting illnesses in decision making regarding care and treatment and suggests an approach to involving children that recognizes their abilities, vulnerabilities, and relationships with others while at the same time ensuring an ethical and meaningful role for children.

Clinical decision making involves a consideration of multiple factors; clinical options are constructed based on the objective clinical data and evidence-based standards. Technologic advances have led not only to life saving interventions, but also to the use of these technologies when benefit to the patient was unclear or unexamined. The cases of Karen Quinlan, Nancy Cruzan, and Terri Schiavo provide a framework for examining the evolution of clinical decision making, including when to use or not to use technologies such as ventilators and artificial nutrition and hydration, and the role of specific questions in the process. Advance directives are a means to convey patient preferences, however, in the absence of advance directives, skilled questioning can elicit patient preferences. Nurses' roles in clinical decision making are often nebulous but can be enhanced by understanding these interrelated processes, as well as by knowing the policies and procedures of their institutions.

Ensuring patient comfort begins with a comprehensive assessment for symptom distress. The dying patient poses unique challenges for assessment because of the high prevalence of declining and impaired cognition that typifies this population. The focus of this paper is on the practical clinical question: How can we recognize respiratory distress when the patient cannot provide a report about dyspnea?

Sickle cell disease is a chronic illness that affects patients physically and emotionally and can do so at an early age. An ecological model of palliative care that involves improved communication among the health care team, patients, and their families can be beneficial. Open and honest communication regarding advance care planning, disease management, relief of pain and other symptoms, and bereavement and grief are all important for the patient, family, and health care team. Given the multiple acute and chronic complications of sickle cell disease, an approach to care that is holistic and comprehensive may help to improve a patient's biologic function and the perceived health, functional status, and quality of life of the patient and family.

The discipline of palliative care is growing rapidly in the United States but, as in many other areas of medical care, multiple barriers exist to providing such care to low-income patients with end-stage cancer and other diseases. Reports vary with regard to definition and scope of these and other barriers. This article briefly reports a pilot study of perceived barriers to palliative care and related issues in an urban cancer clinic, reviews the current literature, and suggest ways to identify and overcome such barriers in low-income patients with cancer.

As the seventh leading cause of death among people aged 25 to 64 years, end-stage liver disease (ESLD) affects many Americans in the most productive years of their lives. Despite the increasing number of individuals who are dying of ESLD, little is documented about their end of life challenges as the disease progresses. The purpose of this article is to highlight specific challenges for people with ESLD, their families, and their implications for health care providers: ascites, spontaneous bacterial peritonitis, hepatic encephalopathy, malnutrition, altered drug metabolism, renal insufficiency and hyponatremia, hepatocellular carcinoma, and pain. The authors also present a case study to illustrate disease progression and difficulties facing patients, family members, and providers.

Life-sustaining therapy (LST) is commonly withdrawn in critical care units. Little is known about the families' perceptions of death when a critically ill patient dies after LST is withdrawn. The purpose of this study was to understand if families perceived that their family members had a good or a bad death when a family member had LST withdrawn after an unexpected, life-threatening illness or injury. Twenty-two family members participated in a hermeneutic phenomenological study. They were interviewed 1 to 2 years after a family member had died after withdrawal of LST. Most family members perceived that their loved ones died a good death. Although the timing and circumstances of a person's death may be bad in many ways, the actual dying and death can be good.

A main hurdle for end of life research is recruitment of patients. Researchers can enroll interested patients and their families for end of life studies by gaining the trust of the hospice staff, who can make valuable referrals of patients nearing the end of life. Participants in the study should be made as comfortable as possible and not be coerced into the interview process. Once the patients have confidence in the researchers, they are more than willing to be a part of the research process because it can prove to be cathartic to many of the patients and their family members.

The diagnosis of advanced illness often brings with it an element of limited time. Being diagnosed with a life-limiting illness and facing death can evoke many painful emotions including anxiety, sadness, and uncertainty. However, it can also create the potential for profound growth and transformation. The end of life is a time-intensive crucible in which patients and family members have important things to express to one another. Embedded in this time are 2 elements of daily functioning: personal relationships and communication. Having conversations about the relationship and communicating love, gratitude, and/or forgiveness may have potential benefits for the dying person and those considered close and important.

American parents of chronically ill children prefer to be involved in decision making about their ill child's end of life care. Parents trust the clinicians involved with their ill child to make reasoned judgments on behalf of the ill child and to consistently look out for the child's best interests. Parents report that having access to understandable information about their child's health status influences their ability to participate in end of life decisions. This information includes the certainty that all reasonable attempts to save the child have been done and in the best possible ways.

This is a personal story of the lived experience of the authors, both nurses, who as partners face ovarian cancer. We describe the initial impact of such a diagnosis and its immediate life-changing consequences, treatment decisions and sequelae, remission and recurrence, and choices about living with a chronic illness and the ever-present specter of death. We recognize that our experience is uniquely ours, yet we believe it has meaning for all patients and caregivers, as well as the many health professionals who treat, care for, guide and comfort those who bear the burden of cancer.

Preface

During the past decade, "palliative care" became a widely used phrase in health care. Often believed to be synonymous with "end of life care" by many health care providers,[1] palliative care is actually a much broader concept. "The goal of palliative care is to prevent and relieve suffering and to support the best possible quality of life for patients and their families, regardless of the stage of the disease or the need for other therapies."[2] Palliative care, then, should be considered and available for many patients, independent of prognosis.

Equating palliative care and end of life care leads many providers to choose not to make palliative care referrals, not wanting to disturb families or "take away hope."[3] Physicians may be reluctant to consult palliative care, believing they know their patients better than other providers and not wanting to relinquish control of patient's care.[4]

It is incumbent on providers to make referrals that optimize patients' options and outcomes, for patients who are likely to recover fully from their disease, for patients who will live for many years with the effects of their disease, and for patients whose death is a proximal reality. Failure to refer means that patients and families may not receive adequate clinical support in each of the dimensions of palliative care, including symptom management, decision making, and end of life care.[5]

Understanding palliative care more precisely and more broadly than end of life care challenges nurses to expand their view of opportunities and responsibilities with patients. The palliative approach offers a novel avenue of care for patients with life-limiting as well as chronic medical conditions.

Several of the articles in this volume describe how palliative care is readily applicable for those *living with* chronic illnesses that may or may not cause a patient's death. Campbell describes ways to recognize respiratory distress in people whose condition leaves them incapable of reporting the symptom. Wilkie and colleagues' descriptions of opportunities for caring for people with sickle cell disease reinforce the notion that palliative care allows people to live well, hopefully into old age. The principles of decision making described in another article apply equally to healthy people and those who are at the end of life; decision making should be based on medical indications before consideration of patient or family preferences and always with consideration of what is in the best interest of the patient.

Palliative care encompasses end of life care, helping people to live well until their deaths. Hinds and Kelly describe decision making in the end of life care of children. This is important not only because optimal decision making maintains a focus on what can benefit children but also because it allows parents to live well after a child has died. Bluebond-Langner and colleagues complement this information by discussing the role and process of including children in the decision-making process.

When palliative care is implemented, the goals of a patient's care may be evolving. Hansen and colleagues describe the processes of considering options as liver disease progresses to end-stage liver disease. Both symptom management and decision making are parts of this process. Bookbinder and McHugh describe the importance of symptom management in meeting the goals of both excellent symptom management as well as its role in end of life care. Still, too frequently, patients in the United

doi:10.1016/j.cnur.2010.04.004

States die in an intensive care unit, most often following the discontinuation of life-prolonging therapies. Wiegand and Petri describe how this process that requires both good symptom management and optimal decision making can leave families believing that their loved one died a good death. Prince-Paul explores the importance of communication in accomplishing the goals of end of life care, allowing a good death and the healthy survival of loved ones.

Palliative care and end of life care are often challenging to implement. Lyckholm and colleagues describe several of the barriers to palliative care in patients with cancer. Sheehan describes challenges to doing the research that has brought the understanding of palliative care to its current state.

Several of the authors in this volume have many years of research that undergird their contributions. Others are newer to research. One of the hallmarks of palliative care is the interdisciplinary team; several of the teams of authors exemplify the strengths of the interdisciplinary team, and their articles are richer for considering these perspectives.

Our greatest teachers are patients and their families. Occasionally, these are also colleagues. Strumpf and Buhler-Wilkerson frame the lessons of this volume by reminding us that illness is not just about tests and procedures, health care encounters, and disease progression. Rather, these factors are road signs in the journey of any illness. Most often, the goal is cure or long life with a disease. Palliative care can be the means to make that living better. Sometimes, however, that goal cannot be achieved. When the goals of care have to shift because of disease progression, it does not represent any kind of failure. Evolving goals of care are a challenge and an opportunity for nurses and other providers, but it is far more than that for patients and families. Living with a disease, dying from a disease are singular journey for each patient and family. Strumpf and Buhler-Wilkerson allow us to share their journeys. All the knowledge and skills of palliative care and end of life care are important only in the context of patient and family centered care.

Margaret M. Mahon, PhD, RN
George Mason University
4400 University Drive ms3c4
Fairfax, VA 22030, USA

E-mail address:
mmahon@gmu.edu

REFERENCES

1. Mahon MM, McAuley WJ. Oncology nurses' personal understandings about palliative care. Oncol Nurs Forum 2010;37:E141–50.
2. National Consensus Project for Quality Palliative Care. Clinical practice guidelines for quality palliative care. 2nd edition. Available at: http://www.nationalconsensusproject.org. 2009. Accessed February 11, 2010.
3. Fadul N, Elsayem A, Palmer L, et al. Supportive versus palliative care: what's in a name? Cancer 2009;115:2013–21.
4. Lawson R, Glajchen M, DeSandre P, et al. A screening protocol to identify unmet palliative care and hospice needs of elderly patients in the ED. Ann Emerg Med 2007;50(3):S95.
5. Mahon MM, Sorrell JM. Palliative care for people with Alzheimer's disease. Nurs Philos 2008;9:110–20.

Dedication

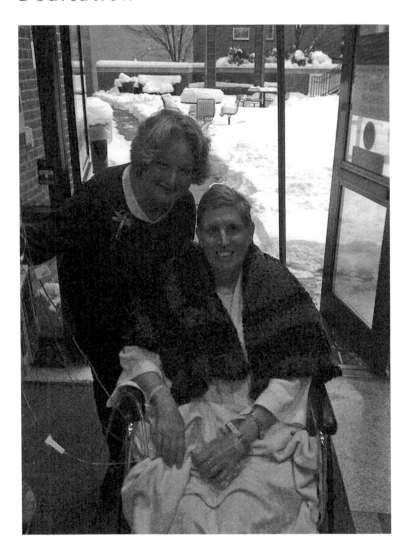

In this issue, Drs Karen Buhler-Wilkerson and Neville Strumpf share the experience of living with Karen's ovarian cancer, which resulted in her death shortly after the article was completed. Nevertheless, readers are privileged to glimpse two lives well lived, even in the face of serious illness. Pascal wrote, "The strength of [one's] virtue should not be measured by [her] special exertions, but by [her] habitual acts." Karen's "habitual acts," as Neville said at the funeral, "set a high bar, without being too serious,

Nurs Clin N Am 45 (2010) xv–xvi
doi:10.1016/j.cnur.2010.04.005
0029-6465/10/$ – see front matter © 2010 Elsevier Inc. All rights reserved.

[whether] with her children, with her students, [or] in her dying." Her standards of excellence, evidenced by myriad accomplishments, worn lightly, included uncovering and telling the stories of our profession, learning from our forebears, and urging us to accept the challenges revealed by our common history. Karen was a generous teacher, mentoring generations of undergraduate, master's, and doctoral students and widely disseminating publications that continue to inform nursing practice and policy. Karen encouraged learning, long before her last testament in the coauthored essay, published here, on her personal experiences of illness. Her commitment to living fully is embodied in her development and implementation, with nursing colleagues at the University of Pennsylvania, of the Living Independently for Elders (LIFE) program, which allows vulnerable elders, all of whom are eligible for nursing home placement, to remain at home. All who knew, loved, and admired Karen remember best her respect for others and her understanding of individual circumstances. Any conversation, in a crowded room or very privately, mattered, and every person with whom she interacted felt highly valued. Karen taught us grace, and at her funeral, the Rev. Thomas Eoyang eloquently summed up her life: "The world has been changed forever because of the work she did here, because of the joy she spread here, because of the love she shared here. We have been forever changed because we knew her, and because we learned from her." In that spirit of work, joy, learning, and love, this volume is dedicated to Karen Buhler-Wilkerson.

Margaret M. Mahon

Symptom Management in Palliative Care and End of Life Care

Marilyn Bookbinder, RN, PhD, FPCN[a],*,
Marlene E. McHugh, DNP, FNP-BC, RN[b,c]

KEYWORDS

- Symptom management • Dyspnea • Constipation
- Fatigue • Pain • Delirium

The literature in the last 2 decades has highlighted the need for generalist- and specialist-level palliative care clinicians proficient in symptom management and care coordination. Major factors contributing to this need include changed disease processes and trajectories, improved medical techniques and diagnostic testing, successful screening for chronic conditions, and drugs that often prolong life. The rapid progressive illnesses and deaths that plagued the first half of the twentieth century (infectious diseases and cancers) have been replaced in the twenty-first century by increased survival rates. Conditions that require ongoing medical care beyond a year define the current chronic illness population. Long years of survival are often accompanied by a reduced quality of life that requires more medical and nursing care and longer home care.

An aging society is another cause of increased chronic conditions. In 1900, life expectancy was less than 50 years of age for men and women; by the year 2007, the average life expectancy in the United States was estimated to be 75 years for men and 81 years for woman. Currently, 12% of the population of the United States is older than 65 years. By 2050, it is estimated that this figure will be approximately 19%.[1] The number of children living with life-threatening diseases and chronic illnesses continues to increase, given improved technology in utero and across the

[a] Department of Pain Medicine and Palliative Care, Beth Israel Medical Center, First Avenue at 16th Street, New York, NY 10003, USA
[b] Palliative Care Service, Montefiore Medical Center, 3347 Steuben Avenue, Second Floor, Bronx, NY 10467, USA
[c] Clinical Nursing, Columbia University School of Nursing, 617 West 168th Street, New York, NY 10032, USA
* Corresponding author.
E-mail address: mbinder@chpnet.org

Nurs Clin N Am 45 (2010) 271–327
doi:10.1016/j.cnur.2010.04.002
0029-6465/10/$ – see front matter © 2010 Elsevier Inc. All rights reserved.

pediatric continuum. **Box 1** lists demographic factors contributing to aging and chronic illness in the United States.[2]

Studies conducted from 1990 to 2009[3] by the Partnership for Solutions: Better Lives for People with Chronic Conditions,[3] a project of the Robert Wood Johnson Foundation (RWJ) and Johns Hopkins University, show that nearly 50% of Americans (133 million) live with a chronic condition. The range of illnesses includes a variety of diagnoses, from heart and respiratory diseases, cancer, and rheumatoid arthritis to conditions such as migraines, arthritis, or back pain from a car accident. Findings from studies performed through the Robert Wood Johnson (RWJ) partnership indicate that the current health care system in the United States is not structured to adequately meet Americans' needs, and that care provided in the current acute, episodic model is not cost-effective and can lead to poor outcomes. Researchers assert that, for treatments to be more effective, services need to be more readily available and better coordinated, with emphasis on early diagnosis and interventions that maintain health status and minimize episodes of acute illness. Nurses can play a major role in reaching these outcomes.

The number of people with chronic illnesses is projected to reach 157 million by 2020. These chronic conditions account for 83% of health care spending: Those with 5 or more chronic conditions have an average of almost 15 physician visits and fill more than 50 prescriptions in a year.[3] Of Americans with chronic illnesses:[2,4]

- 96% live with an illness that is invisible (ie, they do not use a cane or any assistive device and may look perfectly healthy)
- 60% are between the ages of 18 and 64 years

Box 1
Demographics of aging and chronic illness

1. The size of the aging population will reach nearly 20% worldwide by 2050

2. The 65 years and older population has increased worldwide as well as in the United States

3. Improved medical care and illness prevention have increased life expectancy in the twentieth century

4. Mortalities from the young old to oldest old are decreasing

5. The old-age dependency ratio is increasing greatly

6. The aging population is becoming more racially and ethnically diverse

7. There is growing evidence of disparities in health outcomes among older adults, depending on race, ethnicity, and economic status

8. Chronic diseases are the leading causes of death among older adults

9. The pain and disability associated with chronic diseases can diminish quality of life

10. Poor health or functional limitation is not an inevitable result of chronic illness

11. Facilitation of an independent longer life is possible

12. Chronic diseases are responsible for a large percentage of health care costs

13. Psychosocial problems and the effect of chronic conditions are interrelated

14. The American health care system has become more fragmented and challenged by the increasing numbers and complexity of cases of chronic illness

Adapted from Christ G, Sadhna D. Chronic illness and aging. Section 1: the demographics of aging and chronic diseases. The National Center for Gerontologic Social Work Education. Council on Social Work Education. 2008. Available at: http://www.cswe.org/File.aspx?id=24133; with permission.

- 90% of seniors have at least 1 chronic disease but most (77%) have 2 or more chronic diseases
- 11.1 million people are cancer survivors with various side effects from treatment, of whom 65% are expected to live at least 5 years
- The divorce rate among the chronically ill is more than 75%
- Depression is 15% to 20% higher for people who are chronically ill than for the average person.

Nurses, particularly advanced practice nurses, have a critical role in contributing to this goal, and the evolving discipline of palliative care offers great opportunities to influence practice, scholarship, public policy, and research to improve health care for individuals, families, and communities. The World Health Organization (WHO) defines palliative care as the "the active total care of patients whose disease is not responsive to curative treatment... when control of pain, of other symptoms and of psychological, social and spiritual problems is paramount."[5] Since the initial 1989 WHO definition, palliative care experts internationally have worked to clarify the scope of practitioners' roles, and goals of care for recipients. For example, The Palliative Care Subcommittee of the New Zealand Cancer Treatment Working Party[6] developed a working definition of palliative care that targets people of all ages with a life-limiting illness. The goals of care aim to: (1) optimize an individual's quality of life until death by addressing the person's physical, psychosocial, spiritual, and cultural needs, and (2) provide appropriate support to the individual's family and other caregivers, through the illness and after death. The definition delineates the trajectory and appropriateness of palliative care: provided according to an individual's need, whether death is days, weeks, months, or even years away. Palliative care is sometimes considered suitable when treatments are aimed at improving quantity of life.

The definition also outlines the generalist and specialist roles for nurses:

- Generalist palliative care is palliative care provided in the community by general practice teams and in hospitals by bedside staff, as well as disease-specific teams such as oncology, respiratory, renal, and cardiac teams
- Specialist palliative care is provided by those who have undergone specific training or accreditation in palliative care/medicine, working in the context of an expert interdisciplinary team of palliative care health professionals.

In the decades ahead, nurses at all levels of practice will need competencies in palliative care to help manage a large, aging population with the likelihood of chronic illnesses. Alleviation of symptoms is intimately tied to the palliative care goal of maximizing quality of life. Those interested in reading more about generalist- and specialist-level palliative nursing care are referred to http://www.moh.govt.nz/moh.nsf/indexmh/palliativecare-definition.

SELECTION OF THE MOST PREVALENT SYMPTOMS

The selection of 5 symptoms was guided by the results of 2 national nursing surveys targeting research needed in palliative care, including end-of-life care. The Hospice and Palliative Nurses Association Research Agenda for 2009–2012[7] identified dyspnea, fatigue, and constipation as the most prevalent and distressing symptoms for the leading cause of death in the United States: heart failure. The 2008 Oncology Nursing Society[8] (ONS) Research Priorities Survey reported pain, fatigue, and cognitive dysfunction in their top-ranking symptoms for patients living with cancer, the nation's second leading cause of death. Given the results, we selected the symptoms of dyspnea, constipation, fatigue, pain, and delirium.

Our approach to addressing each symptom includes (1) a definition of the symptom, (2) epidemiology of the symptom at the end of life, (3) pathophysiology, (4) screening and assessment tools, (5) treatment and management protocols (medical and nondrug management based on the strongest levels of evidence), (6) translation of evidence into practice (showcasing institutions and systems using best practices to improve outcomes), and (7) questions for future nursing research. Although research on symptom clusters is still in the early stages, we introduce the symptoms with this additional section to increase nurses' awareness of the interaction of multiple symptoms and how they affect prognosis, quality of life, and functional status.

Palliative care experts note that one of the major barriers to providing optimal palliative care is the lack of evidence on which to base that care. A review of the literature revealed that, to date, a few seminal texts provide the most complete accounts of symptom prevalence and evidence-based management.[9–13] We have attempted to provide the strongest evidence available (ie, grade A, randomized controlled trials [RCTs] and meta-analyses [eg, Cochrane Database]; grade B, other evidence such as well-designed controlled and uncontrolled studies). However, if the strength of the evidence is not graded A or B, this does not mean that nurses cannot apply research in practice. If evidence is not clear and convincing and practice implications not definitive, nurses are still encouraged to disseminate the evidence available to the patient care team for discussion of the risks and benefits of the intervention and appropriateness of use in an individual's plan of care. For more about applying research into practice see Wysocki and Bookbinder.[14]

Although experts in palliative care are making progress to move best practices upstream (ie, earlier in the disease trajectory), the literature that influenced our selection of symptoms for this article was centered around end-of-life care practices and research that nurses have championed.

SYMPTOM CLUSTER RESEARCH

The concept of symptom clusters has been defined by oncology nurse researchers as "concurrent and related symptoms that may or may not have a common etiology."[15–17] It is proposed that symptoms can be related and, therefore, share a common variance, thus producing different outcomes than the symptom alone.[18]

The concept is important to mention here because studies have shown that clustering does occur, and, although investigations are in the early stages of testing, nurses need to know more about how symptoms interact and the synergy that produces specific clinical outcomes, as well as the need for multidimensional assessment and early intervention.

Symptom clustering has been examined in several investigations. Nine examples of multiple clusters and pairs relate to fatigue, pain, and difficulty breathing. These include (1) fatigue, nausea, weakness, appetite, altered taste, and vomiting;[19] (2) fatigue and pain;[16,20,21] (3) fatigue and insomnia;[22,23] (4) fatigue, anxiety, insomnia, and depression;[24] (5) pain and depression;[21,25] (6) pain, fatigue, and insomnia;[22,23,26] (7) pain, nausea, and fatigue;[27,28] (8) difficulty breathing and cough;[27] and (9) difficulty breathing, pain, and fatigue.[27]

Fatigue is present in 7 of the 9 examples, suggesting its role as a mediating variable in symptom clusters.[27] The additive effect of symptom clusters is an important clinical phenomenon. In one study, the presence of pain, fatigue, and insomnia together were associated with greater risk of decreased functioning than the presence of fewer or none of these symptoms.[29]

Optimal management of a symptom cluster should include the consistent measurement of parallel dimensions (ie, severity and distress) of each symptom within the same time frame using the same method for measuring responses.[30] This means that clinicians should measure all symptoms independently, at the same time, using the same tools. Two multidimensional scales that nurses commonly use in palliative care practice to identify symptom clusters are the Edmonton Symptom Assessment System[31] (http://www.hospicecare.com/resources/pain-research.htm) and the Condensed Memorial Symptom Assessment Scale (CMSAS) (**Fig. 1**).[32]

MANAGEMENT OF SYMPTOMS IN THE IMMINENTLY DYING

Managing symptoms refractory to treatment in this population can be difficult for palliative specialists. Such symptoms have been called refractory, meaning that they cannot be controlled despite aggressive efforts with standard therapies, and without inducing unacceptable side effects. One approach to management has been palliative sedation. Although there is no universally accepted definition of palliative sedation, it is often defined as the monitored use of nonopioid medications intended to induce varying degrees of unconsciousness, but not death, for relief of refractory and unendurable symptoms in imminently dying patents.[33]

Because of the serious implications of sedation in the imminently dying, its implementation should follow guidelines based on compassion, consideration, and trust.[34] Sedation should be implemented only after clarification of the medical conditions, a thorough discussion with the patient and family has taken place, consent has been obtained, and the goals of care have been clearly established. Once sedation has been activated, ongoing information should be provided to family and staff, questions should be answered, and ethical and legal implications should be clarified.[33,34] For a more comprehensive discussion of palliative sedation, readers are referred to

How much did this symptom bother or distress you in the past 7 days?

Symptom	Present		Not at all	A little Bit	Some what	Quite a bit	Very much
Lack of energy*	Y	N	0	1	2	3	4
Lack of appetite*	Y	N	0	1	2	3	4
Pain*	Y	N	0	1	2	3	4
Dry mouth*	Y	N	0	1	2	3	4
Weight Loss*	Y	N	0	1	2	3	4
Feeling drowsy*	Y	N	0	1	2	3	4
Shortness of breath*	Y	N	0	1	2	3	4
Constipation	Y	N	0	1	2	3	4
Difficulty sleeping*	Y	N	0	1	2	3	4
Difficulty concentrating*	Y	N	0	1	2	3	4
Nausea	Y	N	0	1	2	3	4

How frequently did these symptoms occur during the last week?

Symptom	Present		Rarely	Occasionally	Frequently	Almost constantly
Worrying	Y	N	1	2	3	4
Feeling sad	Y	N	1	2	3	4
Feeling nervous	Y	N	1	2	3	4

The scoring is similar to that for the MSAS Short Form
For the top box (physical symptoms), weights of zero for N, 0.8 for not at all, 1.6 for a little bit, 2.4 for somewhat, 3.2 for quite a bit, and 4.0 for very much. The average of the starred symptoms would be the PHYS subscale.
For the bottom box (psychological symptoms), weights of zero for N, 1 for rarely, 2 for occasionally, 3 for frequently, 4 for almost constantly. The average of the 3 symptoms would be the PSYCH subscale.

Fig. 1. CMSAS. (*From* Chang VT, Hwang SS, Kasimis B, et al. Shorter symptom assessment instruments: the Condensed Memorial Symptom Assessment Scale (CMSAS). Cancer Invest 2004:22(4):526–36; with permission.)

the National Hospice and Palliative Care Organization[33] and the American Academy of Hospice and Palliative Medicine.[35]

DYSPNEA
Definition

Dyspnea is an unpleasant awareness of breathing. It is a subjective experience.[36] Patients often will use the term breathlessness to describe the feeling they experience when they do not think they will be able to draw another breath; this experience is accompanied by fear, panic, and a feeling of tightness in the chest.[37]

Epidemiology

In a 2007 nursing study of symptom prevalence in hospice patients with end-stage heart failure, 75% of patients had dyspnea on exertion and 53% at rest; other studies show prevalence rates ranging from 20% to 60% of all patients with cancer,[38] with dyspnea increasing for patients with end-stage heart[39] and lung diseases in their final years (56%–94%). Patients positive for human immunodeficiency virus (HIV) suffer from dyspnea as a result of comorbid conditions like *Pneumocystis carinii* (now renamed *Pneumocystis jiroveci*) pneumonia, Kaposi sarcoma with lung infiltration, and tuberculosis (41%–68%).[38] Prevalence and intensity increase in patients with cancer (46%–50%) with lung, pleural, and mediastinal involvement.[38,40,41]

Pathophysiology

Understanding the multidimensional nature of dyspnea and the pathophysiologic mechanisms that cause it in patients with advanced disease is important for all nurses.[36] The underlying pathology will determine the most appropriate medical and nursing interventions. The longer the symptom continues, the more likely it is that psychological factors, such as fear, anxiety, depression, and frustration, will influence the patient's perception and the intensity of the symptom. There is consensus in the literature concerning the physiologic response of dyspnea that suggests that the degree of perceived breathlessness is proportional to respiratory effort. Ventilatory demand cannot be met by the body's ability to respond. Dyspnea develops when there is a mismatch between central respiratory motor activity and incoming afferent information from receptors in the airways, lungs, and chest wall structures. The greater the unsuccessful respiratory effort exerted by an individual, the greater the sensation of breathlessness experienced.[42–45]

Extensive research has been done on the pathophysiology and affective components of dyspnea; however, the precise physical mechanism of breathlessness remains elusive. Breathlessness management aims to take into account feelings and physiology and to increase the person's capacity to understand and be understood as a means to improve coping.

Three models that assist in understanding breathlessness can help nurses gain the patient's perspective about the symptom. The models assume that the patient's emotional experience is inseparable from the physical experience. Using a holistic framework, the symptom is assessed in the context of the individual's life, illness experience, and its meaning.[46]

1. The physiologic/neural model addresses neural pathways, biochemical processes, and oxygen starvation. Treatment approaches depend on the capacity of pharmacology to change these processes and responses.
2. The biopsychosocial model includes the physiologic/neural model and adds the person's beliefs, attitudes, and ability to cope. Treatment includes ways to make relevant behavioral and psychosocial changes.

3. The integrative model combines the first 2 models and regards the mental and physical experiences as inseparable.

A report of 10 patient-family units interviewed during an acute episode of living with chronic obstructive lung disease supports nurses' use of an integrative model for nursing assessment. The report describes the dyspnea-anxiety-dyspnea cycle.[47] Patients' understanding of acute dyspnea as an experience was inextricably related to anxiety and emotional functioning. Findings suggest that, given the absence of clear objective measures of illness severity, patient-reported anxiety might provide an important marker during acute exacerbation events. Health care providers are encouraged to recognize anxiety as an important and potentially measurable sign of invisible dyspnea for end-stage patients with chronic obstructive pulmonary disease (COPD) in acute respiratory distress.

Screening and Assessment Measures

Like pain, dyspnea is a subjective experience. The clinical assessment of dyspnea should include a complete history of the symptom. A simple method for obtaining a systematic and thorough assessment of symptoms is the mnemonic device PQRST: P stands for palliative or precipitating factors, Q for quality of dyspnea, R for region or radiation of dyspnea, S for subjective description, and T for timing.[48] **Table 1**[49] shows how the device can be applied for an initial assessment of any symptom in a palliative care patient.

Although dyspnea is a multidimensional phenomenon with an affective component, the standard measurement approach, a simple screen, has also been used. Patients rate a single dimension: the intensity or severity of breathlessness. Three instruments (a numeric rating scale,[50] the 0–10 category ratio scale developed by Borg,[51] and the dyspnea visual analog scale [VAS]) have been used primarily for patients' self-report of breathlessness at rest. Studies of the reliability of these instruments in a cognitively impaired sample or in patients at the end of life could not be found.

The National Institutes of Health[52] Consensus Conference on End-of-Life Research concluded that many existing measures may not be of use among persons with severe cognitive or communication disorders. When patients cannot self-report, observation for signs of respiratory distress has been shown to be more reliable than proxy measures by family members.[53] The Respiratory Distress Scale is an example of a behavioral scale for use with patients who cannot self-report.[54] Further information about assessing dyspnea can be found at http://summit.stanford.edu/pcn/M07_Dyspnea/assess_L1b.html.

Management

Treatment of dyspnea includes pharmacologic and nondrug interventions. For information about other palliative measures, see http://summit.stanford.edu/pcn/M07_Dyspnea/palliation.html. **Box 2** shows an evidence-based plan of care for the patient with dyspnea.[55]

Pharmacologic management

Opioids, most commonly morphine or fentanyl, are the mainstay of pharmacologic management of terminal dyspnea. The effectiveness of this approach has been shown in numerous clinical trials. A meta-analysis of 18 double-blind, randomized, placebo-controlled trials of opioids in the treatment of dyspnea from any cause revealed a statistically positive effect on the sensation of breathlessness.[56] Further analysis indicated a greater effect from oral or parenteral opioids than from nebulized opioids,

Table 1
PQRST. A systematic method for assessing symptoms

P	Q	R	S	T
Provocative(aggravating) or palliative(alleviating)	Quality or quantity	Region or radiation	Severity scale	Timing
What causes the symptom? What makes it better or worse?	How does the symptom feel, look or sound? How much of it are you experiencing now?	Where is the symptom located? Does it spread?	How does the symptom rate on a severity scale of 1 to 10, with 10 being the most extreme?	When did the symptom begin? How often does it occur? Is it sudden or gradual?
First occurrence. What were you doing when you first experienced or noticed the symptoms? What seems to trigger it: stress, position, certain activities, arguments? For a physical symptom such as a discharge: what seems to cause it or make it worse? For a psychological symptom such as the depression occur when you feel rejected? What relieves the symptom: changing diet, position, taking medication, being active? *Aggravation.* What makes the symptom worse?	*Quality.* How would you describe how the symptom. feels, looks, or sounds. *Quantity.* How much are you experiencing now? Is it so much that it prevents you from performing any activities? Is it more or less than you experienced at any other time?	*Region.* Where does the symptom occur? *Radiation.* Does pain travel down your arm, up your neck, or down your legs?	*Severity.* How bad is the symptom at its worst? Does it force you to lie down, sit down, or slow down? *Course.* Does the symptom seem to be getting better, getting worse, or staying about the same?	*Onset.* On what date did the symptom first occur? What time did it begin? *Type of onset.* How did the symptom start? Suddenly or gradually? *Frequency.* How often do you experience the symptom: hourly, daily, weekly, monthly? When do you usually experience it: during the day, at night, in the early morning? Does it awaken you? Does it occur before, during, or after meals? Does it occur seasonally? *Duration.* How long does an episode of the symptom last?

Adapted from Registered Nurses Association of Ontario. Nursing Best Practice Guideline. Assessment & management of pain. Available at: http://www.rnao.org/ Storage/29/2351_BPG_Pain_and_Supp.pdf; 2002. Accessed April 23, 2010; with permission.

with approximately the same results found between patients with COPD and patients with cancer. Doses for treating dyspnea are not definitively established, but are often much smaller than the doses required to alleviate pain.

Because fear or anxiety may be components of the respiratory distress experienced by the dying patient, the addition of a benzodiazepine to the opioid regimen has been successful in patients with advanced COPD[57] and advanced-stage cancer.[58]

Nondrug management

A Cochrane review was performed to determine which nondrug methods relieve shortness of breath and which are the most effective.[59] A total of 47 studies (2532 participants) were categorized into 12 subgroups. The review identified interventions that may help to relieve shortness of breath: vibration of the patient's chest wall, electrical stimulation of leg muscles, walking aids, and breathing training. There were mixed results for the use of acupuncture/acupressure. Other interventions identified were counseling and support, alone or in combination with relaxation/breathing training; music; relaxation; a hand-held fan directed at the patient's face; case management; and psychotherapy. Most studies were conducted in participants with chronic lung disease. Only a few studies included participants with heart failure, cancer or neurologic disease. Currently, there are not enough data to judge the level of evidence for these unique nondrug interventions.

In another Cochrane review,[60] oxygen therapy, administered in a nonacute care setting, provided additional relief of dyspnea in study participants with chronic endstage disease compared with that provided by breathing room air or placebo air as a control. Eight studies meeting the inclusion criteria included a total of 144 participants (cancer, n = 97; cardiac failure, n = 35; kyphoscoliosis, n = 12). Four studies (2 studies with the participants at rest and 2 involving exercise testing) compared oxygen inhalation with air inhalation for dyspnea management in adults with advanced cancer. There was no overall improvement of breathlessness in participants with cancer when oxygen breathing was compared with air breathing, although some patients appeared to feel better breathing oxygen. Three studies compared the use of oxygen inhalation to air inhalation in adults with stable chronic heart failure for dyspnea management during exercise testing. Oxygen breathing slightly reduced breathlessness in 2 of the 3 studies after 6 minutes of exercise, but the effect at peak exercise was uncertain. One study compared ambulatory oxygen therapy with air inhalation on exercise-induced dyspnea for study participants with kyphoscoliosis. The study found that breathing oxygen reduced breathlessness on exercise for study participants. This review highlights the research in progress to test nonpharmacologic approaches but was limited by the small number of studies, the small number of study participants, and by the methods used in the studies.[60]

In a third Cochrane review,[61] investigators assessed the effectiveness of noninvasive interventions delivered by health care professionals to improve symptoms, psychological functioning, and quality of life in patients with lung cancer. Noninvasive interventions were defined as physical treatments not requiring catheterization, skin puncture, intubation, incision, drainage, endoscopy, or pharmacologic intervention, and treatments performed to enhance well-being or quality of life. Nine trials were included; 2 trials of a nursing intervention to manage breathlessness showed benefit for symptom experience, performance status and emotional functioning. Given the heterogeneity of the interventions and outcome measures, a quantitative pooling of results was not performed. Three trials assessed structured nursing programs and found positive effects on delay in clinical deterioration (eg, 6 weeks later compared with standard physician follow-up visits), dependency, and symptom distress

Box 2
Evidence-based plan of care for the patient with dyspnea

Assessment

1. Assess patients at high risk for dyspnea, including medical-surgical patients with acute or chronic conditions, psychiatric patients, obstetric patients, pediatric patients, patients with transplanted organs, patients receiving mechanical ventilation, and patients in palliative care (level VI evidence: clinical studies in a variety of patient populations and situations to support recommendations).

Rationale: Dyspnea affects a wide range of patients.

2. Assess dyspnea from the patient's perspective whenever possible. Use a dyspnea assessment instrument if appropriate.

Assessment should include the following:

(Level V evidence: clinical studies in more than 1 or 2 different patient populations and situations to support recommendations)

- Quality and timing of dyspnea
- Alleviating and precipitating factors
- Associated symptoms
- Physical assessment and pulmonary function measures, as indicated
- Pulmonary factors; for example, hypoxia or increased work of breathing
- Nonpulmonary factors; for example, pain, anxiety, depression, or fluid overload

Rationale: Dyspnea is a subjective symptom that occurs with many conditions and is affected by physiologic, psychological, social, and environmental factors. Because the mechanisms and causes of dyspnea are multifactorial, a good, basic physical assessment is essential.

Treatment of the Underlying Disease Process

3. Treat underlying disease processes as follows:

Level V evidence: clinical studies in more than 1 or 2 different patient populations and situations to support recommendations)

- COPD: inhaled anticholinergic agents and β2 agonists
- Asthma: inhaled steroids
- Malignant airway obstruction: stents
- Pleural effusion: pleurodesis or pleuroperitoneal shunt
- Heart failure: left ventricular unloading, diuretic agents, digoxin, β-blockers, angiotensin-converting enzyme inhibitors

Rationale: Specific cause-focused treatment is always the first line of therapy.

Pharmacologic Interventions

4. Administer opioids orally, subcutaneously, or intravenously, at a dose of 2.5 to 7.5 mg every 4 hours, as needed. Titrate higher as needed to relieve dyspnea. Morphine sulfate (Roxanol SR or MS Contin), with morphine sulfate immediate release (MSIR) to treat breakthrough dyspnea, is commonly given orally.

(Level V evidence: clinical studies in more than 1 or 2 different patient populations and situations to support recommendations).

Rationale: Opioids are believed to decrease dyspnea by blunting the central perception of dyspnea and lowering the ventilatory drive.

5. Administer anxiolytic and other psychoactive agents as follows:
(Level IV evidence: limited clinical studies to support recommendations)

- Diazepam (Valium), 25 mg once a day orally
- Alprazolam (Xanax), 0.5 mg twice a day orally
- Buspirone (BuSpar), 10 mg twice a day orally

Rationale: These agents relieve anxiety or agitation by various actions, depending on the drug class.

Oxygen Administration

6. Administer oxygen for the following indications:

(Level V evidence: clinical studies in more than 1 or 2 different patient populations and situations to support recommendations)

- Hypoxia
- When improvement in functional status is required, especially exercise capacity and social functioning
- Discomfort at end of life (palliative care)
- For patients on ventilation, altering mechanical ventilation settings may reduce dyspnea:

  Lower tidal volumes to 6 to 8 mL/kg

  Increase intermittent mandatory ventilation rates or pressure support

Rationale: Oxygen may relieve dyspnea by depressing the hypoxic drive mediated by peripheral chemoreceptors; however, there is also evidence that oxygen reduces dyspnea by other means, such as by improving respiratory musculature function or by altering the perception of dyspnea. Furthermore, the flow of oxygen over the nasal mucosa may relieve dyspnea by stimulating nonspecific nasal receptors. Oxygen masks generally are poorly tolerated because they are uncomfortable, they must be removed to eat or drink, and heat radiates to the face around the nose and mouth.

7. Use fans to blow cool air across the face.

(Level IV evidence: limited clinical studies to support recommendations)

Rationale: Some believe that this method decreases intensity of dyspnea owing to trigeminal nerve–mediated stimulation of upper-airway receptors.

Other Therapies

8. Adjust the patient's position (to sitting, leaning forward, or resting the arms on a table in front of the patient).
(Level IV evidence: limited clinical studies to support recommendations).

Rationale: Positions that increase abdominal pressure may improve respiratory musculature function. Leaning forward may facilitate excursion of the diaphragm and supports accessory muscles so that they are more available to assist with respiration.

9. Encourage diaphragmatic breathing with pursed lips, and slowed-pace breathing, which may temporarily relieve dyspnea.

(Level IV evidence: limited clinical studies to support recommendations)

Rationale: Pursed-lip breathing slows expiration and raises intra-airway pressure, thereby preventing airway collapse. Diaphragmatic breathing may improve respiratory synchrony of the abdominal and thoracic muscles.

10. Institute complementary treatment modes, such as acupuncture, acupressure, and relaxation techniques (level IV evidence: limited clinical studies to support recommendations).

Rationale: Acupuncture and acupressure use specific pressure points to relieve dyspnea. Relaxation decreases anxiety associated with dyspnea.

Adapted from Spector N, Connolly MA, Carlson KK. Dyspnea. Applying research to bedside practice. AACN Adv Crit Care 2007;18(1):52–5; with permission.

(eg, less breathlessness) and improvements in emotional functioning and satisfaction with care. One trial assessing counseling showed benefit on some emotional components of the illness, but the findings were inconclusive. Another trial assessing an exercise program found a beneficial effect on self-empowerment. A trial of nutritional interventions found positive effects for increasing energy intake, but no improvement in quality of life. One trial of reflexology showed some positive but short-lasting effects on anxiety. This review found that a specialized nursing program to reduce breathlessness using noninvasive interventions was effective in patients with lung cancer whose active treatment had finished.[61]

Translation into Practice

Assessment and management of dyspnea using evidence-based practice protocols has been a priority for nurses. One example of best practice guidelines is available from the Registered Nurses Association of Ontario.[62] This nursing best practice guideline has 30 recommendations: practice (16), education (1), and organization and policy (13). A discussion of the evidence and implications for nurses follows each recommendation. For example, practice recommendation 4.0 states that "Nurses will assess for hypoxemia/hypoxia and administer appropriate oxygen therapy to individuals for all levels of dyspnea." Evidence ranges from strong (1b) to expert opinion (IV).[62]

The discussion of the evidence emphasizes that patients with COPD having an acute exacerbation experience an increase in the work of breathing because of the ongoing disease progression and the acute underlying pathology. Difficulty occurs in maintaining adequate oxygenation. According to the recommendation, the goal of oxygen therapy during an acute event is to reach or maintain arterial blood saturation between 89% and 90% and Pao_2 at 60 mm Hg or greater.[63–68] Oxygen flow rates should be titrated to the lowest optimal oxygenation to minimize respiratory acidosis ($Pco_2 < 45$ mm Hg; $pH > 7.35$).

However, assessing the need for oxygen therapy in individuals with comorbidities such as asthma, heart failure, pneumonia, pleural effusion, pulmonary embolism, pneumothorax, and sleep apnea may require higher concentrations of oxygen therapy. Intense monitoring of their respiratory status is essential.[69] In end-stage disease, oxygen therapy is most often used in conjunction with other therapies, prioritizing comfort with attention to the individual's goals of care.[69]

Research Questions

1. What is the validity and reliability of behavioral assessment tools measuring dyspnea for patients at end of life?
2. When is oxygen indicated and beneficial for patients?
3. What is the efficacy of implementing a nursing protocol for the treatment of dyspnea on level of comfort and family distress in patients with advanced disease?
4. What is the feasibility and clinical usefulness of valid and reliable dyspnea measurements in different settings?

CONSTIPATION
Definition

Constipation is defined as a decrease in the passage of formed stool, characterized by stools that are hard and difficult to pass. Constipation may be accompanied by abdominal pain, nausea, vomiting, abdominal distention, loss of appetite, and headache.[70] Constipation is a common problem that can generate considerable levels of suffering for patients from unpleasant physical symptoms and psychological preoccupations that may arise.[71]

Epidemiology

Constipation is common in palliative care patients, occurring in approximately half of all patients with advanced cancer, 63% of the elderly in hospitals, 22% of the elderly in the home, and nearly 95% of patients receiving opioids.[72]

Pathophysiology

The causes of constipation may be classified into 3 categories:[71]

1. Lifestyle-related or primary constipation associated with low-fiber diet, poor fluid intake, and inactivity, which bring about a reduction in abdominal muscle activity and stimulation, producing a sluggish bowel, also referred to as slow-transit constipation. A slowing of physical activity is also a cause of primary constipation. A lack of privacy or environmental factors, or both (eg, having to use a bedpan or a commode, or sharing a bathroom) can also inhibit bowel function and predispose debilitated patients to constipation.
2. Disease-related or secondary constipation arises from a pathologic condition and includes a variety of disease processes such as abdominal tumor, anal fissure, anterior mucosal prolapse, colitis, diabetes, diverticular disease, hypercalcemia, hemorrhoids, hernia, hypokalemia, hypothyroidism, and rectocele.
3. Drug-induced constipation can occur from a wide range of drugs. These include opioids, anticholinergic-type drugs such as anti-parkinsonian drugs, tricyclic antidepressants, antipsychotic drugs, anticonvulsants, iron or calcium supplements, and antacids (calcium and aluminum compounds).

Screening and Assessment Measures

A nursing assessment of patients with constipation includes a thorough history of the patient's bowel pattern, diet changes, and medications, along with a physical examination. Gathering the history from the patient by asking about his or her most recent bowel movement is not enough. Although a constipation diagnosis may be established with diagnostic tests, such as abdominal radiographs, assessing subjective symptoms by talking to patients is the most efficient and cost-effective way to determine the presence of this common problem.[73]

The patient should be asked a simple screen: "When was your last full, complete, and satisfying bowel movement?" to address the dimensions of effort and relief,[74] and "In what environment would you feel most comfortable moving your bowels?" to address the dimension of privacy and preferences. An accurate descriptive bowel record is essential for determining ongoing assessment and evaluation of intervention and personal comfort.

If constipation is suspected by the nurse, a thorough history and physical examination is indicated. This process would include assessment of the mouth for possible causes of decreased intake of food or fluids (eg, ulcerations or ill fitting dentures); inspection of the abdomen for distension; auscultation for bowel sounds, which may be increased, slow, or absent; palpation of the abdomen for a mass; inspection of the anus for fissures or fecal leakage; and rectal examination, which may reveal a mass, hard stool, or absent stool (may be an indication of an obstructive process higher than the rectum).[75]

The Constipation Assessment Scale (CAS) (**Fig. 2**)[76] is a commonly used tool in palliative care. The scale has 8 items that assess subjective information commonly

Directions: Circle the appropriate number to indicate whether, during the past three days, you have had No problem, Some problem or a Severe problem with each of the items listed below.			
Item	No Problem	Some Problem	Severe Problem
1. Abdominal distension or bloating	0	1	2
2. Change in amount of gas passed rectally	0	1	2
3. Less frequent bowel movements	0	1	2
4. Oozing Liquid stool	0	1	2
5. Rectal fullness or pressure	0	1	2
6. Rectal pain with bowel movement	0	1	2
7. Smaller stool size	0	1	2
8. Urge but inability to pass stool	0	1	2
Patient's Name:	Date:		

Fig. 2. CAS. (*From* McMillan SC, Williams FA. Validity and reliability of the constipation assessment scale. Cancer Nurs 1989;12:183–8; with permission.)

occurring with constipation, including abdominal distention, bloating, change in the amount of gas passed frequently, fewer bowel movements, urgency but inability to pass stool. The CAS has been translated into other languages, including Chinese, Korean, Thai, and Turkish; however, no validity or reliability data are available for the translated versions. Patients with cognitive impairments require more systematic assessments and assistance in performing bowel regimens, including caregiver education when possible.

The ONS Web site offers a comprehensive list of references and instruments to measure constipation in various populations (http://www.ons.org/Research/NursingSensitive/Summaries/media/ons/docs/research/summaries/constipation/references.pdf), and resources for conducting a comprehensive assessment of constipation can be found at http://moffitt.usf.edu/moffittapps/ccj/v6n2/department9.htm.

Management

Because effective palliative care includes aggressive symptom management with the goal of comfort, a preventive approach to symptom management is needed. In the case of constipation, such a preventive regimen involves the dose of laxatives being titrated against the clinical effect. Even if constipation is absent but risk factors are present, a preventive regimen is started. When constipation is present, the findings of the subjective and objective assessment will determine appropriate interventions and the level of urgency.

Prevention and management of primary constipation usually includes increasing fluid and fiber intake; encouragement of physical activities; planning for regular bowel hygiene; and measures to remove factors that may inhibit defecation, such as lack of privacy and poor positioning. Karam and Nies[77] reported use of a bowel management regimen for the elderly that included fluids, exercises, fiber, and a regular toileting time. The program was implemented at 3 levels: mild, moderate, and aggressive. The mild program included a minimum of 1500 mL of fluid per day, abdominal and pelvic exercises, 28 g (1 oz) of fiber supplement daily, 5 to 15 minutes on the commode after each meal, and ambulation of at least 15 m (50 ft) twice per day. The same elements were included in the moderate and aggressive programs, but the amount of fiber supplement was increased to 56 g (2 oz) and 85 g (3 oz) per day, respectively. As a result of this protocol, laxative use was markedly decreased and spontaneous bowel movements significantly increased.

Patients with advanced illness often have multiple factors contributing to constipation. This article discusses the pharmacologic and nondrug management of disease-related and drug-induced constipation. **Table 2** lists medications used for the treatment of chronic constipation.[78]

Pharmacologic management
Laxatives We located 2 Cochrane reviews, one addressing the effectiveness of laxatives for the management of constipation in palliative care patients,[71] and one more specific to those with neurogenic bowel conditions.[79] In the first review, 4 randomized trials involving 280 palliative care patients with constipation were included. Outcomes included patient-reported data measuring changes in stool frequency and ease in passing stools. All of the laxatives used in the trials were ineffective for a significant number of patients, and some patients required multiple rescue laxatives, indicating the severity of the problem and relative lack of treatments to relieve constipation. The report concludes that there is a lack of evidence to support the use of one laxative, or combinations of laxatives, rather than another.[71]

The second review determined the effectiveness of management strategies for fecal incontinence and constipation in people with neurologic diseases affecting the central nervous system (CNS); this population is at higher risk than the general population. This review is relevant to most patients with chronic and advanced illness. Nine randomized trials were identified, all with small samples and mostly of poor quality. Five trials studied the effect of oral medications for constipation. Cisapride did not seem to have clinically useful effects in people with spinal cord injuries (3 trials); psyllium was associated with increased stool frequency in people with Parkinson disease but not altered colonic transit time (1 trial); and prucalopride did not show obvious benefits in this patient group (1 study). Rectal preparations (eg, bulking agents, laxatives, enemas) intended to initiate defecation produced faster results than others (1 trial). Different time schedules for administration of rectal medication produced different bowel responses (1 trial). Mechanical evacuation (eg, digital stimulation, manual evacuation, abdominal massage, rectal irrigation) may be more effective than oral or rectal medication (1 trial). One study revealed that patients may benefit from even 1 educational intervention from nurses (1 trial). The review concludes that there is little research available on this common and, to patients, significant condition, and that recommendations based on the trials could not be drawn. For this palliative care population (neurogenic), bowel management must remain empirical until

Table 2
Medications for treatment of chronic constipation

Agent	Formula/Strength	Adult Dosage
Bulk Laxatives		
Methylcellulose (Citrucel)	Powder, 2 g (mix with 237 mL [8 oz] liquid); tablets, 500 mg (take with 237 mL liquid)	1–3 times daily 2 tablets up to 6 times daily
Polycarbophil (Fibercon)	Tablets, 625 mg	2 tablets 1–4 times daily
Psyllium (Metamucil)	Powder, 3.4 g (mix with 237 mL liquid)	1–4 times daily
Stool Softeners		
Docusate calcium (Surfak)	Capsules, 240 mg	Once daily
Docusate sodium (Colace)	Capsules, 50 or 100 mg; liquid, 150 mg per 15 mL; syrup, 60 mg per 15 mL	50–300 mg[a]
Osmotic Laxatives		
Lactulose	Liquid, 10 g per 15 mL	15–60 mL daily[a]
Magnesium citrate	Liquid, 296 mL per bottle	0.5–1 bottle per day
Magnesium hydroxide (milk of magnesia)	Liquid, 400 mg per 5 mL	30–60 mL once daily[a]
Polyethylene glycol 3350 (Miralax)	Powder, 17 g (mix with 237 mL liquid)	Once daily
Sodium biphosphate (Phospho-soda)	Liquid, 45 mL, 90 mL (mix with 118 mL [4 oz] water, then follow with 237 mL water	20–45 mL daily
Sorbitol	Liquid, 480 mL	30–150 mL daily
Stimulant Laxatives		
Bisacodyl (Dulcolax)	Tablets, 5 mg	5–15 mg daily
Cascara sagrada	Liquid, 120 mL; Tablets, 325 mg	5 mL once daily; 1 tablet daily
Castor oil	Liquid, 60 mL	15–60 mL once daily[a]
Senna (Senokot)	Tablets, 8.6 mg	2 or 4 tablets once or twice daily
Prokinetic Agents		
Tegaserod (Zelnorm)	Tablets, 2 mg, 6 mg	Twice daily[b]

[a] May be taken in divided doses.
[b] Used for constipation related to irritable bowel syndrome in women.
Data from Hsieh C. Treatment of constipation in older adults. Am Fam Physician 2005;72(11):2277–84.

well-designed controlled trials with adequate numbers and clinically relevant outcome measures become available.[79]

Methylnaltrexone In 1 study,[80] subcutaneous methylnaltrexone rapidly induced laxation in 133 patients with advanced illness and opioid-induced constipation for more than 3 days. Patients were randomly assigned to receive subcutaneous methylnaltrexone (at a dose of 0.15 mg per kilogram of body weight) or placebo every other day for 2 weeks. In the methylnaltrexone group, 48% of patients had laxation within 4 hours after the first study dose, compared with 15% in the placebo group; and 52% had laxation without the use of a rescue laxative within 4 hours after 2 or more of the first 4 doses, compared with 8% in the placebo group. Although more research is needed across palliative care settings, these results suggest an additional approach to constipation for patients facing the end of life.[80]

Neostigmine Although not included among standard treatment of constipation failing to respond to usual measures, low-dose subcutaneous neostigmine has been reported to induce a prompt response in acute colonic pseudo-obstruction in patients with advanced cancer. The median neostigmine dose was 0.5 mg (range 0.25–1.25 mg). Four of 8 patients (50%) had evacuation of stools from a few minutes to 10 hours after the neostigmine injection. No drug-related secondary effects were observed. The results suggest that subcutaneous low-dose neostigmine represents a parenteral alternative approach that can easily palliate severe and refractory constipation in a percentage of patients with cancer.[81] Case reports of the usefulness of neostigmine for the management of severe constipation or fecal impaction not responding to conservative measures have also been published.[82] Further studies are needed to confirm the effectiveness of neostigmine as a salvage therapy in patients with severe and refractory constipation.

Nondrug management
In addition to pharmacologic interventions, nondrug approaches continue to be tested.

Abdominal massage A systematic review of the evidence to support abdominal massage for chronic constipation was published in 1999.[83] Four trials, with a total of 54 patients with chronic constipation, were evaluated. Control groups received an active treatment phase of abdominal massage compared with a control phase of no massage or treatment with laxatives. Outcomes included total gastrointestinal (GI)/colonic transit time, stool frequency, number of days with bowel movements, episodes of fecal incontinence, number of enemas given, stool consistency, and patient well-being. The 4 trials included 1 randomized study of 32 patients: no significant differences were shown in outcomes (GI transit time, stool frequency and consistency, number of enemas given, patient well-being) between the different treatment phases (3-week run-in, regular massage for 7 weeks, 1-week wash-out, laxatives for 7 weeks). Two additional trials of 21 patients found no significant difference between massage and control phases for total colonic transit time and stool frequency, although 1 trial found massage therapy to cause significant improvement in the number of days with bowel movements, episodes of fecal incontinence, and number of enemas given. One N-of-1 (1 patient) trial reported improved stool frequency and consistency with abdominal massage compared with the control phase. Results indicate that there is insufficient evidence of the effect of abdominal massage for chronic constipation. The trials were small and of poor methodological quality. No sound scientific evidence exists to determine whether massage is effective in patients with chronic constipation.

A 2009 RCT studied the effectiveness of abdominal message,[84] indicating the positive effects of this intervention. Sixty Swedish participants, with constipation based on criteria set for functional constipation, were recruited from the general population. Subjects were randomized to the intervention group (abdominal massage in addition to an earlier prescribed laxative) or the control group (those receiving laxatives alone). GI function was assessed with the Gastrointestinal Symptoms Rating Scale (GSRS) on 3 occasions: at baseline, week 4, and week 8. Abdominal massage significantly decreased the severity of GI symptoms assessed with the GSRS according to total score ($P = .003$), constipation syndrome ($P = .013$), and abdominal pain syndrome ($P = .019$). The intervention group also had a significant increase in bowel movements compared with the control group ($P = .016$). There was no significant difference in the change of the amount of laxative intake after 8 weeks. The massage did not lead to a decrease in laxative intake, indicating that abdominal massage could be a complement to, rather than a substitute for, laxatives.

Caregiver education Caregiver education has been targeted as another means to assist patients with constipation. McMillan and Small[85] completed a large RCT in which the caregivers of patients with advanced-stage cancer in hospices (n = 329) were taught symptom assessment and management, including that of constipation. Family involvement in symptom management significantly alleviated patients' symptom burden, although constipation intensity remained unchanged.

Translation into Practice

The United States National Guideline Clearinghouse, an initiative of the Agency for Health care Research and Quality (AHRQ), US Department of Health and Human Services,[86] supports the Registered Nurses Association of Ontario best practice guideline in the prevention and management of constipation in the older adult.[87] The guideline has 18 recommendations: practice (15), education (1), and organization and policy (2). Levels of evidence range from level Ia (strongest evidence, that is obtained from meta-analysis or systematic review of RCTs) to level IV (evidence obtained from expert committee reports or opinions or clinical experiences of respected authorities). Eleven recommendations were level IV and 7 practice recommendations were rated level III, defined as evidence obtained from well-designed nonexperimental descriptive studies, such as comparative studies, correlation studies, and case studies. No recommendations were rated levels I or II, highlighting the need for more research in this area to support practices. Level III recommendations can be described in 4 groups.

The first group of recommendations focus on the need for a comprehensive assessment for those at high risk, including patients on chronic laxative use and those taking anticholinergic medications such as antihypertensives, analgesics, and antidepressants.[88] Screening for polypharmacy, including duplication of prescription and over-the-counter drugs and their adverse effects, is often overlooked.[89] History taking needs to include bowel patterns, toileting habits, as well as a detailed health assessment, and medical and medication history.

A second group of recommendations highlight the importance of identifying the patient's functional abilities; mobility, eating and drinking, and cognitive status. Problems in communicating and following simple instructions are common in those with diminished functional and cognitive ability and the frail elderly, increasing their risk for constipation.[89,90]

A third group recommends that fluid intake should be between 1500 and 2000 mL per day, minimizing caffeinated and alcoholic beverages, and that dietary fiber gradually be increased to 25 to 30 g per day once a consistent fluid intake of 1500 mL per 24 hours is achieved.

The fourth set of recommendations promote regular and consistent toileting each day based on the client's triggering meal, with safeguards to protect the patient's visual and auditory privacy when toileting. Evidence shows that the sitting or squat position should be used to facilitate the defecation process. For those unable to use the toilet (eg, bed-bound) and squat position, it is recommended to place the patient in a left-side lying position while bending the knees and moving the legs toward the abdomen.[87]

In summary, evidence supporting interventions to treat constipation is weak. Constipation is a potentially serious problem, is highly prevalent, and yet is still often overlooked and undermanaged. Nurse experts promote the need for ongoing assessment of bowel function change across the trajectory of illness. Given the lack of evidence, nurses' assessments should include a careful evaluation of the causes of patients' constipation, a review of the literature, and a discussion with the health care team about the evidence and benefit/harm ratio of specific interventions appropriate to patients in need.[91] Nurses should be vigilant about medications that can increase the risk of constipation, especially for those patients treated with long-term opioids. Although it may seem a minor complication compared with a life-threatening illness, constipation can have major negative effect on patients' quality of life.

Research Questions

1. What strategies (including assessment tools) are nurses using to assess constipation in the cognitively impaired at the end of life across settings: home, hospice, long-term care, and acute care?
2. Will an opioid rotation (such as methadone or transdermal fentanyl) decrease the incidence of constipation in patients with advanced disease?[74]
3. What are the effects of complementary therapies such as acupuncture, positioning, abdominal massage, and reflexology in alleviating constipation in patients?
4. What is the amount of dietary fiber needed to prevent constipation in people with cancer across disease and treatment trajectories?

FATIGUE
Definition

Fatigue is a complex, multidimensional, subjective sensation involving impaired physical, cognitive, and affective functioning. The term is broadly used to describe a state of extreme tiredness, exhaustion, weariness, or lethargy, which is usually unrelieved by rest; however, there is no universal agreement on the definition of fatigue.[92] Fatigue is qualitatively different from feeling tired, and is not relieved merely by more sleep.

Fatigue may be classified as acute or chronic. Acute fatigue has a recent onset and is temporary in duration. It is usually related to excessive physical activity, lack of exercise, insufficient rest or sleep, poor diet, dehydration, increase in activity, or other environmental factors. Acute fatigue can be a protective body function, alerting a person to rest. It is anticipated to end in the near future, with interventions such as rest or sleep, exercise, and a balanced diet. However, chronic fatigue persists, and recovery is not anticipated quickly. Chronic fatigue may be associated with numerous illnesses, such as cancer, acquired immune deficiency syndrome (AIDS), heart, lung or kidney problems, multiple sclerosis (MS), and other medical conditions. Fatigue can also accompany psychological problems, such as depression, or result from the use of medications.[93]

Cancer-related fatigue (CRF) is now an accepted diagnosis in the International Classification of Diseases 10th Revision-Clinical Modification (ICD-10-CM).[94] There are set criteria to define this clinically relevant syndrome (**Box 3**).[95] CRF develops over time, diminishing energy, mental capacity, and the psychological condition of patients with cancer.

Epidemiology

Fatigue is one of the most frequent symptoms resulting from cancer treatment. Fatigue (84%), weakness (66%), and lack of energy (61%) were 3 of the 5 most frequent symptoms in a study of 1000 patients in a palliative care program in the United States,[96] and has been reported in up to 99% of patients following radiotherapy or chemotherapy.[97,98] Long-term cancer survivors (17%–56%) report fatigue as one of the major symptoms impairing quality of life even months after treatment has ended.[97] In interviews with parents whose child died of cancer, fatigue was the most common symptom, affecting 57% of patients.[99]

Box 3
Proposed criteria for CRF

The following symptoms have been present every day, or nearly every day, during the same 2-week period in the past month:

Significant fatigue, diminished energy, or increased need to rest, disproportionate to any recent change in activity level

Plus 5 (or more) of the following:

Complaints of generalized weakness or limb heaviness

Diminished concentration or attention

Decreased motivation or interest in engaging in usual activities

Insomnia or hypersomnia

Experience of sleep as unrefreshing or nonrestorative

Perceived need to struggle to overcome inactivity

Marked emotional reactivity (eg, sadness, frustration, or irritability) to feeling fatigued

Difficulty completing daily tasks attributed to feeling fatigued

Perceived problems with short-term memory

Postexertional malaise lasting several hours

The symptoms cause clinically significant distress or impairment in social, occupational, or other important areas of functioning.

There is evidence from the history, physical examination, or laboratory findings that the symptoms are a consequence of cancer or cancer-related therapy.

The symptoms are not primarily a consequence of comorbid psychiatric disorders such as major depression, somatization disorder, somatoform disorder, or delirium.

From Portenoy RK, Itri LM. Cancer-related fatigue: guidelines for evaluation and management. Oncologist 1999;4(1):1–10; with permission.

Pathophysiology

The pathophysiology of fatigue in patients in palliative care is not fully understood, but may be related to a variety of medical, physical, and psychological factors.[100] Primary fatigue has been said to be related to high cytokine load (release of large amounts of cytokines from the tumor or antineoplastic therapy). Secondary fatigue is associated with disease-related symptoms such as sleep disturbances, infections, malnutrition, hypothyroidism, and anemia. Identification and treatment of the underlying cause is the first step in treating patients with secondary fatigue. Medical prognosis, patient and family goals of care, and quality-of-life concerns need to be considered when weighing the possible risks and potential benefits of causal therapies.

Fatigue at the end of life may provide protection and shielding from suffering for the patient, and thus treatment to relieve fatigue may be detrimental. Identification of the time in the final phase of life at which treatment of fatigue is no longer indicated is important to optimize comfort and alleviate distress.[101]

Screening and Assessment Measures

Most patients with CRF do not receive adequate treatment.[102] A study involving 576 outpatients revealed that patients who experience fatigue do not report it to their doctors because they believe it is inevitable (43%), unimportant (34%), or untreatable (27%).[103] Patients do not regard fatigue as a valid problem to report unless a health care provider specifically asks.[94,104] This makes assessment of fatigue crucial.

Fatigue assessment begins with a detailed description of its history, development, symptoms, and causes. This information is acquired from the patient's self-report, medical history, physical examination, and review of laboratory tests such as a complete blood count, thyroid function, and imaging studies (computed tomography [CT] or magnetic resonance imaging [MRI] scan). The onset of fatigue, course of the symptoms, severity or intensity, level of distress, and degree of interference with daily activities (eg, grooming, shopping) should be assessed. Factors that relieve fatigue or make it worse should also be elicited. These factors may be emotional (eg, moods), social (relationships with family and friends), and psychological (effect on thought process), and can be assessed using a verbal rating scale (none, mild, moderate, and severe) or a 0 to 10 scale (0, no fatigue; 10, the worst fatigue imaginable). One scale is usually adopted and consistently used. **Fig. 3**[101] shows an algorithm for clinicians and illustrates the multifactorial nature of fatigue assessment in patients in palliative care and highlights the need to thoroughly assess a variety of medical and physical conditions, psychosocial factors, and disease states and symptoms.

As with other subjective symptoms that produce distress, fatigue measurement remains inconsistent. Efforts to conceptualize fatigue have considered patient perceptions of fatigue and changes in performance; to date, there is no gold standard instrument for the measurement of fatigue.[101]

Screening tools, such as the 1-item Visual Analog Scale-Fatigue, provide a clinically convenient but one-dimensional assessment of fatigue using a 0 to 10 self-report scale to indicate severity; however, such a tool has limited validity for evaluating a patient before and after any intervention. To address this deficit, several self-report scales have been developed to provide a more nuanced assessment of patient fatigue. **Table 3**[101] provides a list of commonly used assessment tools in the measurement of fatigue.

Experts note the challenges faced when discussing fatigue (eg, definitions and assessment tools) among varying languages. Although the term fatigue is immediately understandable by English and French speakers, the concept translates poorly

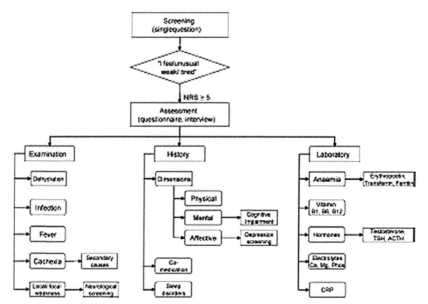

Fig. 3. Algorithm for the diagnosis of fatigue in palliative care patients. (*From* Radbruch L, Strasser F, Gonçalves JF, et al. Fatigue in palliative care patients - an EAPC approach. Palliat Med 2008;22:21; with permission.)

into other languages. Patients in a German validation study related fatigue more with cognitive and affective dimensions than with physical exhaustion, and cutoff points for worst fatigue differed in the German and English versions of the Brief Fatigue Inventory.[105] Translating "fatigue" into other languages requires care and careful methods. Radbruch and colleagues[105] propose a differentiated assessment of fatigue depending on the setting. They recommend that screening for fatigue in non-specialized settings, such as oncology departments or general practice, be done with a single-item question such as "Do you feel unusually tired or weak?" Using a 0 to 10 scale (0, no fatigue; 10, overwhelming fatigue), patients with high scores (severe weakness/tiredness >4) should receive special attention and assessment by specialists.

No standardized tool to measure fatigue is currently available for children. School-age children can use adult tools, but children who may not be able to self-assess, special populations, and adults with moderate to severe cognitive impairment will lack the ability for abstract thinking. Experts recommend assessment by caregivers or staff for these patients, taking into account that family carers tend to overestimate, and staff tend to underestimate, fatigue severity.

Management

A thorough assessment of fatigue should (1) clarify the nature of the fatigue; (2) identify the existence of potentially treatable causes; (3) determine comorbidities (such as pain), treatment of which could result in less fatigue; and (4) determine the patient's goals for treatment. Once causative factors of fatigue are identified, a multimodal treatment approach can be established. More specific assessment of underlying causes may be needed, such as nutritional status, sleep patterns, depression, deconditioning, activities of daily living, and cognitive status.[95] This article presents evidence for pharmacologic and nonpharmacologic interventions for the management fatigue.

Pharmacologic management

There have been trials evaluating drug interventions to improve CRF, but results have been conflicting, depending on the population studied and the outcome measures used. A Cochrane review[106] assessing the efficacy of drugs for the management of CRF identified 45 trials meeting inclusion criteria, but only 27 (6746 participants) were deemed suitable for detailed analysis. Results were mixed, with some drugs showing an effect on fatigue; mostly drugs that stimulate red blood cell production and those drugs that improve levels of concentration. Methylphenidate, a stimulant drug that improves concentration, is effective for the management of CRF, but the small samples mean that more research is needed to confirm its efficacy in improving fatigue outcomes. Erythropoietin and darbopoetin, drugs that improve anemia, are effective in the management of CRF in patients who are anemic as a result of chemotherapy. However, these drugs have side effects, and they should be used under expert supervision and their effect closely monitored.

New drug therapies for non-CRF A Cochrane systematic review[107] evaluating the use of amantadine for fatigue in MS is the only published review on drug treatment of fatigue in noncancer palliative care patients. Four of 12 publications met the criteria for inclusion in the review: 1 trial was a parallel-arm study, and 3 were crossover trials. The number of randomized participants ranged from 10 to115, and a total of 236 MS patients were studied. The 4 studies reported small and inconsistent improvements in fatigue. The clinical relevance of these findings and the effect on patient functioning and health-related quality of life remain undetermined. Participants reporting side effects during amantadine therapy ranged from 10% to 57%, without significant differences between treatment and placebo. The side effects reported were generally mild, and discontinuation of the drug because of side effects occurred in less than 10% of patients. The Cochrane review team concluded that amantadine treatment is well tolerated; however, its efficacy in reducing fatigue in people with MS is poorly documented and there is insufficient evidence to make recommendations to guide prescribing.

Although the evidence base is small at this time, promising results from trials of L-carnitine, a micronutrient that helps the body turn fat into energy, show that fatigue decreased significantly with carnitine supplementation, but without a significant effect on sleep quality. L-Carnitine is usually produced by the body in the liver and kidneys and stored in the skeletal muscles, heart, brain, and sperm, and is found in meat and dairy products that translocate long-chain fatty acids into the cell, where it can be converted into energy. Some patients may become deficient in carnitine because their bodies cannot make enough or transport it into tissues so it can be used. Certain chemotherapeutic agents, such as cisplatin, specifically impair carnitine reabsorption by the kidney. Carnitine deficiency is found in about half of patients with cancer. In preliminary trials,[108] carnitine deficiency was defined as free carnitine levels less than 35 μM/L for men and less than 25 μM/L for women. Supplementation at up to 3 g per day was inexpensive, safe, and well tolerated in patients with cancer, and relieved CRF with no toxicities and no side effects. Total carnitine levels increased from 32.8 μM/L to 54.3 μM/L and free carnitine levels increased from 26.8 μM/L to 44.1 μM/L. A double-blind, placebo-controlled trial of 4 weeks of carnitine supplementation in patients with cancer or

Table 3
Assessment instruments for fatigue in palliative care

Instrument	Items	Example	Scales	
EORTC QLQ C30 V2.0	30 items, among them 3 questions on fatigue	Did you need to rest? Have you felt weak? Were you tired?	4-step VRS: not at all, a little, quite a bit, very much	Translated and validated in many languages
FACT-An and -F	13 items (FACT-F), 7 items (FACT-An), used together with the 27 items of the FACT-G	I feel fatigued I feel weak all over I am frustrated with being too tired to do the things I want to do	5-step NRS: 0, not at all; 4, very much	Translated and validated in many languages
Piper fatigue scale	27 items, behavioral/severity (6 items), affective meaning (5 items), sensory (5 items), cognitive/mood (6 items), 5 additional items	To what degree is the fatigue that you are feeling now causing you distress? To what degree are you now feeling lively/listless?	Adjective wording scales (22 items), open questions (5 items)	Only in English language
BFI	10 items; intensity (3 items), impairment (6 items)	Have you felt unusually tired or fatigued in the last week? (yes, no) Please rate your fatigue (weariness, tiredness) by circling 1 number that best describes your fatigue right now	11-step NRS: 0, no fatigue; 10, as bad as you can imagine	English, German and Japanese languages Other translations in the process of validation
Fatigue symptom inventory	13 items; intensity (4 items), duration (2 items), interference with functional status (7 items)	Rate the level of fatigue on the day you felt most fatigued during the past week Rate how much, in the past week, fatigue interfered with your general level of activity	11-step NRS: 0, not at all fatigued; 10, as fatigued as I could be	English and Italian language versions

Multidimensional fatigue symptom inventory	83 items, short form with 30 items (currently tested): general dimension (6 items), physical dimension (6 items), emotional dimension (6 items), mental dimension (6 items), vigor (6 items)	I feel sluggish My arms feel weak I feel tense	5-step VRS: not at all, a little, moderately, quite a bit, extremely	English, Estonian, Finnish, French for Canada, Hebrew, and Lithuanian language versions
Multidimensional fatigue inventory	20 items; general fatigue, physical fatigue, reduced activity, reduced motivation, mental fatigue	I feel fit physically I feel only able to do a little I feel very active	7-step Likert scale: 1, yes that is true; 7, no that is not true	English, Dutch, French, German, Danish, and Swedish language versions
Fatigue assessment questionnaire	23 items; intensity (3 items), physical dimension (11 items), affective dimension (5 items), cognitive dimension (3 items), sleeping problems (single item)	Did you experience weakness, loss of strength? Did you experience difficulties in concentrating? Did you feel sad?	4-step VRS: not at all, a little, quite a bit, very much VAS for intensity: I did not feel unusually tired at all; I felt extremely tired, exhausted	English and German language versions
"I get tired for no reason"	Single item	I get tired for no reason	4-step VRS (none or a little of the time to most or all of the time)	English language only
Rhoten fatigue scale	Single item		10-point NRS (0, not tired, peppy; 10, total exhaustion)	

Abbreviations: NRS, numerical rating scale; VAS, visual analogue scale; VRS, verbal rating scale.
From Radbruch L, Strasser F, Gonçalves JF, et al. Fatigue in palliative care patients – an EAPC approach. Palliat Med 2008;22:21; with permission.

patients with other chronic illnesses and severe fatigue is nearing completion, and L-carnitine's efficacy in the treatment of fatigue will be better answered with the study's results.

Nonpharmacologic management

Exercise A Cochrane review by Cramp and colleagues[109] evaluated the effect of exercise on CRF during and after cancer treatment. A total of 28 RCTs were included in the review (n = 2083 participants), with most trials involving patients with breast cancer (n = 16 studies; n = 1172 participants). A meta-analysis was conducted, incorporating 22 comparisons that provided data for 920 participants who received an exercise intervention and 742 control participants. At the end of the intervention period, exercise was statistically more effective than the control intervention. Results suggest that physical exercise may be beneficial and help to reduce fatigue during and after treatment of cancer; however, the evidence is not sufficient to show the best type or intensity of exercise for reducing the symptom of fatigue.

Psychosocial interventions Another Cochrane systematic review[110] evaluated the effectiveness of psychosocial interventions and the types of interventions that are most effective in reducing fatigue in patients receiving active treatment of cancer. The review found only a limited number of studies, and these were restricted to patients with advanced cancer, or to patients undergoing radiotherapy. Twenty-seven studies met the inclusion criteria, with a total of 3324 participants; 7 studies reported significant effects of the psychosocial intervention on fatigue. In 3 studies, the effectiveness of interventions specific for fatigue was significantly higher (80%) compared with interventions not specific for fatigue (14%). In 5 of 27 studies specifically focused on fatigue, 4 were effective. The interventions comprised 3 individual sessions provided by oncology nurses, educating participants about fatigue, teaching self-care or coping techniques, and stressing activity management. Of the remaining 22 studies, only 3 were effective in reducing fatigue; these interventions addressed psychological distress, mood, and physical symptoms, and varied greatly in duration and content. The Cochrane reviewers concluded that, although evidence is limited, psychosocial interventions are effective in reducing fatigue during active treatment in patients with cancer. Most promising are psychosocial interventions specifically designed to treat fatigue. These include education about fatigue, self-management and coping techniques, and managing daily activities. Interventions that did not specifically focus on fatigue were rarely effective in reducing fatigue.

Other studies of psychosocial support, therapy, and complementary treatments, such as mindfulness meditation, resulted in levels of CRF compared with control treatments among patients undergoing treatment and cancer survivors with different cancer diagnoses. The lack of detailed descriptions of interventions and large variety of psychosocial support interventions limit the ability to make a generalized assessment of efficacy.[74]

Nutrition Research shows that L-carnitine can be effective in increasing energy, sometimes greatly, in people with a wide variety of conditions commonly requiring palliative interventions, including chronic fatigue syndrome, fibromyalgia, MS, kidney disease, cancer, and advanced age.[108] However, most oncologists recommend complete avoidance of all dietary supplements during chemotherapy and radiation, despite the evidence that there is a high rate of dietary supplement use by patients throughout all phases of cancer care. Hardy[111] points out how this exclusion contributes to patients' negative perceptions of physicians and to the widespread nondisclosure of use by patients. The author's review of the clinical literature shows that some evidence for harm does exist; however, data also show benefit from using specific supplements. As other researchers have concluded, clinicians need to increase their knowledge base about dietary supplement use and assess deficiencies in L-carnitine levels with blood and urine diagnostics.[108]

Translation into Practice

Clinicians should begin routinely to assess the phenomenon of fatigue and offer guidelines for management. Increased awareness will encourage better assessment and consideration of available therapeutic options. Management will improve as new research clarifies the prevalence and nature of the problem, yields validated assessment tools, and evaluates specific treatment strategies. Nurses will need to work with patients and families to develop routines that can be incorporated into daily life. Examples might be sleep hygiene diaries, using reminders for when to set time for bedtime and wake time, routine rest periods, and rest after exertional activities. For some patients, exercise has been shown to decrease fatigue, whereas in others it may exacerbate the symptom. Nurses and other health care professionals are critical in helping patients recognize and report fatigue to health care providers, and in facilitating discussions that support fatigue management strategies. In patients with chronic fatigue syndrome and known deficiencies (eg, L-carnitine deficiency), L-carnitine has been recommended as a safe and well-tolerated treatment that can improve function and quality of life.

Practice protocol

In a recent study in one institution, nurses evaluated process and outcome indicators following implementation of the National Comprehensive Cancer Network (NCCN) Fatigue Guidelines.[102] The Fatigue-Intensity Scale (FIS), an investigator-developed, 11-item numeric rating scale that measures subjective fatigue on a 0 (no fatigue) to 10 (overwhelming fatigue) scale, was used. The FIS is similar to the screening tool recommended by the NCCN guidelines. It has face, content, and strong concurrent validity estimates when correlated with the standardized Piper Fatigue Scale (PFS) ($r = 0.83$, $P \leq .001$) and strong criterion validity ($r = 0.95$, $P \leq .0001$) when tested with a comparable single-item FIS in patients with cancer undergoing chemotherapy, radiation therapy, hormonal therapy, and biologic therapies (Bookbinder M, Piper BF. Unpublished data from the Memorial Sloan-Kettering Cancer Center Fatigue Study Group).

The FIS was completed by patients as a screening tool to ensure that patients had moderate to severe levels of fatigue (≥ 4–10) to be eligible for the study. In this study, the FIS was modestly correlated with the PFS total score ($r = 0.37$; $P = .002$), indicating that the FIS was a simple but valid measure of fatigue.

Research Questions

1. What are the barriers and facilitators to successful implementation of routine fatigue assessment?
2. What nonpharmacologic strategies are available for patients in palliative care and their caregivers with fatigue?
3. Can screening and assessment protocols reduce patient-reported fatigue in palliative care patients?
4. What is the feasibility of using various screening and assessment tools with palliative care patients at varying disease points?

PAIN
Definition

Pain has been defined as an unpleasant sensory and emotional experience associated with actual or potential tissue damage, or described in terms of such damage.[112] Pain is always subjective and always unpleasant and, therefore, also an emotional experience. **Table 4**[112] provides a taxonomy of common pain terms used in clinical practice. Understanding these terms is important to assist nurses in their assessment and management of various types of pain.

Epidemiology

Pain is one of the most feared and incapacitating symptoms among patients facing the end of life. Pain is common in people with advanced cancer and other chronic diseases. Pain prevalence was reported to be 35% to 96% in 19 trials involving 10,379 patients with cancer; 63% to 80% in 3 trials, including 942 patients with AIDS; 41% to 77% in 4 trials of 882 patients with heart disease; 34% to 77% in 3 trials of 372 patients with COPD; and 47% to 50% in 2 trials with 370 patients with renal disease.[113]

Pathophysiology

Pain as a physiologic response is a normal consequence of tissue injury or intense stimuli that produce tissue injury. Peripheral nerves then transmit this information from the body tissues to the spinal cord, where neurons relay the information to the brain and simultaneously trigger reflexes that withdraw the body part involved in the painful stimulus.[114] Understanding the physiology of pain is key to targeting the most appropriate assessment and treatment. Close monitoring of side effects is needed to evaluate the potential additive or synergistic effects of using analgesic medications that act on different pain mechanisms.[115]

Several pathophysiologic approaches can be used to identify the cause of the pain stimulus. This article briefly describes 3 types of pain that nurses frequently encounter: acute pain, chronic pain, and cancer-related pain. An overall image that can assist in understanding the mechanism of acute and chronic pain and its processes is to think of acute pain as fast and chronic pain as slow, based on nerve fiber responses. The speed of the pain is based on the speed of transmission of the communication signals from the origination site to the brain. Acute pain signals are communicated to the brain along different nerves than chronic pain signals. In an acute pain event, A-δ fibers detect thermal and mechanical injury and transmit information that allows quick localization of pain and a rapid protective response. In chronic pain, C-fibers slowly detect mechanical, thermal, or chemical stimuli, and are poorly localized, typically resulting in aching or burning pain.[116] Whether fast or slow, both types of nerve fibers travel on the spinothalamic tract, the main pathway for nerve fibers that communicate pain to the brain.

Acute pain is described as transient in nature, having a sudden or recent onset, and can usually be linked to an injury, surgical procedure, or other identifiable cause. Pain serves as a warning. Patients in acute pain may seem anxious or restless, have tachycardia, hypertension, and diaphoresis, and have the appearance of being in pain. They may also exhibit pain behaviors such as guarding of the painful site, moaning, rubbing, and splinting the affected area. Examples of acute pain include postoperative pain, fractures, and infections.[116]

Chronic pain is pain without apparent biologic value that has persisted beyond the normal tissue healing time (usually 3 months).[112] It can persist for extended periods;

Table 4
A taxonomy of common pains terms used in clinical practice

Allodynia	Pain caused by a stimulus that does not normally provoke pain
Analgesia	Absence of pain in response to stimulation that would normally be painful
Anesthesia dolorosa	Pain in an area or region that is anesthetic
Causalgia	A syndrome of sustained burning pain, allodynia, and hyperpathia after a traumatic nerve lesion, often combined with vasomotor and sudomotor dysfunction and later trophic changes
Central pain	Pain initiated or caused by a primary lesion or dysfunction in the central nervous system (CNS)
Dysesthesia	An unpleasant abnormal sensation, whether spontaneous or evoked
Hyperalgesia	An increased response to a stimulus that is normally painful
Hyperesthesia	Increased sensitivity to stimulation, excluding the special senses. Allodynia is suggested for pain after stimulation that is not normally painful. Hyperesthesia includes allodynia and hyperalgesia, but the more specific terms should be used wherever they are applicable
Hyperpathia	A painful syndrome characterized by an abnormally painful reaction to a stimulus, especially a repetitive stimulus, as well as an increased threshold
Hypoalgesia	Diminished pain in response to a normally painful stimulus produces pain
Hypoesthesia	Decreased sensitivity to stimulation, excluding the special senses
Neuralgia	Pain in the distribution of a nerve or nerves
Neuritis	Inflammation of a nerve or nerves
Neurogenic pain	Pain initiated or caused by a primary lesion, dysfunction, or transitory perturbation in the peripheral or CNS
Neuropathic pain	Pain initiated or caused by a primary lesion or dysfunction in the nervous system
Neuropathy	A disturbance of function or pathologic change in a nerve: in 1 nerve, mononeuropathy; in several nerves, mononeuropathy multiplex; if diffuse and bilateral, polyneuropathy
Nociceptor	A receptor preferentially sensitive to a noxious stimulus or to a stimulus that would become noxious if prolonged
Noxious stimulus	A noxious stimulus is one that is damaging to normal tissues
Pain	An unpleasant sensory and emotional experience associated with actual or potential tissue damage, or described in terms of such damage
Pain threshold	The least experience of pain that a subject can recognize
Pain tolerance level	The greatest level of pain that a subject is prepared to tolerate
Paresthesia	An abnormal sensation, whether spontaneous or evoked
Peripheral neurogenic pain	Pain initiated or caused by a primary lesion or dysfunction or transitory perturbation in the peripheral nervous system
Peripheral neuropathic pain (NP)	Pain initiated or caused by a primary lesion or dysfunction in the peripheral nervous system

Adapted from The International Association for the Study of Pain (IASP) Pain Terminology.

weeks, months, and even a lifetime. Chronic pain can be subclassified into malignant and nonmalignant pain. Chronic pain may accompany a chronic disease process such as HIV, AIDS, COPD, and arthritis. It also can be pain associated with an injury that has not resolved in an expected period of time, such as phantom limb pain, low back pain, and trauma. Patients living with chronic pain may exhibit signs of lassitude, depression, anorexia, weight loss, insomnia, and loss of libido. However, a patient's appearance or behavior may not always reflect whether he/she is experiencing pain.[116]

The clinical presentation of cancer pain varies depending on the pathophysiologic mechanism, which further depends on the characteristics and progression of disease and the sites of metastases. The causes of pain in advanced cancer have been grouped into 4 categories: the cancer itself, anticancer or other treatments, cancer-related debilities such as constipation or muscle spasms, and a concurrent disorder such as osteoarthritis.

Pain can also be understood by its inferred pathophysiology: (1) nociceptive (somatic, visceral), and (2) neuropathic pain (NP; stimuli abnormally processed by the nervous system) (**Table 5**).[48] The types of NP are often divided into categories according to the basis of the mechanism believed to be primarily responsible for causing the pain (ie, peripheral or CNS activity). For further reference and explanation of the physiologic process, readers are referred to McCaffrey and Pasero[116] or Fishman and colleagues.[117]

Screening and Assessment Measures

Optimal pain management is predicated on an assessment of what the patient is experiencing. Because nurses are responsible for assessing, monitoring, and intervening to keep the patient as comfortable as possible, it is critical that they understand the multidimensional nature of pain and how other factors may be contributing to the pain experience. For example, evidence of ethnic group differences in response to pain is quickly growing;[118,119] it is important for the health care provider to increase cultural awareness and sensitivity to pain to make the best assessment.

The term total pain, coined by Dame Cicely Saunders, is frequently used to educate nurses about the need for comprehensive pain assessment, including the physical, psychological, social, and spiritual domains. Pain intensity measures alone are viewed

Table 5
Defining characteristics of nociceptive pain and neuropathic pain

| Nociceptive Pain | | Neuropathic Pain |
Somatic Pain	Visceral Pain	Neuropathic Pain
Arises from the musculoskeletal system	Arises from the visceral organs such as the gastrointestinal tract and pancreas	Injury to the central or peripheral nervous system
Achy, dull, throbbing, sore	Gnawing, squeezing, cramping	Shooting, burning, electriclike sensation, tingling, stabbing
Localized	Can be diffuse and poorly localized; often referred pain to distant sites	Can follow a nerve path or be poorly diffuse
Example: fracture, postoperative, infection	Example: pancreatitis	Example: phantom limb pain, complex regional pain syndrome

Data from McCaffrey M, Pasero C. Pain: clinical manual. 2nd edition. St. Louis (MO): Mosby, 1999.

as a simple screen and should not be confused with a comprehensive assessment, performed by nursing professionals.[120] Research continues to show that one of the main barriers to optimal pain management is inadequate assessment.[121] Given the complexity of patient care delivery systems, professional nurses will need to collaborate with other members of the health care team to perform screening and multidimensional assessments. The goal is to improve early access to specialist-level care.

Screening for pain

A simple screen of pain intensity (0, no pain; 10, worst pain) is used in many settings to elicit basic information, but is not sufficient for any patient with advanced disease; a full assessment of the multidimensional aspects are needed. Some nurses continue to rely on their own observations rather than asking patients to describe their pain.[121] This approach does not allow for an adequate assessment of a patient's total pain and lacks consideration of the patient's perspective or spiritual, psychological, and social aspects that may be contributing to pain and suffering.[122] It fails to capture the complexity of their pain experience. The mnemonic PQRST (see **Table 1**) is a frequently used approach to obtaining a full assessment.

Nonverbal measures Most dying patients are not able to self-report about their pain. Thus, it is essential for critical and long-term care health professionals, at times with the assistance of the patient's family members, to screen for pain without a self-report from the patient. Behavioral pain scales with sufficient validity testing are available for use with these patients. Two examples, the Behavioral Pain Scale[123] and the Critical-Care Pain Observation Tool,[124] are frequently used in intensive care unit (ICU) settings. Descriptors of specific observations could indicate that the patient is experiencing pain. In addition, nurses are using a brief behavior observation tool, known to correlate in research with patients' self-reports of pain: grimacing, rigidity, wincing, shutting of eyes, clenching of fists, verbalization, and moaning.[125]

Proxy measures For those who are unable to self-report, a close family member's assessment of pain should not be overlooked. Although the evidence regarding the validity of surrogates' reports is equivocal, some findings are promising enough that they should be considered in situations such as when a patient in an ICU is close to death. In the Study to Understand Prognosis and Preference for Outcomes and Risks of Treatment (SUPPORT) and in a cohort of 2645 patients and their surrogates, surrogates had a 73.5% accuracy rate in estimating presence or absence of the patient's pain, with a tendency for the surrogates to overestimate patient pain.[126] In a review of pain management in ICUs of patients receiving palliative and end-of-life care, surrogates' accuracy in estimating the exact level of patients' pain was poorer (53%) than patient self-report, but specific factors increased the level of accuracy, including (1) when patients' levels of pain (0–10 rating scale) were at the lowest and highest extremes, (2) estimating within 1 level of the patients' pain, and (3) providers completing their pain assessment on the same day as the patient pain reports.[127] Research has also shown that agreement about symptoms was not dependent on the type of proxy rater (ie, family member, nurse, or physician), suggesting that one type of rater is not preferable to another.[128] Investigators agree that erring on the side of treatment and symptom control is a priority and may help reduce patient and family suffering.[127] Data suggest that an integrated approach that incorporates multiple proxy raters of patients' symptoms may be the most valuable in accurately assessing pain.[128]

Bispectral monitoring Innovative technologies offer nurses opportunities to measure patient responses with increased sensitivity and specificity. Nurses in ICU settings are challenged to measure comfort in patients who may be unresponsive and have complex symptom management needs, including intractable pain and suffering. Providers who are not confident in assessing and managing pain can experience this as an anxiety-producing event. Objective tools are needed to provide rapid feedback for managing comfort in the unresponsive patient. One case report[129] describes a promising measure: the Bispectral (BIS) Index Monitor. The BIS measures muscular and cortical activity using a single, small, flexible sensor that is applied to the forehead and temporal region. The BIS was found to be useful in the titration of sedatives and analgesics for the patient and was also beneficial for the family members involved in the dying process.

In a larger study,[130] the BIS was compared with the COMFORT scale in measuring the level of sedation in 75 pediatric patients on ventilation. In 869 paired observations, a correlation coefficient between COMFORT scores and BIS values averaged 0.61 ($P<.0001$). Although more research is needed, BIS results suggest that it may be an objective monitor for patients who are nonverbal and can aid in symptom management. The ability of the BIS monitor to distinguish between deep levels of sedation may be useful to prevent oversedation of children and adults and useful to help clarify the appropriate target level of sedation, and the pharmacologic management of pain and suffering.

Assessment of pain

Tools for assessment Although a variety of pain scales[131] have been used in different patient populations, little research has been done on the appropriateness of pain scales for patients at the terminal phase of life, especially when self-report becomes a less reliable source in the patient with fluctuating cognitive impairment. Cognitive and language skills are needed by patients to use pain assessment scales such as the VAS and the verbal descriptor scale (VDS). In dying patients and the elderly, simple pain scales, such as the Faces Scale or a numerical rating scale (NRS), may be more appropriate and useful.[132] In a convenience sample of 50 inpatients, 50% preferred the NRS, 38% preferred the VDS, and the VAS was selected by 12%.[133] Twenty percent of patients had difficulty completing the VAS (difficulty sitting, unable to hold the pencil, slash marks too wide, and asking for instructions repeatedly).[133] Each of the commonly used rating scales seems to be adequately valid and reliable as a measure of pain intensity in patients with cancer and the elderly. As patients become nonverbal or cognitively impaired, specific behavioral cues can be used for assessing pain. Herr and colleagues[134] provide an extensive list of tools for this subset of patients, including validity and reliability estimates, scoring, and outlining strengths and weaknesses for readers.

A description of tools for assessment can be found at http://prc.coh.org/pain_assessment.asp.[131] **Box 4**[135] shows a strategy for assessing pain from advanced cancer in the palliative care setting.

Management

A comprehensive multimodal strategy for managing pain in palliative care and end-of-life care integrates analgesic pharmacotherapy with nondrug approaches. Readers are referred to Paice[136] for an extensive review of state-of-the art pharmacologic and nonpharmacologic management of pain at the end of life.

Box 4
Assessment of patients with advanced cancer

1. Assess the pain (persistent and breakthrough)

   Pain intensity

   - Use a standardized scale (eg, numeric or VAS, Wisconsin Brief Pain Inventory) to assess pain relief and pain effect on 0 to 10 scale
   - Response to prior analgesia

   Pain quality

   - Location
   - Description (sharp, dull, stabbing, aching, burning, stinging, pins and needles)
   - Onset and temporal pattern
   - Aggravating and relieving factors
   - Effect of pain

2. Assess the cancer

   Disease location

   - Location of primary and metastatic lesions
   - Response to prior anticancer therapy
   - Cancer-related organ damage

   Benefit or burden of further anticancer therapy

   - Local: palliative surgery or radiation therapy
   - Systemic: hormones, chemotherapy, targeted therapy, immunotherapy

   Prognosis

   - Final hours
   - Hours to days
   - Days to weeks
   - Weeks to months

   Goals of cancer care

3. Assess concurrent medical conditions

   Constraints on further anticancer therapy

   Constraints on analgesic and coanalgesic therapy

   Prior or new sources of pain

4. Assess psychosocial status

   Preexisting psychopathology

   Adjustment to cancer

   Adjustment to pain

   History of substance abuse

   Effectiveness of support system

From Ferrell B, Levy M, Paice J. Managing pain from advanced cancer in the palliative care setting. Clin J Oncol Nurs 2008;12(4):575–81; with permission.

Pharmacologic management

The extensively validated WHO analgesic ladder[5] offers a stepwise approach to the use of analgesic drugs. It suggests starting with a nonopioid drug (acetaminophen or a nonsteroidal antiinflammatory drug [NSAID]), and, if pain is insufficiently controlled, progressing to a combination opioid (eg, oxycodone plus acetaminophen). If required, the next step indicates a strong opioid (eg, morphine, hydromorphone, buprenorphine, hydrocodone, tramadol, fentanyl, methadone). Analgesics may be combined with adjuvant drugs, such as corticosteroids, anticonvulsants, tricyclic antidepressants, or bisphosphonates, for specific pain syndromes. If used correctly, the WHO ladder has been shown to lead to adequate control of cancer-related pain in 70% to 100% of patients.[137] Acetaminophen is contraindicated in patients with liver disease and 4 g/d is the dose limit for prolonged use. NSAIDs increase the risk of renal failure and GI bleeding and are particularly risky in the elderly, for whom opioid analgesics are usually a safer option. Meperidine, once a widely used opioid analgesic, is gradually being restricted in hospital formularies. Meperidine is not recommended in the treatment of chronic pain. Normeperidine (an active metabolite of meperidine and a CNS stimulant) may accumulate and precipitate anxiety, tremors, or seizures. Consultation with a palliative care specialist or anesthesiologist is recommended for patients for whom the WHO ladder does not lead to effective pain relief.[138]

NSAIDs NSAIDs are frequently used in the management of various chronic pain syndromes. However, evidence is accumulating on the potential toxicities and efficacy of NSAIDs; clear recommendations are lacking to guide the appropriate use of these drugs. Major toxicities typically occur within the early months of treatment. Cardiovascular and GI adverse events are the most frequent. Educating patients and carers in astute screening and monitoring for this adverse effect is a critical patient-education activity. Consensus recommendations have been published.[139] **Box 5**[135] suggests several coanalgesics, including NSAIDs, for cancer pain management. Researchers caution clinicians to err on the side of conservatism before selecting any analgesic, weighing patient benefits, on a case-by-case basis.

Opioid analgesics Because the first-line treatment of severe pain is opioid medication, expertise in the management of opioid analgesics is the single most important factor in the successful treatment of the patient's pain. Onset and duration of action vary based on the medication and route of administration, and the nurse needs to be knowledgeable about both. An understanding of the type of pain medication, its action, duration, and side effects can improve the patient's pain management, as can knowing the most efficacious route to use.

Nurses need to be aware of several important concepts regarding opioid use. One is the concept of breakthrough pain, which typically refers to a transitory flare-up of pain. Two types of breakthrough pain are incident pain and end-of-dose failure. Incident pain occurs spontaneously without warning, or as a result of an identifiable event, such as coughing, movement onto a stretcher, or turning in bed. The pain varies in duration and frequency. It may be slow or sudden in onset. End-of-dose failure occurs when pain returns at the end of the dosing interval. This pain is common with patients receiving around-the-clock (ATC) analgesics.

Next is the concept of scheduled ATC dosing, rather than dosing as needed. This dosing is intended to maintain stable analgesic blood levels. Consideration of the duration of the opioid effect, for short- and long-acting opioids, is essential in managing chronic pain. Short-acting opioids are useful when immediate relief of pain is needed, such as in the management of acute, severe pain, and episodes of breakthrough pain. With long-acting opioids, oral drugs allow dosing 1 to 3 times

---

Box 5
Coanalgesic therapy for common cancer pain syndromes

Oral NSAIDs

- Choline magnesium trisalicylate 1500 mg orally twice a day
- Ibuprofen 800 mg orally three times a day
- Naproxen 500 mg orally three times a day

Parenteral or enteral NSAIDs

- Ketorolac 15 to 30 mg intravenously every 6 hours (<5 days)
- Indomethacin 50 mg via the rectum every 6 to 8 hours

Corticosteroids

- Dexamethasone 4 to 8 mg orally 2 to 3 times a day
- Methylprednisolone 16 to 32 mg orally 2 to 3 times a day
- Dexamethasone 10 to 20 mg intravenously every 6 hours
- Methylprednisolone 40 to 80 mg intravenously every 6 hours

Tricyclic antidepressants

- Nortriptyline 100 to 150 mg orally at bedtime
- Desipramine 100 to 300 mg orally at bedtime

Anticonvulsants

- Gabapentin 300 to 900 mg orally 3 to 4 times a day
- Carbamazepine 200 mg orally 2 to 4 times a day
- Clonazepam 0.25 to 0.5 mg orally 3 times a day

Antispasticity drug

- Baclofen 5 to 30 mg orally 2 to 3 times a day

Local anesthetic

- Topical lidocaine 1 to 3 patches every day, 12 hours on and 12 hours off

Pamidronate 90 mg intravenously every 3 to 4 weeks

Zoledronic acid 4 mg intravenously every 4 to 6 weeks

Calcitonin 200 IU intravenously or intranasal twice a day

Scopolamine 0.4 mg intravenously or subcutaneously every 4 hours

Octreotide 50 to 100 μg subcutaneously 2 to 3 times a day

From Ferrell B, Levy M, Paice J. Managing pain from advanced cancer in the palliative care setting. Clin J Oncol Nurs 2008;12(4):575–81; with permission.

---

per day; transdermal drugs allow dosing every 2 to 3 days. Usually, steady state is approached with these formulations within a few days and dose adjustments are best made in this time frame.

Third is the concept of rescue doses. Short-acting or immediate-release opioids are usually used for a limited period to treat acute pain or to help identify a useful starting dose for a long-acting drug. These short-acting drugs are often the same medications that are used for acute pain management. They can be useful as supplemental doses given as needed to patients who are receiving a concomitant long-acting drug. This episodic use for breakthrough or other acute pain is an approach known as rescue dosing. The rescue dose is usually in the range of 5% to 15% of the total daily dose.[140]

A fourth concept is gradual adjustment, or titration, of the dose until a favorable balance between pain relief and side effects is attained. If this favorable balance is not possible with one drug, a rotation to another opioid might be considered. Nurses are critical to the process of reaching this balance efficiently and effectively through monitoring and providing feedback about pain relief and dose-limiting side effects. Once the opioid dose has been titrated to maximal analgesic effect, a nonopioid analgesic or an adjuvant medication may be added if necessary.

It is imperative that the nurse thoroughly assess the patient to be able to intervene when pain is not controlled. Patients are often undertreated with opioids because the clinician may not order enough, the assessing RN may not give the opioid frequently enough, and the patient may not request it enough. Nursing assessment of the patient's pain, the response to treatment, and documentation of these are ongoing. Collaboration with the prescriber to adjust the medication as needed is also ongoing.[116] Information about determining dose calculations for ongoing pain management, rescue doses, and titrating of opioids can be found at http://stoppain. org/pcd/content/forpros/other.asp.

Other concepts encountered in clinical practice when caring for patients with chronic pain receiving opioids are tolerance, physical dependence, and opioid addiction or addiction disease. McCaffrey and Pasero[116] provide an expert resource for nurses caring for patients with pain across the trajectory of illness and across settings. Clinicians have become increasingly aware of the need to assess for an active or previous history of substance use in palliative care and end of life. Caring for patients with addiction disease and their families can be extremely challenging. A comprehensive history of the patient and family and a patient physical examination are required. Nurses need to be knowledgeable about these terms when working with patients on opioid therapy, especially at the end of life. The investigators emphasize that tolerance to opioids and physical dependence on opioids are not the same as addiction to opioids.

Tolerance is a normal physiologic response that occurs with regular administration of an opioid; tolerance consists of a decrease in 1 or more effects of the opioid (eg, decreased analgesia, sedation, or respiratory depression). It cannot be equated with addictive disease. In contrast, pseudotolerance is the misconception that the need for increasing doses of a drug is the result of tolerance rather than other factors.

Physical dependence is a normal response that occurs with repeated administration of the opioid for more than 2 weeks; it cannot be equated with addictive disease. Physical dependence is a state of adaptation that is manifested by the occurrence of withdrawal symptoms when the opioid is suddenly stopped, rapidly reduced, or an antagonist is given.

Opioid addiction, or addictive disease, is a chronic neurologic and biologic disease. Its development and manifestations are influenced by genetic, psychosocial, and environmental factors. No single cause of addiction, such as taking an opioid for pain relief, has been found. Addiction is characterized by behaviors that include 1 or more of the following: impaired control of drug use, compulsive use, continued use despite harm, and craving.[116] In contrast, pseudoaddiction is the false assumption of addiction in a patient who is seeking pain relief.

Special populations, such as individuals with histories of substance abuse and those participating in methadone maintenance programs, are at risk for being undertreated. A key concept for nurses caring for those with active or previous histories of substance abuse is that pain and all of its dimensions cannot be proven. The phrase "pain is what the patient says it is," coined by Margo McCaffrey decades ago, remains a core principle for nurses and all providers caring for patients with pain, and especially patients at the end of life. Patients must be believed for therapeutic relationships to be effective.

Oral morphine for cancer pain   Oral morphine is an effective opioid for the relief of cancer pain and is considered the gold standard for relieving moderate to severe pain. A Cochrane review of 54 studies (3749 participants)[141] of immediate-release and modified-release morphine revealed that, despite design limitations related to the formulations being tested and comparator drugs, morphine gives good relief for cancer pain. As with other opioids, morphine has unwanted effects, mainly constipation, and nausea and vomiting. The review reinforced the view that it is possible to use modified-release morphine to titrate to analgesic effect. There is limited evidence to suggest that transmucosal fentanyl provides more rapid pain relief for breakthrough pain compared with morphine.

Methadone for cancer pain   Like morphine, methadone is an opioid drug that can be given by mouth as liquid, tablet, or capsule, via the rectum as a suppository, or injected into the vein, muscle, or under the skin. A Cochrane review[142] of 9 RCTs was performed to determine how effectively methadone relieves cancer pain and how well tolerated this treatment is for patients with cancer. The investigators concluded that methadone has a similar efficacy to morphine in treating cancer pain; methadone is no more effective than morphine for cancer-related, nerve-related pain; and methadone has a similar side effect profile; but these side effects may become more prominent with repeated dosing.

Patients receiving methadone for chronic pain require increased monitoring of side effects. Although the half-life of methadone, 24 to 36 hours or longer, which allows for longer dosing intervals, an 8-hour dosing schedule is recommended for pain control. Despite the advantages of lower cost and its long-acting properties, much is unknown about the dosing ratio between methadone and morphine, the gold standard equivalent, or the safest and most effective time course for conversion from another opioid to methadone. With methadone, drug accumulation can occur before achieving steady state, putting patients at high risk for oversedation and respiratory depression. It is recommended that methadone be prescribed by experienced pain specialists. The nurses' role in understanding the mechanism and side effects of methadone administration and of close monitoring of these potentially life-threatening side effects is essential in providing safe and effective pain management.[136]

Adjuvant analgesics   Adjuvant analgesics are drugs for which the initial use was not for pain but for other conditions. They are a diverse group of drugs that includes antidepressants and anticonvulsants (see **Box 5**).[135,136] They may be added to pharmacologic regimens to enhance analgesia or may be trialed alone. Readers are referred to http://www.StopPain.org for more information about these options.

Local anesthetics   Local anesthetics can be given orally, topically, intravenously, subcutaneously, or spinally. Systemic administration of local anesthetic agents to relieve NP has shown promising results. Efficacy and safety were evaluated in a Cochrane review of 27 randomized trials.[143] Nineteen trials had data suitable for meta-analysis (n = 706 patients in total). Lidocaine and mexiletine were superior to placebo and equal to morphine, gabapentin, amitriptyline, and amantadine for NP. The therapeutic benefit was more consistent for peripheral pain from trauma and diabetes and central pain. The most common adverse effects of lidocaine and mexiletine were drowsiness, fatigue, nausea, and dizziness. The investigators concluded that lidocaine and mexiletine produced no major adverse events in controlled clinical trials, were superior to placebo to relieve NP, and were as effective as other analgesics used for this condition.

Nurses at the bedside and management levels are needed to offer patients these opportunities. Nurses can promote these therapies by assisting in careful preparation of policies and procedures, including monitoring guidelines and patient education, for opioid administration of epidural and intrathecal lidocaine or bupivacaine trials aimed at reducing NP.[136]

Ketamine Ketamine, an anesthetic agent, is used by pain specialists to improve analgesia when opioids alone are ineffective; however, evidence for its effectiveness is limited. Two small trials suggest that when ketamine is given with morphine it may help to control cancer pain, but the benefits and harms (eg, cognitive changes) of adding ketamine to strong opioids such as morphine are not yet established, and data are insufficient to assess the effectiveness of ketamine in oncology settings.[144]

As palliative care treatment begins closer to time of diagnosis to improve quality of life rather than end of life alone, drugs such as ketamine show promise. In outpatient settings, ketamine is beginning to show its usefulness as an analgesic to treat nonresponsive NP; however, it is not widely administered because of fear of side effects such as hallucinations and other cognitive disturbances. A retrospective chart review was conducted of 13 outpatients with NP receiving low-dose intravenous or subcutaneous ketamine infusions for up to 8 weeks under close supervision by home health care personnel.[145] Using a 10-point VAS, 11 of 13 patients (85%) reported a significant decrease in pain from the start of infusion treatment to the end. Side effects were minimal and not severe enough to deter treatment. Prolonged analgesic doses of ketamine infusions were safe for the small sample studied. The results suggest that ketamine may provide a reasonable alternative treatment of nonresponsive NP in ambulatory outpatients.

Bisphosphonates Bisphosphonates affect the way bone develops, and they are proving useful in treating pain in patients with bone metastases. They can reduce pain, hypercalcemia, and skeletal morbidity associated with breast cancer and multiple myeloma. A review by Wong and Wiffen[146] showed that bisphosphonates have some effect but are not as useful as strong analgesics (such as morphine) or radiotherapy. Although there is insufficient evidence to recommend bisphosphonates for immediate effect as a first-line therapy, they should be considered when analgesics or radiotherapy are inadequate for the management of painful bone metastases.

Palliative care patients may be candidates, throughout the disease trajectory, for various multimodal therapies, including opioids, adjuvants, bisphosphonates, and nondrug approaches. Nurses seeking more information on these topics are referred to http://www.aspmn.org.

Nondrug approaches
Single fraction versus multifraction radiotherapy Metastasis to the bone is common with many malignancies. These conditions may be associated with severe pain, compression of the spinal cord, and the potential for bone fracture. A Cochrane review team performed a meta-analysis evaluating whether a single fraction of radiotherapy is better than multifractions of radiotherapy for alleviating the symptoms.[147] The primary sites of disease were prostate, breast, or lung. The investigators concluded that single-fraction radiotherapy was as effective as multifraction radiotherapy in relieving metastatic bone pain. Spinal cord compression rates were similar for both arms.

Transcutaneous electrical nerve stimulation The use of transcutaneous electrical nerve stimulation (TENS) in the management of chronic pain is widespread; however, the analgesic effectiveness of TENS remains uncertain. A Cochrane review identified 124 studies using TENS; 25 met the inclusion criteria for evaluation in the review, but data were insufficient for a meta-analysis.[148] New studies of rigorous design and adequate size are needed before any evidence-based recommendations can be made.

Cognitive behavioral techniques Palliative care patients who are cognitively intact and can participate in treatment may experience improved pain control with cognitive behavioral techniques (CBT). In a review by Devine and Westlake,[149] psychoeducational care was shown to benefit adults with cancer in relation to pain; however, the reviewers could not determine the most effective of the various types of psychoeducational care. Two RCTs in 368 patients with cancer with and without chemotherapy showed that standard CBT and profile-tailored CBT reduced pain severity compared with usual therapy. Tailored CBT was better in the short-term (at 1 month), and patients reported less pain interference with physical symptoms, activities, and relationships, but standard CBT proved to be more effective at 6 months, with patients reporting significant improvements in symptom distress and mental quality of life.[150] In another meta-analysis of CBT techniques with patients with breast cancer, 7 studies found that CBT reduced pain in 69% of participants compared with control groups. Interventions included relaxation (±visualization, cognitive restructuring, coping skills training, problem solving, or imagery) and hypnosis. Individual versus group CBT did not produce larger effect sizes, and the amount of patient contact was not significantly correlated with effect size on distress and pain outcomes.[150–152]

Music for pain relief Integrating music with supportive care of the dying is becoming more common in hospice and palliative care programs. The use of music as an adjunct support service is an example of how the multidisciplinary teams are addressing the total person and the family. Music is being used at different stages of the support continuum, ranging from stress relief for the healthy, to bedside support for the acutely dying, at memorial services, and as part of supportive care for grief recovery.

A Cochrane review[153] of 51 studies, involving 1867 subjects, was conducted to evaluate the effect of music on acute, chronic, or cancer pain intensity, pain relief, and analgesic requirements. Reviewers found that music reduced pain, increased the number of patients who reported at least 50% pain relief, and reduced requirements for morphinelike analgesics. However, because the magnitude of these positive effects is small, the clinical relevance of music for pain relief in clinical practice is unclear. The reviewers concluded that music should not be considered as a primary mode for pain relief and that clinicians should be aware of music's limited usefulness to decrease pain or analgesic requirements. Because the review was limited to assessing only the effect of music on pain indicators and opioid requirements, the effect of music on other outcomes, such as anxiety, is not known and needs to be investigated. In addition, the combination of music and other nonpharmacologic therapies could have a synergistic effect to produce clinically important benefits on pain intensity or analgesic requirements, thus deserving further evaluation.

Reminders A large RCT (more than 300 nurses managing 637 people with cancer in a home care setting) found that nurse-targeted, patient-specific, 1-time e-mail reminders, highlighting 6 pain-specific clinical recommendations, significantly improved patients' pain intensity scores compared with controls.[154] Although this large RCT shows promise that evidence-based reminders may improve pain management, further research is needed to establish the validity of reminder features to reliably predict clinically worthwhile improvements in care. More recently, a review of 32 studies[155] reported that computer reminders achieved small to modest improvements in care, with a median improvement of 4.2% (interquartile range [IQR] 0.8%–18.8%). Even using the best outcome from each trial, the median improvement was only 5.6% (IQR 2.0%–19.2%). These changes are less than the thresholds for clinically significant improvements specified in most trials, and they are smaller than the improvements generally expected from computerized order entry and electronic medical record systems. These improvements are also no larger than those observed for paper-based reminders.

Complementary and alternative medicine Complementary and alternative medicine (CAM) may help decrease pain, anxiety, and other symptoms at the end of life, thereby enhancing patients' and family members' quality of life. CAM services include massage, music therapy, and energy healing. Volunteers typically provide these services, because hospice benefits do not pay for them. The National Center for Complementary and Alternative Medicine has not specified end-of-life guidelines; however, it supports auricular acupuncture, therapeutic touch, and hypnosis as useful in managing cancer-related symptoms and for palliative care.[156]

Massage Systematic reviews and additional RCTs found promising results for massage with or without aromatherapy, reflexology, hypnosis, imagery, support groups, acupuncture, healing touch, and electromyogram biofeedback-assisted relaxation sessions. However, the overall quality of these studies was too low to draw definite conclusions.[157–160]

Chinese herbal therapies Traditional Chinese medicine (TCM), including herbal therapies, is becoming increasingly popular in the West and elsewhere. In another systematic review of 41 RCTs, no significant differences between Chinese herbal medicines and analgesic drug treatment were found.[161] Results suggest that Chinese herbal medicine may be useful for managing cancer pain, at least for short-term application. The products evaluated seem safe, with no serious adverse effects reported. There seems to be a widely applied and established practice and a significant body of practical clinical experience for the use of herbal preparations for the TCM treatment of cancer pain, which is not limited to oral application. The investigators of the review concluded that most of the studies reviewed had poor methods and designs and advocated for better designed and conducted clinical trials to establish the efficacy of Chinese herbal medicine for cancer pain.

Those interested in more information on herbs, botanicals, and other products are referred to http://www.mskcc.org/mskcc/html/11790.cfm?Disclaimer_Redirect=%2Fmskcc%2Fhtml%2F69296.cfm.

Patients report a reluctance to disclose their use of CAM to their physicians. Nurses need to elicit discussions about CAM to develop an open and honest patient-doctor-nurse relationship, encourage adherence to conventional palliative treatment, and monitor adverse effects and interactions with medications. Advanced practice nurses working in palliative care are piloting the use of tools that might identify patients' receptiveness to various CAM approaches that could be used in addition to traditional pharmacologic therapies (Reich and colleagues, Assessing patient preferences for use of complementary therapies in symptom management. Unpublished instrument. Department of Pain Medicine and Palliative Care, Beth Israel Medical Center, New York, NY). Those interested in reading more in this area are referred to the Holistic Nurses Association (http://www.aspmn.org/).

Translation into Practice

Neuropathic pain has been the focus of advanced-practice nurses at Dartmouth Hitch-cock Medical Center for nearly a decade.[162] Using a translation-into-practice quality improvement methodology, nurse practitioners led a 5-year study to improve NP screening at a comprehensive cancer center. In phase I, nurses and assistants participated in educational sessions about screening, assessment, and treatment. Clinical systems using electronic records were used to facilitate documentation of NP severity scores and treatment approaches. Pre- and post-test score results showed competency of new knowledge. A 90% NP screening adherence rate was achieved (n = 3831). Patients with cancer who reported no general pain (n = 291) were found to have moderate to severe NP. Successful achievement of the initial screening and assessment phase of the study has contributed to (1) health care professional education and periodic reinforcement of learning, and (2) system infrastructure changes. In phase II, early results for 20 patients support the use of a standardized NP assessment and evidence-based treatment algorithm to improve symptom severity, function, and patient satisfaction.[163] Findings suggest the value of systematic screening and assessment by nursing assistants and nurses, and nurse practitioner use of an evidence-based treatment algorithm for NP to improve patient outcomes.[163]

Research Questions

1. Is an integrated approach to pain assessment that incorporates multiple proxy raters more accurate in assessing patients' symptoms and distress than unique assessments by professional caregivers?
2. What is the validity and reliability of the BIS Index Monitor with unresponsive patients?
3. What is the relationship among patients' treatment options for chronic pain management, quality of life, and health economic outcomes?

DELIRIUM
Definition

Delirium is a cognitive disturbance resulting from an altered mental state, described in terms of disrupted consciousness and impaired cognition.[164] Based on criteria from the *Diagnostic and statistical manual of mental disorders, 4th edition* (DSM-IV),[165] delirium is defined as an acute and fluctuating organic brain syndrome characterized by global cerebral dysfunction that includes disturbances in attention, the level of consciousness, and basic cognitive functions (thinking, perception, and memory). Features also include decreased psychomotor activity, disturbances in the sleep/wake cycle, and emotional lability.[165]

Delirium is frequently confused with dementia. Delirium is characterized by an acute confusional state, dementia by a slow, insidious, and progressive chronic state of confusion. This distinction is crucial, as the causes and treatment of each differ. **Table 6**[166] lists the distinguishing characteristics of delirium and dementia. Delirium is accompanied by agitation and hallucinations, delusions, or paranoia, and must be distinguished from a psychosis caused by a psychiatric disorder, such as manic-depressive illness or schizophrenia. Those with a psychosis caused by a psychiatric disorder do not have confusion or memory loss; the level of consciousness does not change. A psychosis that begins during old age usually indicates delirium or dementia.[167]

Table 6
Differentiating delirium and dementia

	Delirium	Dementia
Onset	Acute or subacute, occurs in a short period of time (hours/days)	Insidious, often slow and progressive
Course	Fluctuates in the course of the day, worsens at night. Resolves in days to weeks	Stable in the course of the day; is progressive
Duration	If reversible, short-term	Chronic and nonreversible
Consciousness	Impaired and can fluctuate rapidly. Clouded, with a reduced awareness of the environment	Clear and alert until the later stages. May become delirious
Cognitive defects	Impaired short-term memory, poor attention span	Poor short-term memory; attention span less affected until later stage
Attention	Reduced ability to focus, sustain, or shift attention	Unaffected in the earlier stages
Orientation	Disoriented regarding time and place	Intact until months or years with the later stages. May have anomia (difficulty recognizing common objects) or agnosis (difficulty recognizing familiar people)
Delusions	Common, fleeting, usually transient and poorly organized	Often absent
Hallucinations	Common and usually visual, tactile, and olfactory	Often absent
Speech	Often uncharacteristic, loud, rapid, or slow (hypoactive)	Difficulty in finding words and articulating thoughts; aphasia
Affect	Mood lability	Mood lability
Sleep-wake cycle	Disturbed; may be reversed	Can be fragmented
Psychomotor activity	Increased, reduced, or unpredictable; variable depending on hyper/hypodelirium	Can be normal; may exhibit apraxia

From Kuebler KK, Heidrich DE, Vena C, et al. Delirium, confusion and agitation. In: Ferrell B, Coyle N, editors. Textbook of palliative nursing. 2nd edition. New York: Oxford University Press; 2006. p. 405; with permission.

Epidemiology

In the SUPPORT study,[168] delirium affected 20% to 30% of people with cancer, COPD, and end-stage liver disease. Its prevalence increases to 44% in patients with terminal cancer, and eventually to 83% of patients during their final days.[169] Delirium is associated with a higher rate of mortality during and following hospitalization.[170]

The prevalence of delirium on all hospital admissions ranges from 14% to 24%, and the incidence of delirium increases during hospitalization to 56% among general hospital populations.[171,172] Delirium is the most frequent complication in the hospitalized elderly. Delirium rates vary depending on patient factors, the setting of care, and the sensitivity of the measurement tool. Postoperative delirium occurs in 15% to 53% of older patients,[171] and in 70% to 87% of those in ICUs.[173] Nursing homes or post-acute care settings report delirium in up to 60% of patients[174,175] and in up to 83% of all patients at the end of life.[176,177]

The overall prevalence of delirium in the community is 1% to 2%;[178,179] however, this rate increases with age, rising to 14% among those more than 85 years old. In 10% to 30% of older patients presenting to emergency departments, delirium often signals the presence of life-threatening conditions.[171]

The mortalities among hospitalized patients with delirium range from 22% to 76%;[180] as high as the rates among patients with acute myocardial infarction or sepsis. The 1-year mortality associated with cases of delirium in hospitals is 35% to 40%.[181,182]

Pathophysiology

Delirium has many potential underlying causes, varying in specific populations. In a prospective study of delirium in patients with advanced cancer in a tertiary palliative care center, investigators found a median of 3 (range 1–6) precipitating factors for each episode of delirium.[183] Common causes of delirium in patients with cancer are summarized in **Box 6**.[184]

Patients with delirium can generally be classified into 1 of 3 diagnostic categories depending on the clinical features that are present: a hyperactive/agitated delirium, a hypoactive delirium, or a mixed delirium (features of hyper- and hypoactive). The hallmark of delirium is an acute change in the level of arousal, characterized by an altered sleep/wake cycle, mumbling speech, disturbance of memory and attention, and perceptual disturbances, with delusions and hallucinations.

Some investigators have suggested that various subtypes of delirium are associated with specific pathophysiologic changes, resulting from various causes. Delirium has hypoactive and hyperactive forms. The hypoactive form of delirium is more common among older persons and often goes unrecognized. Hyperactive delirium is characterized by obvious agitation and vigilance, whereas hypoactive delirium is characterized by lethargy, with a markedly decreased level of motor activity.

Another approach to understanding the pathophysiology of delirium is to consider the extent of underlying brain dysfunction: global and nonspecific, or more limited and specific. Delirium may stem from a heterogeneous group of disorders caused by different pathophysiologic mechanisms that result in different symptom complexes.[185,186]

With improved understanding of the pathophysiology of delirium, treatment targeted at specific underlying abnormalities will hopefully improve management of this condition.

Screening and Assessment Measures

The National Quality Measures Clearinghouse of the AHRQ (www.qualitymeasures. ahrq.gov/) currently includes delirium as a marker of the quality of care and patient

---

Box 6
Common causes of delirium in patients with cancer

- Sepsis
- Metabolic problems (renal failure, hepatic failure, hypercalcemia, hyponatremia)
- CNS involvement (brain metastases, leptomeningeal disease)
- Opioid medication
- Other drugs (eg, tricyclic antidepressants, anticholinergics, benzodiazepines, corticosteroids, antiemetics)
- Withdrawal syndromes (opioids, benzodiazepines, alcohol)
- Chemotherapeutic agents (eg, ifosfamide)
- Dehydration
- Hypoxia
- Paraneoplastic syndromes
- Nutritional deficiencies (vitamins)
- Endocrine problems (eg, thyroid or adrenal dysfunction)

Data from Bruera E, Sweeney C. Delirium research questions. In: Max MB, Lynn J. Interactive textbook on clinical symptom research. Available at: http://symptomresearch.nih.gov/chapter_5/.

---

safety, highlighting the importance for nurses in recognizing and managing this acute symptom early. The Assessing Care of Vulnerable Elders Project has ranked delirium among the top 3 conditions for improved quality of care.[187] Total national costs related to preventable adverse events are estimated to be between $17 billion and $29 billion per year; delirium may account for at least a quarter of these costs.[188–191] Greater impetus for addressing delirium comes in the decade ahead, as health care costs will be allocated based on performance. Pay for performance, currently targeted at prevention of pressure ulcers,[192] is likely to spread to other highly prevalent conditions for the aged that have quality, safety, and cost implications.[193]

Delirium is a clinical diagnosis. Delirium is often unrecognized by physicians and nurses,[165,194,195] in part because of its fluctuating nature, its overlap with dementia, lack of formal standardized cognitive assessment tools, and underappreciation of its clinical consequences to the patient's and family's quality of life. In addition, delirium may be superimposed on dementia, depression, and anxiety, making the diagnosis even more difficult.

The most commonly used measures by clinicians who need to rapidly screen for cognitive impairment include the Delirium Rating Scale-Revised,[196] Confusion Assessment Method,[197] NEECHAM Confusion Scale (NCS),[198] and The Memorial Delirium Assessment Scale (MDAS) (**Box 7**).[199] The MDAS has been validated in inpatient palliative care settings, with a sensitivity of 97% and a specificity of 95% at a cutoff score of 13 on a maximum possible score of 30.[199,200] Clinicians also use the Mini-Mental State Examination (MMSE)[201] (downloadable copy available from http://www.nia.nih.gov/health/pubs/clinicians-handbook/test.pdf).

For further information about assessment tools to aid nurses in assessing delirium, see http://www.rnao.org/Storage/12/645_BPG_DDD.pdf.

Management

Pharmacologic management

A review[9] of the international literature and RCTs of pharmacotherapies for the treatment of delirium in patients with terminal illness yielded only 1 small study with 30 participants. The sample consisted of patients with AIDS and delirium who were receiving 1 of 3 different agents: chlorpromazine, haloperidol, or lorazepam. Chlorpromazine and haloperidol were found to be equally effective, although those receiving chlorpromazine showed slightly worse cognitive function over time, but this result was not statistically significant. Excessive sedation occurred using lorazepam, forcing this arm of the study to be stopped early. The review suggests that haloperidol is the most suitable drug therapy for the treatment of patients with delirium near the end of life, although chlorpromazine may be an acceptable alternative (if a small risk of slight cognitive impairment is not a concern). There is insufficient evidence to draw any conclusions about the role of pharmacotherapy in terminally ill patients with delirium.

Management of terminal delirium at end of life is focused on symptomatic control and relief of the distress of the patient and the family. Benzodiazepines or sedating neuroleptics are usually effective at settling the patient.[202]

Box 7
Assessment instruments for cognitive impairment and delirium

Instruments that can be administered and rated by a minimally trained observer:

Cognitive impairment screening tools

    Mini-Mental State Examination

    Cognitive Capacity Screening Examination

    Short Portable Mental Status Questionnaire

Psychomotor skill tests

    Trail-making test

    Hand-held tachistoscope

    Clock drawing

Instruments that require administration and rating by a more highly trained observer

Delirium diagnostic instruments

    ICD-10

    DSM-IV

    Confusion Assessment Method

    Delirium Symptom Interview

NRSs

    Delirium Rating Scale

    Saskatoon Delirium Checklist

MDAS

Data from Bruera E, Sweeney C. Delirium research questions. In: Max MB, Lynn J. Interactive textbook on clinical symptom research. Available at: http://symptomresearch.nih.gov/chapter_5/.

Nonpharmacologic management

Holistic measures that prioritize hands-on care as a primary strategy is increasing in nursing homes and for the hospitalized elderly. Hospitalized elderly patients with escalating delirium may be placed on sleep protocols that increase uninterrupted sleep. Protocols, promoting non-pharmacological sleep intervention (ie, an alternative to a sleeping pill), may include a five minute back rub, warm milk or herbal tea, and recorded relaxation materials).[182]

In nursing home residents, programs such as Namaste Care, designed to offer meaningful activities to those with advanced dementia or those who cannot be engaged in traditional activities are also being tested. Specially trained nursing assistants provide activities of daily living in an unhurried manner, with a "loving touch" approach to care. The program takes place in a room with lowered lighting, soft music playing, and the scent of lavender. In one study of 86 seniors in resident centers, results of Minimum Data Set data before the program were implemented and after residents were involved in the program for at least 30 days showed a decrease in residents' withdrawal, social interaction, delirium indicators, and trend for decreased agitation. Families of patients receiving Namaste Care reported feeling that in spite of the many losses experienced because of the disease process, something special can still help their loved one to feel comforted, cared for, and cared about in a unique loving environment.[203]

Translating Research into Practice

Delirium is a serious and frequently occurring disorder with increased morbidity and mortality in patients who are critically ill with prolonged intensive care stays. Without the use of a screening instrument, more than 60% of patients with delirium are missed by ICU nurses and more than 70% by physicians.[204,205] Unrecognized delirium is untreated delirium.

In a recent quality improvement study,[206] ICU nurses evaluated the implementation of the Confusion Assessment Method-ICU (CAM-ICU) and the relationship between use of the CAM-ICU and the frequency and duration of haloperidol use. Using a tailored implementation strategy focused on potential barriers and facilitators to screening, the team measured CAM-ICU compliance, interrater reliability, and knowledge level about delirium. They also compared haloperidol use, as a proxy for delirium incidence, before and after the implementation of the CAM-ICU.

The tailored strategy was implemented in a 4-month period in 2006. This strategy included staff education, education outreach, reminders, audit and feedback, and leadership activities, and a delirium assessment tool was successfully introduced in a 40-bed ICU. Data were collected and compared during the following 3 years. By year 3 (2008), 641 patients had been assessed. Of these, 147 (22.9%) were identified as delirious. Of these, 25 (17%) had a hyperactive type, 47 (32%) a hypoactive type, and 74 patients (50.3%) had a mixed-type delirium. Adherence to the assessment protocol and delirium knowledge significantly increased from 77% to 92%, ($P<.0001$). Interrater reliability in using the CAM-ICU increased from 0.78 to 0.89. More patients were treated with haloperidol (9.9%–14.8%, $P<.001$); however, they were treated with a lower dose (18 mg to 6 mg, $P = .01$) and for a shorter time period (from 5 [IQR 2–9] to 3 [IQR 1–5] days, $P = .02$).

This quality improvement study is an exemplar for nursing and illustrates methods for translating research into practice. Early detection of delirium in critically ill patients increases the number of patients who receive treatment with haloperidol, with a lower dose and for a shorter time period.

Research Questions

1. What is the feasibility of implementing a standard screen and assessment for delirium in geriatric populations with advanced illness?
2. Does early recognition and treatment of delirium affect outcomes (patient comfort and family distress)?

REFERENCES

1. Federal interagency forum on aging-related statistics. 2008 older Americans: key indicators of well-being. Available at: http://www.agingstats. gov/agingstatsdotnet/Main_Site/Data/2008_Documents/Population.aspx; 2008. Accessed October 1, 2009.
2. Christ G, Sadhna D. Chronic illness and aging. Section 1: the demographics of aging and chronic diseases. The National Center for Gerontologic Social Work Education. Council on Social Work Education; 2008. Available at: http://www. cswe.org/File.aspx?id=24133. Accessed October 15, 2009.
3. Partnership for Solutions. Chronic care in America: a 21st century challenge. Prepared for the Robert Wood Johnson Foundation. Baltimore (MD): Johns Hopkins University; 2004. Available at: http://www.rwjf.org/pr/product.jsp? id=14685. Accessed October 15, 2009.
4. Statistics – chronic illness. National Invisible Chronic Illness Awareness Week Newsletter. Available at: http://invisibleillnessweek.com/?p=69; May 6, 2009. Accessed December 12, 2009.
5. World Health Organization. Cancer pain relief and palliative care. Geneva (Switzerland): WHO; 1989.
6. Palliative Care Subcommittee of the New Zealand Cancer Treatment Working Party. A working definition of palliative care in New Zealand. Available at: http://www.moh.govt.nz/moh.nsf/indexmh/palliativecare-definition.   Accessed March 3, 2010.
7. Hospice and Palliative Nurses Association. Research agenda for 2009–2012. Available at: http://www.hpna.org/DisplayPage.aspx?Title=Research. Accessed March 3, 2010.
8. Oncology Nursing Society. 2008 ONS research priorities survey. Available at: http://ons.metapress.com/content/b4m4103372233t25/fulltext.html.   Accessed March 3, 2010.
9. Lipman AG, Jackson KC, Tyler LS. Evidence-based symptom control in palliative care: systematic reviews and validated clinical practice guidelines for 15 common problems in patients with life-limiting disease. Binghamton (NY): Pharmaceutical Products Press; 2000.
10. Twycross R, Wilcock A, Stark Toller C. Symptom management in advanced cancer. 4th edition. Oxford (UK): Radcliffe Publishing; 2009.
11. Ferrell BR, Coyle N, editors. Oxford textbook of palliative nursing. 3rd edition. New York: Oxford University Press; 2010.
12. O'Connor M, Aranda S, editors. Palliative care nursing: a guide to practice. Oxford (UK): Radcliffe Publishing Ltd; 2003.
13. Hanks G, Cherny NI, Christakis NA, et al, editors. Oxford textbook of palliative medicine. Oxford (UK): Oxford University Press; 2009.
14. Wysocki A, Bookbinder M. Implementing clinical practice changes: a practical approach. Home Health Care Manag Pract 2005;17(3):164–74.
15. Dodd M, Janson S, Facione N, et al. Advancing the science of symptom management. J Adv Nurs 2001;33:668–76.

16. Dodd M, Miaskowski C, Paul SM. Symptom clusters and their effect on the functional status of patients with cancer. Oncol Nurs Forum 2001;28:465–70.
17. Dodd MJ, Miaskowski C, Lee KA. Occurrence of symptom clusters. J Natl Cancer Inst Monogr 2004;32:76–8.
18. Miaskowski C, Dodd M, Lee K. Symptom clusters: the new frontier in symptom management research. J Natl Cancer Inst Monogr 2004;32:17–21.
19. Gift AG, Jablonski A, Stommel M, et al. Symptom clusters in elderly patients with lung cancer. Oncol Nurs Forum 2004;31:203–12.
20. Loge JH, Abrahamsen AF, Ekeberg, et al. Fatigue and psychiatric morbidity among Hodgkin's disease survivors. J Pain Symptom Manage 2000;19:91–9.
21. Gaston-Johansson F, Fall-Dickson JM, Bakos AB, et al. Fatigue, pain, and depression in preautotransplant breast cancer patients. Cancer Pract 1999;7:240–7.
22. Miaskowski C, Lee KA. Pain, fatigue, and sleep disturbances in oncology outpatients receiving radiation therapy for bone metastasis: a pilot study. J Pain Symptom Manage 1999;17(5):320–32.
23. Beck SL, Schwartz AL. Unrelieved pain contributes to fatigue and insomnia [abstract]. Oncol Nurs Forum 2000;27:350.
24. Redeker NS, Lev EL, Ruggiero J. Insomnia, fatigue, anxiety, depression, and quality of life of cancer patients undergoing chemotherapy. Sch Inq Nurs Pract 2000;14:275–90 [discussion: 291–8].
25. Cleeland CS. The impact of pain on the patient with cancer. Cancer 1984;54: 2635–41.
26. Winningham ML, Nail LM, Burke MB, et al. Fatigue and the cancer experience: the state of the knowledge. Oncol Nurs Forum 1994;21:23–36.
27. Kurtz ME, Kurtz JE, Given CW, et al. Symptom clusters among cancer patients and effects of an educational symptom control intervention. Cancer Ther 2007;5: 105–12.
28. Fan G, Filipczak L, Chow E. Symptom clusters in cancer patients: a review of the literature. Curr Oncol 2007;14(5):173–9.
29. Given B, Given C, Azzouz F, et al. Physical functioning of elderly cancer patients prior to diagnosis and following initial treatment. Nurs Res 2001;50:222–32.
30. Barsevick AM, Whitmer K, Nail LM, et al. Symptom cluster research: conceptual, design, measurement, and analysis issues. J Pain Symptom Manage 2006;31: 85–95.
31. Bruera E, Kuehn N, Miller MJ, et al. The Edmonton symptom assessment system (ESAS): a simple method of the assessment of palliative care patients. J Palliat Care 1991;7:6–9.
32. Chang VT, Hwang SS, Kasimis B, et al. Shorter symptom assessment instruments: the Condensed Memorial Symptom Assessment Scale (CMSAS). Cancer Invest 2004;22(4):526–36.
33. Kirk TW, Mahon MM. Palliative Sedation Task Force of the National Hospice and Palliative Care Organization Ethics Committee. National Hospice and Palliative Care Organization (NHPCO) position statement and commentary on the use of palliative sedation in imminently dying terminally ill patients. J Pain Symptom Manage 2010;39(5):914–23. Available at: http://www.jpsmjournal.com/article/S0885-3924(10)00213-7/pdf. Accessed May 12, 2010.
34. Cherny N, Coyle N, Foley K. Guidelines in the care of the dying cancer patient. Hematol Oncol Clin North Am 1996;1:261–86.
35. American Academy of Hospice and Palliative Medicine. Statement on palliative sedation. Available at: http://www.aahpm.org/positions/sedation.html. Accessed March 3, 2010.

36. Dudgeon D. Dyspnea, death rattle, and cough. In: Ferrell BR, Coyle N, editors. Textbook of palliative nursing. New York: Oxford University Press; 2001. p. 164–74.

37. Corner J, O'Driscoll M. Development of a breathlessness assessment guide for use in palliative care. Palliat Med 1999;13(5):375–84.

38. End of Life Online Curriculum Project. Prevalence of dyspnea. End of life curriculum project, a joint project of the US Veterans Administration and SUMMIT, Stanford University Medical School. Available at: http://summit.stanford.edu/pcn/M07_Dyspnea/prev.html. Accessed October 15, 2009.

39. Anderson H, Ward C, Eardley A, et al. The concerns of patients under palliative care and a heart failure clinic are not being met. Palliat Med 2001;15(4):279–86.

40. Reuben DB, Mor V. Dyspnea in terminally ill cancer patients. Chest 1986;89(2): 234–6.

41. Dudgeon DJ, Kristjanson L, Sloan JA, et al. Dyspnea in cancer patients: prevalence and associated factors. J Pain Symptom Manage 2001;21(2):95–102.

42. Campbell EJ, Howell JB. The sensation of dyspnea. Br Med Bull 1963;19:36–40.

43. el-Manshawi A, Killian KJ, Summers E, et al. Breathlessness during exercise with and without resistive loading. J Appl Physiol 1986;61(3):896–905.

44. Jones PW. Breathlessness perception in airway obstruction. Eur Respir J 1992; 5(9):1035–6.

45. Jones PW, Wilson R. Cognitive aspects of breathlessness. In: Adams L, Guz A, editors. Respiratory sensation. New York: Marcel Dekker; 1996. p. 311–35.

46. Corner J, Plant H, Warner L. Developing a nursing approach to managing dyspnoea in lung cancer. Int J Palliat Nurs 1995;1:5–10.

47. Hill PH. The dyspnea-anxiety-dyspnea cycle–COPD patients' stories of breathlessness: "it's scary/when you can't breathe". Qual Health Res 2004;14(6):760–8.

48. Registered Nurses Association of Ontario. Assessment and management of pain. Nursing best practice guideline. Available at: http://www.rnao.org/Storage/29/2351_BPG_Pain_and_Supp.pdf; 2002. Accessed March 3, 2010.

49. Registered Nurses Association of Ontario. Nursing Best Practice Guideline. Assessment & management of pain. Available at: http://www.rnao.org/Storage/29/2351_BPG_Pain_and_Supp.pdf; 2002. Accessed December 20, 2009.

50. Gift AG, Narsavage G. Validity of the numeric rating scale as a measure of dyspnea. Am J Crit Care 1998;7:200–4.

51. Borg G. Perceived exertion as an indicator of somatic stress. Scand J Rehabil Med 1970;2-3:92–8.

52. National Institutes of Health. State of the science conference statement on improving end-of-life care. Paper presented at: NIH State of the Science Conference, Bethesda (MD); December 6–8, 2004.

53. Campbell MI. Terminal dyspnea and respiratory distress. Crit Care Clin 2004; 20(3):403–17.

54. Campbell MI. Psychometric testing of a respiratory distress observation scale. J Palliat Med 2008;11(1):44–50.

55. Spector N, Connolly MA, Carlson KK. Dyspnea. Applying research to bedside practice. AACN Adv Crit Care 2007;18(1):45–60.

56. Jennings AL, Davies AN, Higgins JP, et al. A systematic review of the use of opioids in the management of dyspnoea. Thorax 2002;57(11):939–44.

57. Light RW, Stansbury DW, Webster JS. Effect of 30 mg of morphine alone or with promethazine or prochlorperazine on the exercise capacity of patients with COPD. Chest 1996;109:975–81.

58. Navigante AH, Cerchietti LC, Castro MA, et al. Midazolam as adjunct therapy to morphine in the alleviation of severe dyspnea perception in patients with advanced cancer. J Pain Symptom Manage 2006;31(1):38–47.

59. Bausewein C, Booth S, Gysels M, et al. Non-pharmacological interventions for breathlessness in advanced stages of malignant and non-malignant diseases. Cochrane Database Syst Rev 2008;2:CD005623.

60. Cranston JM, Crockett A, Currow D. Oxygen therapy for dyspnoea in adults. Cochrane Database Syst Rev 2008;3:CD004769.

61. Solà I, Thompson E, Subirana M, et al. Non-invasive interventions for improving well-being and quality of life in patients with lung cancer. Cochrane Database Syst Rev 2004;4:CD004282.

62. Registered Nurses Association of Ontario. Nursing care of dyspnea: the 6th vital sign in individuals with chronic obstructive pulmonary disease (COPD). Available at: http://www.rnao.org/Storage/11/604_BPG_COPD.pdf; 2005. Accessed December 20, 2009.

63. Denniston A, O'Brien C, Stableforth D. The use of oxygen in acute exacerbations of chronic obstructive pulmonary disease: a prospective audit of pre-hospital and hospital emergency management. Clin Med 2002;2(5):449–51.

64. Goldstein RS. Supplemental oxygen in chronic respiratory disease. In: Bach JR, editor. Pulmonary rehabilitation: the obstructive and paralytic conditions. Philadelphia: Hanley and Belfus; 1996. p. 65–83.

65. Gorecka D, Gorzelak K, Sliwinski P, et al. Effect of long-term oxygen therapy on survival in patients with chronic obstructive pulmonary disease with moderate hypoxaemia. Thorax 1997;52(8):674–9.

66. Medical Research Council Working Party. Long term domicillary oxygen therapy in chronic hypoxic cor pulmonale complicating chronic bronchitis and emphysema. Lancet 1981;1(8222):681–6.

67. Wedzicha J. Ambulatory oxygen in chronic obstructive pulmonary disease. Monaldi Arch Chest Dis 1996;51(3):243–5.

68. Wijkstra PJ, Guyatt GH, Ambrosino N, et al. International approaches to the prescription of long-term oxygen therapy. Eur Respir J 2001;18(6): 909–13.

69. Murphy R, Driscoll P, O'Driscoll P. Emergency oxygen therapy for the COPD patient. Emerg Med J 2001;18(5):333–9.

70. Oncology Nursing Society. Definition of constipation. Available at: http://www.ons.org/Research/NursingSensitive/Summaries/media/ons/docs/research/summaries/constipation/definitions.pdf. Accessed March 3, 2010.

71. Miles C, Fellowes D, Goodman ML, et al. Laxatives for the management of constipation in palliative care patients. Cochrane Database Syst Rev 2006;(4):CD003448.

72. Hartford Institute for Geriatric Nursing. Constipation in palliative care. Available at: http://consultgerirn.org/topics/palliative_care/want_to_know_more#item_8. Accessed October 28, 2009.

73. Chambers K, McMillan SC. Measuring bowel elimination. In: Frank-Stromberg M, Olsen S, editors. Instruments for clinical health-care research. 3rd edition. Sudbury (MA): Jones and Bartlett; 2004. p. 487–97.

74. Campbell ML, Happ MB, Hultman T, et al. The HPNA research agenda for 2009–2012. J Hosp Palliat Nurs 2009;11(1):10–8.

75. Bailey B. Constipation. In: O'Connor M, Aranda S, editors. Palliative care nursing: a guide to practice. 2nd edition. Oxford (UK): Radcliffe Publishing; 2003. p. 156–71.

76. McMillan SC, Williams FA. Validity and reliability of the Constipation Assessment Scale. Cancer Nurs 1989;12:183–8.
77. Karam SE, Nies DM. Student/staff collaboration: a pilot bowel management program. J Gerontol Nurs 1994;20:32–40.
78. Hsieh C. Treatment of constipation in older adults. Am Fam Physician 2005; 72(11):2277–84.
79. Coggrave M, Wiesel P, Norton CC. Management of faecal incontinence and constipation in adults with central neurological diseases. Cochrane Database Syst Rev 2006;(2):CD002115.
80. Thomas J, Karver S, Cooney GA, et al. Methylnaltrexone for opioid-induced constipation in advanced illness. N Engl J Med 2008;358(22):2332–43.
81. Rubiales AS, Hernansanz S, Gutiérrez C, et al. Neostigmine for refractory constipation in advanced cancer patients [letter]. J Pain Symptom Manage 2006; 32(3):204–5.
82. Ong SP, Choong CF. Neostigmine in the treatment of severe constipation. Intern Med J 2007;37(12):836–7.
83. Ernst E. Abdominal massage for chronic constipation: a systematic review of controlled clinical trials. Forsch Komplementarmed 1999;6:149–51. Available at: http://www.medicine.ox.ac.uk/bandolier/booth/alternat/AT043.html. Accessed October 1, 2009.
84. Lamas K, Lindholm L, Stenlund H, et al. Effects of abdominal massage in management of constipation. A randomized controlled trial. Int J Nurs Stud 2009;46:759–67.
85. McMillan SC, Small BJ. Using the COPE intervention for family caregivers to improve symptoms of hospice homecare patients: a clinical trial. Oncol Nurs Forum 2007;34(2):313–21.
86. United States National Guideline Clearinghouse. Prevention of constipation in the older adult population. Available at: http://www.guideline.gov/summary/summary.aspx?doc_id=7004#s23. Accessed February 20, 2010.
87. Registered Nurses Association of Ontario. Prevention of constipation in the older adult population. Available at: http://www.rnao.org/Page.asp?PageID=924&ContentID=809. Accessed December 20, 2009.
88. Hert M, Huseboe J. Guideline – management of constipation. Research-based protocol. Iowa City (IA): University of Iowa Gerontological Nursing Interventions Research Center, Research Dissemination Core; 1996.
89. Folden S, Backer JH, Maynard F, et al. Practice guidelines for the management of constipation in adults. Rehabiltiation Nursing Foundation; 2002. Available at: http://www.rehabnurse.org/pdf/BowelGuideforWEB.pdf. Accessed April 14, 2010.
90. Campbell AJ, Busby WJ, Horvath CC. Factors associated with constipation in a community based sample of people aged 70 years and over. J Epidemiol Community Health 1993;47(1):23–6.
91. Economou DC. Bowel management: constipation, diarrhea, obstruction, and ascites. In: Ferrell BR, Coyle N, editors. Textbook of palliative nursing. New York: Oxford University Press; 2001. p. 139–55.
92. Dean GE, Anderson PD. Fatigue. In: Ferrell BR, Coyle N, editors. Textbook of palliative nursing. 2nd edition. New York: Oxford University Press; 2006. p. 91–100.
93. Department of Pain Medicine and Palliative Care. What is fatigue? Available at: http://www.stoppain.org/palliative_care/content/fatigue/default.asp. Accessed October 1, 2009.

94. Cella D, Peterman A, Passik S, et al. Progress toward guidelines for the management of fatigue. Oncology (Williston Park) 1998;12(11A):369–77.

95. Portenoy RK, Itri LM. Cancer-related fatigue: guidelines for evaluation and management. Oncologist 1999;4(1):1–10.

96. Walsh D, Donnelly S, Rybicki L. The symptoms of advanced cancer: relationship to age, gender, and performance status in 1,000 patients. Support Care Cancer 2000;8:175–9.

97. Lawrence DP, Kupelnick B, Miller K, et al. Evidence report on the occurrence, assessment, and treatment of fatigue in cancer patients. J Natl Cancer Inst Monogr 2004;32:40–50.

98. Servaes P, Verhagen C, Bleijenberg G. Fatigue in cancer patients during and after treatment: prevalence, correlates and interventions. Eur J Cancer 2002; 38:27–43.

99. Wolfe J, Grier HE, Klar N, et al. Symptoms and suffering at the end of life in children with cancer. N Engl J Med 2000;342:326–33.

100. Radbruch L, Elsner F, Krumm N, et al. Drugs for the treatment of fatigue in palliative care. Cochrane Database Syst Rev 2007;4:CD006788.

101. Radbruch L, Strasser F, Gonçalves JF, et al. Fatigue in palliative care patients – an EAPC approach. Palliat Med 2008;22:13–22. Available at: http://www.eapcnet.org/publications/research.html#fatigue. Accessed October 1, 2009.

102. Borneman T, Piper BF, Chih-Yi Sun V, et al. Implementing the fatigue guidelines at one NCCN member institution: process and outcomes. J Natl Compr Canc Netw 2007;5(10):1092–101. Available at: http://www.ncbi.nlm.nih.gov/pmc/articles/PMC2515169/?tool=pubmed. Accessed October 1, 2009.

103. Stone P, Richardson A, Ream E, et al. Cancer-related fatigue: inevitable, unimportant and untreatable? Results of a multi-centre patient survey. Cancer Fatigue Forum. Ann Oncol 2000;11:971–5.

104. Schwartz AL, Nail LM, Chen S, et al. Fatigue patterns observed in patients receiving chemotherapy and radiotherapy. Cancer Invest 2000;18:11–9.

105. Radbruch L, Sabatowski R, Elsner F, et al. Validation of the German version of the brief fatigue inventory. J Pain Symptom Manage 2003;25:449–58.

106. Minton O, Stone P, Richardson A, et al. Drug therapy for the management of cancer related fatigue. Cochrane Database Syst Rev 2008;1:CD006704.

107. Pucci E, Branãs P, D'Amico R, et al. Amantadine for fatigue in multiple sclerosis. Cochrane Database Syst Rev 2007;1:CD002818. [Update of Taus C, Giuliani G, Pucci E, et al. Cochrane Database Syst Rev 2007;1:CD002818].

108. Cruciani R, Dvorkin E, Homel P, et al. Safety, tolerability and symptom outcomes associated with L-carnitine supplementation in patients with cancer, fatigue, and carnitine deficiency: a phase I/II study. J Pain Symptom Manage 2006;32(6): 551–9.

109. Cramp F, Daniel J. Exercise for the management of cancer-related fatigue in adults. Cochrane Database Syst Rev 2008;2:CD006145.

110. Goedendorp MM, Gielissen MF, Verhagen CA, et al. Psychosocial interventions for reducing fatigue during cancer treatment in adults. Cochrane Database Syst Rev 2009;1:CD006953.

111. Hardy ML. Dietary supplement use in cancer care: help or harm. Hematol Oncol Clin North Am 2008;22(4):581–617. Available at: http://www.mdconsult.com/das/article/body/174488071-2/jorg=journal&source=MI&sp=20850229&sid=0/N/651864/1.html?issn=#h080006460207. Accessed November 1, 2009.

112. International Association for the Study of Pain. IASP pain terminology. Available at: http://www.iasp-pain.org/AM/Template.cfm?Section=Pain_Definitions&

Template=/CM/HTMLDisplay.cfm&ContentID=1728;   2009.   Accessed November 1, 2009.

113. Solano JP, Gomes B, Higginson IJ. A comparison of symptom prevalence in far advanced cancer, AIDS, heart failure, chronic obstructive pulmonary disease, and renal disease. J Pain Symptom Manage 2006;31:58–69.

114. Mercadante S. Pathophysiology of chronic pain. In: Bruera E, Higginson IJ, Ripamonti C, et al, editors. Textbook of palliative medicine. New York: Hodder Arnold; 2006. p. 357.

115. Miaskowski C. Recent advances in understanding pain mechanisms provide future directions for pain management. Oncol Nurs Forum 2004;31(Suppl 4): 25–35.

116. McCaffrey M, Pasero C. Pain: clinical manual. 2nd edition. St. Louis (MO): Mosby; 1999.

117. Fishman SM, Ballantyne JC, Rathmell JP. Bonica's management of pain. 4th edition. Philadelphia: Lippincott Williams & Wilkins; 2009.

118. Hastie BA, Riley JL, Fillingim RB. Ethnic differences and responses to pain in healthy young adults. Pain Med 2005;6(1):61–71.

119. Rahim-Williams FB, Riley JR III, Herrera D, et al. Ethnic identity predicts experimental pain sensitivity in African Americans and Hispanics. Pain 2007;129(1–2): 177–84.

120. Saunders C. Introduction: history and challenge. In: Saunders C, Sykes N, editors. The management of terminal malignant disease. London: Hodder and Stoughton; 1993. p. 1–14.

121. Gunnarsdottir S, Donovan HS, Ward S. Interventions to overcome clinician- and patient-related barriers to pain management. Nurs Clin North Am 2003;38(3): 419–34.

122. Mehta A, Chan L. Understanding of the concept of total pain: a prerequisite for pain control. J Hosp Palliat Nurs 2008;10(1):26–32.

123. Mularski RA, Puntillo K, Varkey B, et al. Pain management within the palliative and end-of-life care experience in the ICU. Chest 2009;135(5):1360–9.

124. Gelina C, Fillion C, Puntillo KA, et al. Validation of the critical-care pain observation tool in adult patients. Am J Crit Care 2006;15:420–7.

125. Puntillo KA, Morris AB, Thompson CL, et al. Pain behaviors observed during six common procedures: results from Thunder Project II. Crit Care Med 2004;32: 421–7.

126. Desbiens NA, Mueller-Rizner N. How well do surrogates assess the pain of seriously ill patients? Crit Care Med 2000;28:1347–52.

127. Lobchuk MM, Kristjanson L, Degner L, et al. Perceptions of symptom distress in lung cancer patients: I. Congruence between patients and primary family caregivers. J Pain Symptom Manage 1997;14:136–46.

128. Nekolaichuk CL, Maguire TO, Suarez-Almazor M, et al. Assessing the reliability of patient, nurse, and family caregiver symptom ratings in hospitalized advanced cancer patients. J Clin Oncol 1999;17:3621–30.

129. Gambrell M. Using the BIS monitor in palliative care: a case study. J Neurosci Nurs 2005;37(3):140–3.

130. Twite M, Zuk J, Gralla J, et al. Correlation of the bispectral index monitor with the COMFORT scale in the pediatric intensive care unit. Pediatr Crit Care Med 2005; 6(6):648–53.

131. City of Hope Pain & Palliative Care Resource Center. III. Pain and symptom management. A. Pain assessment tools. Available at: http://prc.coh.org/pain_assessment.asp. Accessed March 3, 2010.

132. Paice JA, Cohen FL. Validity of a verbally administered numeric rating scale to measure cancer pain intensity. Cancer Nurs 1997;20(2):88–93.

133. Fink R, Gates R. Pain assessment. In: Ferrell BR, Coyle N, editors. Textbook of palliative care nursing. New York: Oxford University Press; 2001. p. 53–75.

134. Herr K, Bjoro K, Decker S. Tools for the assessment of pain in non-verbal older adults with dementia: a state of the science review. J Pain Symptom Manage 2006;31:170–92.

135. Ferrell B, Levy M, Paice J. Managing pain from advanced cancer in the palliative care setting. Clin J Oncol Nurs 2008;12(4):575–81.

136. Paice JA. Pain at end of life. In: Ferrell BR, Coyle N, editors. Textbook of palliative nursing. 3rd edition. New York: Oxford University Press; 2010. p. 161–85.

137. Quigley C. The role of opioids in cancer pain. BMJ 2005;331:825–9.

138. Fine PG. The evolving and important role of anesthesiology in palliative care. Anesth Analg 2005;100:183–8.

139. Herndon CM, Hutchison RW, Berdine HJ, et al. Management of chronic nonmalignant pain with nonsteroidal antiinflammatory drugs. Joint opinion statement of the Ambulatory Care, Cardiology, and Pain and Palliative Care Practice and Research Networks of the American College of Clinical Pharmacy. Pharmacotherapy 2008;28(6):788–805.

140. Indelicato RA, Portenoy RK. Opioid rotation in the management of refractory cancer pain. J Clin Oncol 2003;21(Suppl 9):87s–91.

141. Wiffen PJ, McQuay HJ. Oral morphine for cancer pain. Cochrane Database Syst Rev 2007;4:CD003868.

142. Nicholson AB. Methadone for cancer pain. Cochrane Database Syst Rev 2007; 4:CD003971.

143. Challapalli V, Tremont-Lukats IW, McNicol ED, et al. Systemic administration of local anesthetic agents to relieve neuropathic pain. Cochrane Database Syst Rev 2005;4:CD003345.

144. Bell RF, Eccleston C, Kalso EA. Ketamine as an adjuvant to opioids for cancer pain. Cochrane Database Syst Rev 2003;1:CD003351.

145. Webster LR, Walker MJ. Safety and efficacy of prolonged outpatient ketamine infusions for neuropathic pain. Am J Ther 2006;13:300–5.

146. Wong RKS, Wiffen PJ. Bisphosphonates for the relief of pain secondary to bone metastases. Cochrane Database Syst Rev 2002;2:CD002068.

147. Sze WM, Shelley M, Held I, et al. Palliation of metastatic bone pain: single fraction versus multifraction radiotherapy. Cochrane Database Syst Rev 2002;1: CD004721.

148. Nnoaham KE, Kumbang J. Transcutaneous electrical nerve stimulation (TENS) for chronic pain. Cochrane Database Syst Rev 2008;3:CD003222.

149. Devine EC, Westlake SK. The effects of psychoeducational care provided to adults with cancer: meta-analysis of 116 studies. Oncol Nurs Forum 1995;22: 1369–81.

150. Dalton JA, Keefe FJ, Carlson J, et al. Tailoring cognitive-behavioral treatment for cancer pain. Pain Manag Nurs 2004;5:3–18.

151. Given C, Given B, Rahbar M, et al. Effect of a cognitive behavioral intervention on reducing symptom severity during chemotherapy. J Clin Oncol 2004;22: 507–16. Available at: http://jco.ascopubs.org/cgi/content/full/22/3/507?ck=nck. Accessed May 10, 2008.

152. Tatrow K, Montgomery GH. Cognitive behavioral therapy techniques for distress and pain in breast cancer patients: a meta-analysis. J Behav Med 2006;29: 17–27.

153. Cepeda MS, Carr DB, Lau J, et al. Music for pain relief. Cochrane Database Syst Rev 2006;2:CD004843.
154. McDonald MV, Pezzin LE, Feldman PH, et al. Can just in time, evidence-based "reminders" improve pain management among home health care nurses and their patients? J Pain Symptom Manage 2005;29:474–88.
155. Shojania KG, Jennings A, Mayhew A, et al. Effect of point-of-care computer reminders on physician behaviour: a systematic review. CMAJ 2010;182(5): E216–25.
156. Horowitz S. Complementary therapies for end-of-life care. Altern Complement Ther 2009;15(5):226–30.
157. Fellowes D, Barnes K, Wilkinson S. Aromatherapy and massage for symptom relief in patients with cancer. Cochrane Database Syst Rev 2004;3:CD002287.
158. Bardia A, Barton DL, Prokop LJ, et al. Efficacy of complementary and alternative medicine therapies in relieving cancer pain: a systematic review. J Clin Oncol 2006;24:5457–64.
159. Stephenson NL, Swanson M, Dalton J, et al. Partner-delivered reflexology: effects on cancer pain and anxiety. Oncol Nurs Forum 2007;34:127–32. Available at: http://ons.metapress.com/content/k477114620185x62/fulltext. html. Accessed May 10, 2008.
160. Tsai PS, Chen PL, Lai YL, et al. Effects of electromyography biofeedback assisted relaxation on pain in patients with advanced cancer in a palliative care unit. Cancer Nurs 2007;30:347–53.
161. Xu L, Lao LX, Ge A, et al. Chinese herbal medicine for cancer pain. Integr Cancer Ther 2007;6:208–34.
162. Lavoie-Smith D, Whedon M, Bookbinder M. Quality improvement of painful peripheral neuropathy. Semin Oncol Nurs 2002;18(1):36–43.
163. Rutledge D, Bookbinder M. Process and outcomes of evidence-based practice. Semin Oncol Nurs 2002;18(1):3–10.
164. Jackson KC, Lipman AG. Drug therapy for delirium in terminally ill adult patients. Cochrane Database Syst Rev 2004;2:CD004770.
165. American Psychiatric Association. Diagnostic and statistical manual of mental disorders. 4th edition. Washington, DC: American Psychiatric Association; 2000.
166. Kuebler KK, Heidrich DE, Vena C, et al. Delirium, confusion and agitation. In: Ferrell B, Coyle N, editors. Textbook of palliative nursing. 2nd edition. New York: Oxford University Press; 2006. p. 401–20.
167. Huang J. Delirium. Whitehouse Junction (NJ): Merck Sharp & Dohme; 2008. Available at: http://www.merck.com/mmhe/sec06/ch083/ch083b.html. Accessed February 20, 2010.
168. A controlled trial to improve care for seriously ill hospitalized patients. The study to understand prognoses and preferences for outcomes and risks of treatments (SUPPORT). The SUPPORT Principal Investigators. JAMA 1995;274(20):1591–8 [erratum in: JAMA 1996;275(16):1232].
169. Lorenz K, Lynn J, Dy SM, et al. Evidence for improving palliative care at the end of life: a systematic review. Ann Intern Med 2008;148:147–59.
170. Leslie DL, Zhang Y, Holford TR, et al. Premature death associated with delirium at 1-year follow-up. Arch Intern Med 2005;165:1657–62.
171. Agostini JV, Inouye SK. Delirium. In: Hazzard WR, Blass JP, Halter JB, et al, editors. Principles of geriatric medicine and gerontology. 5th edition. New York: McGraw-Hill; 2003. p. 1503–15.
172. Inouye SK. Delirium in hospitalized older patients. Clin Geriatr Med 1998;14: 745–64.

173. Pisani MA, McNicoll L, Inouye SK. Cognitive impairment in the intensive care unit. Clin Chest Med 2003;24:727–37.
174. Kiely DK, Bergmann MA, Jones RN, et al. Characteristics associated with delirium persistence among newly admitted postacute facility patients. J Gerontol A Biol Sci Med Sci 2004;59:344–9.
175. Roche V. Etiology and management of delirium. Am J Med Sci 2003;325: 20–30.
176. Breitbart W, Strout D. Delirium in the terminally ill. Clin Geriatr Med 2000;16: 357–72.
177. Casarett D, Inouye SK. Diagnosis and management of delirium near the end of life. Ann Intern Med 2001;135:32–40.
178. Folstein MF, Bassett SS, Romanosski AJ, et al. The epidemiology of delirium in the community: the Eastern Baltimore Mental Health Survey. Int Psychogeriatr 1991;3:169–76.
179. Rahkonen T, Eloniemi-Sulkava U, Paanila S, et al. Systematic intervention for supporting community care of elderly people after a delirium episode. Int Psychogeriatr 2001;13:37–49.
180. American Psychiatric Association. Practice guideline for the treatment of patients with delirium. Am J Psychiatry 1999;156(Suppl):1–20.
181. Moran JA, Dorevitch MI. Delirium in the hospitalized elderly. Aust J Hosp Pharm 2001;31:35–40.
182. Inouye SK. Delirium in older persons. N Engl J Med 2006;354:1157–65.
183. Lawlor PG, Gagnon B, Mancini IL, et al. Occurrence, causes, and outcome of delirium in patients with advanced cancer: a prospective study. Arch Intern Med 2000;160(6):786–94.
184. Bruera E. Delirium research questions: assessment of delirium. In: interactive textbook on clinical symptom research. Available at: http://symptomresearch. nih.gov/chapter_5/cebauthorbio.htm. Accessed October 16, 2009.
185. Ross CA, Peyser CE, Shapiro I, et al. Delirium: phenomenologic and etiologic subtypes. Int Psychogeriatr 1991;3(2):135–47.
186. Smith MJ, Breitbart W, Platt M. A critique of instruments and methods to detect, diagnose, and rate delirium. J Pain Symptom Manage 1995;10(1):35–77.
187. Sloss EM, Solomon DH, Shekelle PG, et al. Selecting target conditions for quality of care improvement in vulnerable older adults. J Am Geriatr Soc 2000;48:363–9.
188. Rothschild JM, Bates DW, Leape LL. Preventable medical injuries in older patients. Arch Intern Med 2000;160:2717–28.
189. Gillick MR, Serrell NA, Gillick LS. Adverse consequences of hospitalization in the elderly. Soc Sci Med 1982;16:1033–8.
190. Kohn LT, Corrigan JM, Donaldson MS, editors. Institute of Medicine Committee on Quality of Health Care in America. To err is human: building a safer health system. Washington, DC: National Academy Press; 2000. p. 26–48.
191. Thomas EJ, Studdert DM, Newhouse JP, et al. Costs of medical injuries in Utah and Colorado. Inquiry 1999;36:255–64.
192. Centers for Medicare and Medicaid Services. Present on Admission (POA) indicator reporting by Acute Inpatient Prospective Payment System (IPPS) hospitals. Available at: http://www.cms.hhs.gov/HospitalAcqCond/Downloads/ poa_fact_sheet.pdf; 2007. Accessed November 1, 2009.
193. Inouye SK, Schlesinger MJ, Lydon TJ. Delirium: a symptom of how hospital care is failing older persons and a window to improve quality of hospital care. Am J Med 1999;106:565–73.
194. Cole MG. Delirium in elderly patients. Am J Geriatr Psychiatry 2004;12:7–21.

195. Inouye SK, Foreman MD, Mion LC, et al. Nurses' recognition of delirium and its symptoms: comparison of nurse and researcher ratings. Arch Intern Med 2001; 161:2467–73.
196. Trzepacz PT. The delirium rating scale: its use in consultation-liaison research. Psychosomatics 1999;40(3):193–204.
197. Inouye SK, van Dyck CH, Alessi CA, et al. Clarifying confusion: the confusion assessment method. A new method for detection of delirium. Ann Intern Med 1990;113:941–8.
198. Neelon VJ, Champagne MT, Carlson JR, et al. The NEECHAM confusion scale. Nurs Res 1996;45(6):324–30.
199. Breitbart W, Rosenfeld B, Roth A, et al. The memorial delirium assessment scale. J Pain Symptom Manage 1997;13(3):128–37.
200. Lawlor PG, Nekolaichuk C, Gagnon B, et al. Clinical utility, factor analysis, and further validation of the Memorial Delirium Assessment Scale in patients with advanced cancer: assessing delirium in advanced cancer. Cancer 2000; 88(12):2859–67.
201. Folstein MF, Folstein SE, McHugh PR. "Mini-mental state". A practical method for grading the cognitive state of patients for the clinician. J Psychiatr Res 1975; 12(3):189–98.
202. Resource for End of Life Care Education. Module 12: last hours of living. Part I: physiological changes and symptom management during the dying process. Available at: http://www.endoflife.northwestern.edu/last_hours_of_living/dysfunction.cfm#TerminalDelirium. Accessed November 9, 2009.
203. Simard J, Volicer L. Effects of Namaste Care on residents who do not benefit from usual activities. Am J Alzheimers Dis Other Demen 2010;25(1):46–50.
204. Immers HE, Schuurmans MJ, Bijl JJ. Recognition of delirium in ICU patients: a diagnostic study of the NEECHAM confusion scale in ICU patients. BMC Nurs 2005;4:7.
205. Inouye SK. Masterclass delirium: a clinical overview. Amsterdam, April 22, 2008.
206. van den Boogaard M, Pickkers P, van der Hoeven H, et al. Implementation of a delirium assessment tool in the ICU can influence haloperidol use. Crit Care 2009;13:R131.

"I Want to Live, Until I don't Want to Live Anymore": Involving Children With Life-Threatening and Life-Shortening Illnesses in Decision Making About Care and Treatment

Myra Bluebond-Langner, PhD[a,b,*], Jean Bello Belasco, MD[c], Marla DeMesquita Wander, MS[d]

KEYWORDS

- Decision making • Ethics • Life-limiting illnesses
- Life-threatening illnesses • Child participation
- Physician-patient relationship

Sections of this article have been adapted from Bluebond-Langner M, DeCicco A, Belasco JB. Involving children with life-shortening illnesses in decisions about participation in clinical research: a proposal for shuttle diplomacy and negotiation. In: Kodish E, editor. *Ethics and Research with Children*. Oxford: Oxford University Press; 2005. p. 323–43.

The authors would like to thank Johnson & Johnson Family of Companies, Stanley Thomas Johnson Foundation, Olivia Hodson Foundation, National Endowment for the Humanities, REACH Fund of Great Ormond Street Hospital, Fannie E. Rippel Foundation, and ELS counselors for their support of Bluebond-Langner's work on children's participation in decision making about care, treatment, and research participation.

[a] Department of Sociology, Anthropology and Criminal Justice, Rutgers University, 405-407 Cooper Street, Camden, NJ 08102, USA

[b] Louis Dundas Centre for Children's Palliative Care, UCL Institute of Child Health - Great Ormond Street Hospital, 30 Guilford Street, London, England WC1N 1EH, UK

[c] Division of Oncology, Children's Hospital of Philadelphia, 34th & Civic Center Boulevard, Philadelphia, PA 19104, USA

[d] Department of Childhood Studies, Rutgers University, 405-407 Cooper Street, Camden, NJ 08102, USA

* Corresponding author. Department of Sociology, Anthropology and Criminal Justice, Rutgers University, 405-407 Cooper Street, Camden, NJ 08102.

E-mail address: bluebond@camden.rutgers.edu

INTRODUCTION AND OVERVIEW

Over the past 25 to 30 years there have been significant changes in the care of children with chronic life-threatening and life-limiting conditions. There has been a major shift in approach to care and treatment from an almost exclusive focus on the physical aspects of a child's condition and management of the disease and its sequelae to a consideration of the impact of the illness on the whole person—physically, socially, emotionally, and spiritually.[1,2] There has been a burgeoning of services and programs dedicated to providing holistic care to children and their families from diagnosis through to death and thereafter.

Along with these changes has come an increasing interest and concern about a child's role in decisions about care and treatment. Pediatric societies in North America as well as in the United Kingdom and Europe take the position that children should be part of the decision-making process.[3–11] Less clear, however, is how that should be accomplished. How is an ethical and meaningful role for children in the decision-making process ensured? How should the role of a child compare with that of a physician or parent?

This article outlines what needs to be considered when taking on the challenge of involving children with life-threatening and life-limiting illnesses in decision making regarding care and treatment. An approach is suggested for involving children that recognizes the abilities and vulnerabilities of children and the realities of their relationships with their parents who are charged with their care and still looks to treat children in an ethical manner. Discussion of the issues that need to be considered and recommendations for involving children in decision making derive from empiric studies by the first author (MB-L) and colleagues as well as a review of articles pertaining to the involvement of children and adolescents with life-limiting and life-threatening illnesses in decision making about care and treatment and participation in medical research. Work on a child's role in decision making about participation in medical research is included, because clinical trials are often part of the palliative care and end-of-life experiences for these children.

Many of the studies referred to in this article include in their findings children, adolescents, and young adults (18 years and older) but do not differentiate among them. Unless otherwise noted, what is discussed regarding children applies to adolescents and young adults. To set the stage for the discussion, there are 5 cases: 1 case from a study of children with cystic fibrosis, 1 case from a cystic fibrosis transplant center meeting, and 3 cases from a study of decision making for children with cancer when cure is not likely.[12–15]

CASES
Case 1

Casey is 8 years old. His cystic fibrosis is far more advanced than is typical for a child his age. He has multiple resistant organisms growing out of all of his sputum cultures, and he is refusing any sort of chest physiotherapy. He is not eligible for a heart-lung transplant. Casey's parents want him to remain in the hospital, but Casey wants to go home. Casey does not talk much about his disease, but his questions show that he understands the seriousness of his condition. One afternoon, lying in his bed watching TV just after rounds, he asked his mother, who was standing by the bed looking up at the TV, "Am I going to die?" She squatted down, took hold of the guardrail, inclined her head so that her eyes were looking into his, and replied, "You don't have to but you have to fight." Casey turned over in the bed, turned up the volume on his TV, and screamed, "Get away! Go away!" How should Casey be involved in decisions about his treatment? What role should he play in the decision to go home?

Case 2

Stephanie is 15 years old with advanced lung disease as a result of cystic fibrosis. She adheres to a complex regimen of chest physiotherapy, antibiotics, enzymes, and nebulizer treatments while "managing to have a life, which my doctor says you have to do too." Stephanie's parents want her to have a heart-lung transplant. When asked about being a transplant candidate, Stephanie said, "I do not want to trade one disease for another. Besides, everyone I know died." She later told the psychologist that, "I don't want to let my parents down. They've done everything for me." How should Stephanie be involved in the decision of a heart-lung transplant? Should the decision to have a transplant be Stephanie's decision to make?

Case 3

Jeremy is 14 years old. He was diagnosed and treated 14 months earlier with radiation and chemotherapy for a partially resected thalamic anaplastic astrocytoma that has now recurred. Treatment has taken a cognitive and a physical toll on Jeremy. Once athletically talented and academically gifted, he now walks with a brace and has learning issues, with particular difficulty in language, specifically, significant expressive and receptive aphasia. Despite his cognitive deficits, his questions show that he knows that his tumor has grown and he is concerned about dying. During an outpatient examination while undergoing radiation and chemotherapy, he said to the neuro-oncologist, "If this tumor doesn't shrink, I'm going to die, right?"

Jeremy's parents want him to be enrolled in experimental phase I-II clinical trials. They are not interested in palliative chemotherapy or hospice care. They believe that the decisions about treatment are not Jeremy's to make. They also do not want the physician to tell Jeremy that this is a phase I-II trial. How should Jeremy be involved in the decision-making process? Should he be told about the other treatment options? Can the physician not tell Jeremy that this is a phase I-II trial and consider Jeremy's willingness to take the drug as an assent to participate, which is a requirement to participate in the trial?

Case 4

Evan is 14 years old with recurrent anaplastic astrocytoma in the thalamic region of his brain. During Evan's last outpatient visit with severe neuropathic pain and waxing and waning of consciousness, Evan's parents signed a do-not-resuscitate (DNR) order. On discharge, he was reported to have episodes of dementia and confusion, slurred speech, sensory loss, and extremity weakness. This, however, did not stop Evan from driving around the neighborhood on a motorized power lawnmower or from freely voicing what he thinks is best for him, which includes, "Not eating that health food that my mom makes me eat, I need junk food. It keeps my weight up." When Evan was asked what he would wish for if he had 3 wishes, he said, "To live until I don't want to live anymore." When asked to describe his brain tumor, he said, "I still have a little, like a one percent power, so I want to take the medicine and I ask the Lord to take it away if it is still there. The tumor can grow and I don't want to take any chances."

Evan's parents have asked that he be considered for a clinical research trial if a slot became available. Once at home, Evan's parents were asked if they wanted the DNR order to remain in place. They did, but they did not want Evan told. How should Evan be involved in the decision to participate in the trial should a slot become available? Should Evan be asked if he wants to remain a DNR?

Case 5

Hamid is 8 years old with Philadelphia chromosome-positive acute lymphoblastic leukemia. When he relapsed after a bone marrow transplant, he responded to chemotherapy. His hematologist and bone marrow transplant specialist suggested a donor lymphocyte infusion (DLI) from his matched sibling donor, Nazneen, age 12. Hamid said, "Her bone marrow didn't help, that's why the leukemia came back." Although Nazneen does not think the DLI will work and is concerned that her brother will get sicker; she has agreed. When asked about her willingness to donate, she told the psychologist, "I will do it."

Hamid and Nazneen's parents do not see the decision about whether or not Hamid has the DLI as Hamid's or Nazneen's to make. They also see the DLI as "the only way to go." Although the parents had agreed to a DNR order when Hamid relapsed with complications that put him in the pediatric intensive care unit, now that he is responding to treatment, they want to go forward with the DLI and whatever else may be offered in the way of chemotherapy. What role should Hamid and his sister Nazneen play in the decision-making process?

WHAT NEEDS TO BE CONSIDERED WHEN INVOLVING CHILDREN IN DECISIONS ABOUT CARE AND TREATMENT

Children's Knowledge and Understanding: Age and Stage of Development, Experiences, Views of the Illness, and Options for Care and Treatment

A basic assumption in involving individuals in decision making is that an individual understands the options: the risks, the benefits, and the likely outcomes. If children are involved, then the question that needs to be asked is, "Can they understand the options before them?" Some use a child's age or level of development as the indicator of whether or not a child is capable. Using age and stage of development is problematic for many reasons, not least among them that "there is considerable difference in the rate of development of each [developmental] trend in each individual."[16] Children do not develop evenly. Some children, for instance, can be described as "socially immature but gifted in math." These variations make it difficult to speak of a certain age or stage at which a particular minor or cohort of minors have or do not have the cognitive capacity for decision making. Adults, including parents, do not always know or understand all of the options that are before them or the elements of the study for which they have just signed up.[17,18]

Age is not necessarily predictive of what children know.[13,19–24] For example, in studies of children who attended cancer camp, the number of years that children attended camp was a better predictor of knowledge than age or several other factors. In all of the children who attended camp, there was a significant increase in their knowledge about cancer, treatment protocols, and investigative procedures post camp, regardless of age, gender, diagnosis, years since diagnosis, condition, or hospital where treated.[23]

Children's experiences with their illnesses play a major role in their understanding, especially children who have been living with the illness for some time, because these children their lived experiences leading to increased understanding.[3,25–30] In some cases, although the illness can lead to cognitive deficits, it does not necessarily lead to decreased understanding, as in the cases (discussed previously) of Jeremy (case 3) and Evan (case 4). These cases illustrate that it is possible to have some understanding, however incomplete, of the condition and options available and to offer a considered and reasonable justification for choices[31–38] even in the face of some cognitive deficits that come as a result of the disease and treatment.

Experiences of relapses and recoveries and all that comes with living with a serious illness from tests to overheard discussions to the ministrations of family, friends, and clinicians are critical to children's acquisition of information and to their integration of that information into their views of themselves.[3,19,22–24,30] As such, the 8 year old who has undergone a transplant can know far more than a newly diagnosed 12 year old.

Also making it difficult to determine what any child knows about a given therapy or intervention, let alone how any particular child views an illness or treatment options, is that children demonstrate different understandings and present different views to different individuals on different occasions. For example, although a child might acknowledge that other children with the same disease and treated in the same way have died, that does not necessarily indicate that that child believes that he or she will die. Children with chronic, life-threatening illnesses hold out hope and for a very long time may believe, sometimes until within days and weeks of death, that there are things that can be done to make them better.[12,15] In on-going review and analysis of a previously published study,[14] the first author [MB-L] found concurring results as the following exchange exemplifies.[15] While Lakshmi, age 5, and Bluebond-Langner were coloring in a hospital playroom, Lakshmi casually remarked, "Leah died. You don't know her. She had JMML [juvenile myelomonocytic leukemia] like me, but I'm going to get more cells," and continued to color. Knowing that Lakshmi did not like it when asked too many questions, Bluebond-Langner did not pursue her remark. Finishing the section of the page she was coloring when she first spoke, Lakshmi added, "…from my mother [the cells]. Then I'm going to get better."[15]

Children are not alone in separating what will happen to them from what has happened to others, so too do their parents. For example, 2 days after Lakshmi died, her mother said,

> *It wasn't until we were in the hospital again this last time that it hit me that all of the other children had died. It wasn't until Lakshmi asked if she was going to the same place as Leah that I realized that all the time, all the treatments, we were just buying time. She wasn't going to be cured. I knew that, well, sort of, it was just too scary, or I just didn't want to think that she wouldn't be cured. But I knew deep down that she wouldn't be.[15]*

Children, like their parents, hold on to the possibility of a cure[39] (through medical or divine intervention or both), stabilization, or, at least, a reasonable amount of time even in the face of phase I trials, despite explanations to the contrary.[14,15,40]

Parents and children can hold on to several views of an illness and efficacy of treatment at once.[15,19,41] The particular view that is dominant at any point in time can vary. As one child put it,

> *My friends' relapses worry me sometimes, because they thought that one day they could be sure and that they could go on with their lives and it didn't turn out that way. So, once in a while I think maybe I will relapse and I won't be around very long. It makes me wonder if I should just give up chemotherapy altogether and live my life the best I can for a couple of months or whatever. Or maybe I should just go out and have a good time, because you really don't know what the future holds.[24]*

Mutual Pretense: Interaction Between Adults and Children

Another obstacle in assessing or eliciting what children want or know is that they may not express their knowledge directly to an adult.[32] Adults and children, in particular parents and children, are often acting in what Glaser and Strauss[42] described for ill adults as the "context of mutual pretense." Mutual pretense, where each party in the interaction knows the prognosis but does not openly acknowledge with the other parties can become the dominant mode of interaction between parents and ill children, especially as the disease progresses and a child's condition deteriorates.[12,15,22]

In mutual pretenses, difficult issues are evaded, avoided, and not met head on. When difficult topics emerge, such as the likelihood of a given drug stopping tumor growth or shrinking the tumor, care is taken so that neither party breaks down.[22] For example, in response to a doctor's statement, "The tumor is growing again," the boy looked to his mother and said, "Yes, but it grew before and the chemotherapy helped. So maybe this new medicine will work."[15]

Children do not necessarily reveal their awareness that the chances for recovery are minimal to none. In part this reflects their desire, not unlike adults for that matter, to try something in the way of further disease-directed therapy.[15,19,43] A child's decision not to reveal awareness of the minimal chances for recovery is also often indicative of awareness of how important a new therapy is to their parents and their effort to protect their parents from their fears and doubts.[15,22] As one child said of a phase I trial of STI-571, for example, "I don't think the drug is working, but I want to try something and my mom thinks it will work."[15]

Even in cases where there is open communication, it is not necessarily there all of the time. For example, although one 16 year old and his parents had had conversations about death when he was diagnosed, sharing what they would like when they died, when the tumor had progressed and various options were presented, including hospice care, neither the parents nor the child discussed death or funeral arrangements.[15]

Societal Roles and Responsibilities: Parents and Children

Children are not autonomous beings. They are certainly not autonomous decision makers in matters of medical care and treatment.[37] That right and that responsibility, legally and some would argue morally as well, belong to parents, who, absent evidence to the contrary, are assumed to act beneficently toward their children.[44] Hence, any approach taken to involve children in decision making must take into account the parents' perspective, what they see as their role in the care and treatment of their children.[26,45,46] Researchers indicate that parents of ill children see themselves not only as decision-makers but also as nurturers, protectors, advocates, and caregivers for their children.[12,15,22,40,47] Illness becomes the context that defines what it means to be a parent.[14,47] Their identity as parents is forged in and through this experience.[48]

In a study of decision making for children with cancer when standard therapy had failed and cure was not likely, Bluebond-Langner and colleagues[14] found that for parents, their task and their responsibility, as they perceived and enacted them, was to leave no stone unturned. Regardless of differences between the US and British health care systems, as well as differences in parents' ethnic, religious, and educational backgrounds, parents on both sides of the Atlantic came to participate in a common practice of parenting.[14,15]

Parents considered cancer-directed options as well as symptom-directed options and wanted further investigative procedures, such as MRIs and laboratory tests. Seeking cancer-directed therapy, being in contact with a child's oncologist, and continuing with further scanning and procedures, symptom-directed treatments, and supportive interventions emerged as primary features of the parental role.

The quest for further cancer-directed therapy was as much a part of parents' relentless efforts as sleepless nights, exhausting days of care and treatment, and trips to the hospital all the while trying to maintain family life despite separations, keep a job, and, in the case of US parents, hold on to insurance. Parents came to understand their roles and responsibilities as parents as keeping options open for their child. They were not necessarily committed to cure. They knew that cure was not possible. They bargained and traded for time. Parents chose treatment options with infinitesimal odds because the prize they sought was of immeasurable worth.[14] Parents saw decisions about their child's care treatment as theirs to make whether or not a child was 6 months, 6 years, or 16 years old.[15,40] This is not to say that parents were insensitive to what their child needed, thought, or understood. As Jeremy's mother (Case 3) explained,

> Jeremy knows he has cancer. He knows people have died from cancer, but we try to have him rely on faith. You have people praying for you, you pray for yourself. It doesn't necessarily have to mean that you know, but that he knows.[13]

Parents felt that to ask children to participate in certain decisions placed too heavy a burden on the children.[45] They wanted to shield their children from what they saw as "painful," "harsh," or "discouraging information." As Jeremy's mother said,

> We felt like telling him it's a clinical trial, but that sounds so harsh. We never did use the word trial. We didn't want him to think that it was some kind of experiment. You know, sometimes experiments don't work. He is only 13, 14 in three weeks. We just felt like this was something that he didn't have to know.[13]

Children are not always present when a physician first tells the parents the results of diagnostic procedures or when options for further care and treatment are first discussed.[40] As is often the case with children with brain tumors, for example, recognition that the tumor had recurred can come from the report on a routine scan. Parents often are back at home when an oncologist receives the report. When a physician calls the parents, it is often left to them to decide whether or not to bring the child with them when they come to review the scans and discuss options for care and treatment. In other cases, a child is in the hospital or clinic when the results of a scan, laboratory findings, or physical examination indicate a change in the child's condition, which warrants discussion of changes in care and treatment. At such times, parents may or may not be offered the opportunity to talk without the child present. Sometimes discussion gets under way without notice or consideration of a child's presence. When parents are offered the option of continuing discussion separately from the child, some choose to have a separate discussion, others do not.[13]

Not surprisingly then, children do not necessarily have the same information as their parents. For example, when Nazneen (Case 5) agreed to be a donor for the DLI, she had not been told, as had her parents had, that "there was less than one in twenty chance of the disease being cured," that "it would in all likelihood come back," that "people are increasingly giving up donor lymphocytes for relapsed acute lymphoblastic leukemia after bone marrow transplant," and that the only reason why the bone marrow transplant and hematology-oncology teams were considering it was because there "was one boy who surprised us by staying well for a long time [following a DLI]."[15]

In a study of informed consent conferences for children diagnosed with acute leukemia, Olechnowicz and colleagues[37] found that parents asked fewer questions when an older child was present and that "most of the children did very little talking." That did not mean, however, that the children did not want "specific information about care and treatment."[37] Studies of adolescents with chronic illness and the physicians who treat them found that adolescents wanted technical information given and explained as well as "straight talk when delivering bad news."[31,33,49,50] Yet, for the most part, they did not want to take the lead in decision making or make the final decision.[31,33] Only 16.9% of the adolescents "preferred patient led decision making."[31] Knopf and colleagues[33] suggest that adolescents' desire for greater parental and physician-led decision may be rooted in their realization of the complexity of the issue at hand.

Some studies suggest that children's decisions to participate in research are based heavily on their parents' wishes.[51,52] When questioned about their deference to "parental influence," Scherer's[51] study participants gave "reasons that fall into four categories: they feel coerced, or that they have no choice; they wish to avoid family tension and conflict with parents; they respect parental judgment and feel that parents know more about these matters; or they feel a need for parental support, emotionally, physically, and/or financially."

Scherer[51] found that children are not likely to dissent from a parent-sanctioned decision even when given the opportunity to do so. This may in part reflect the trust or faith children have in their parents' decisions as evidenced in the study by Broome and Richards on the influence of parental relationships in children with cancer, diabetes, and sickle cell disease in children's decision making regarding participation in clinical trials.[32] Or, perhaps a child's failure to dissent may be indicative of nothing more than the child, after careful consideration, is in agreement with the parents[39] and chooses to have the parents make decisions.[32,35] Or perhaps, as suggested in Case 2 and in the previous discussion of mutual pretense, at the root of a child's reluctance to dissent is a desire not to disappoint or challenge parents or physicians.

Children are socialized to respect the role of parents and other adults as authorities. As Leiken points out, "Even when [children] have a personal reservation, and the offer is made in a form of request, they may still agree to participate in the research simply because they believe that they should be compliant."[16] According to Leiken[16] the situation is not very different in preadolescents, albeit for different reasons. "Preadolescents, to avoid negative consequences, are prone to defer to authority figures."[16]

Leiken[16] states, "This lack of assertiveness in voicing their authentic choices... [raises] serious questions about whether one can justifiably speak of 'assent' when children or young adolescents are concerned." Lest one think that this precludes children from participating in a meaningful way in the decision-making process, Leiken[16] takes care to point out that adults also defer to social pressures when making decisions regarding care, treatment, and participation in clinical trials. Kuther and Posada,[27] echoing Leiken's sentiments, write, "The ability of minors & adults to provide voluntary consent may vary with contextual factors, such as decision at hand, the desires of authority figures & significant others, & personal experience." In short, social and cultural factors are as much a part of decision making involving adults as they are part of those involving children (for a summary of what needs to be considered in decisions about care and treatment see **Box 1**).

SHUTTLE DIPLOMACY: AN APPROACH TO INVOLVING CHILDREN WITH CHRONIC, LIFE-THREATENING, AND LIFE-LIMITING ILLNESSES IN DECISION MAKING ABOUT CARE, TREATMENT, AND RESEARCH PARTICIPATION

The authors propose an approach for involving children in decision making that formally and respectfully recognizes 3 participants: child/patient, parents, and physician. This approach is consistent with the recommendations of others who have worked in the area of involving children with chronic, life-threatening illnesses and life-limiting illnesses in decision making about care, treatment, and research participation.[19,26,28,43,46,53–55] It also shares with others who work in this area a movement away from using a bright line of a particular age as a primary or determining factor

---

Box 1
What needs to be considered when involving children with life-threatening and life-limiting illnesses in medical decisions

- The child
- The parents
- The parent-child relationship

- With regard to the child:
  1. The child's age or stage of development
  2. The child's experiences over the course of the illness
  3. The child's view of the illness and options for care and treatment
  4. The child's participation in the "context of mutual pretense"
  5. The child's actions to protect his or her parents
- With regard to the parents:
  1. The parents' legal and moral responsibility for their child
  2. The parents' positions regarding:

     Their child's care and treatment

     Their child's place in this decision-making process

     What their child should/can be told
- With regard to the parent-child relationship:
  1. Children are not autonomous beings
  2. Parents and their child have their usual decision-making routines
  3. Parents and their child are likely to have different information about the illness and treatment options
  4. Children are prone to defer to authority figures
  5. The likelihood of the child's dissent from parents' sanctioned decisions
  6. The role of social and cultural factors in care and treatment for all ill people—adults and children

---

in a child's eligibility or ineligibility for participation in decision making about care and treatment or research participation.[21,27,30,35,54,56–66] Moreover, it satisfies Crisp and colleagues'[30] and Broome and colleagues's[39] recommendations with regard to involving children in medical research in that it calls for proceeding without assumptions about how children wish to be involved or what they may know or have the capacity to understand.

The approach proposed does not do violence to the parent-child relationship. Central to the approach is the recommendation of recognition and respect for the reality of children's relation to their parents and other adults.[34,35,46] As Hinds and colleagues[19] point out from their study of end-of-life care preferences in children and adolescents with cancer, "decision making factors most frequently reported by patients were relationship based." As Kon[34] writes, "family and other social interactions are often central to a child's understanding of his or her experience and any policy that is blind to the social characteristics of children will not serve them well."

It follows then that the process of decision making about a child's care and treatment should also then be consistent with the ways in which decisions are made about other aspects of the child's life.[34,35] Parents typically make several major decisions concerning their children's lives—from where they will live and go to school to when they must be home. If important decisions (eg, schooling or church attendance) have not been a child's to make in the past, this is not the time to change that. This is not to say, however, that children do not have a role in the decision-making process nor that their concerns, views, and desires should not be taken account (how this is addressed in the proposed model is discussed later).

Finally and not insignificantly, the approach outlined builds in a level of protection,[27] because it recognizes the complexities of children's abilities and vulnerabilities,[28] their relationships with their parents, and the complex medical and moral issues children and parents face in living with chronic life-threatening and life-limiting illnesses.[44,67]

The value of a requirement to involve children in decision making about their care and treatment underscores the importance of talking to and listening to a child at a time when it can be extraordinarily difficult to do so. Parents and physicians are, although they typically try to control them, beset by profound feelings of sorrow and grief when there is, as in these cases, only the faintest chance that what is available will extend a child's life, and then only briefly. To explain this to children, to bring them to understand this, and to ask children to make what some might call a "choiceless choice" are excruciating for parents and doctors. The pain they feel does not come just from empathy or sympathy. It also derives from their roles as physicians and parents—to care for and protect. The directive to involve children in the decision-making process requires physicians to say and hear things that are, to say the least, difficult. It is the value that is implicit in this talking and listening to a child, which needs to be preserved and expanded, without the focus on a particular result.

There are several values that need to be respected in the decision-making process with children. One is that it should be conducted without deceit. Second, participants should be free from coercion. Finally, children, like any other patients, have a right (if they wish to exercise it) to know about the procedures that they undergo.[28] The challenge in creating a role for children in decision making is to balance these values with the social fabric of family life and the rights that are accorded to parents in light of their responsibilities for their children.[53]

A framework for involving children and others in the decision-making process, which addresses these requirements, is one that in the political realm is often referred to as shuttle diplomacy. In political shuttle diplomacy, a diplomat (eg, Henry Kissinger, Christopher Dodd, or George Mitchell) conducts discussions with each of the parties (eg, nation-states, factions within states, and political groups) separately before moving on to negotiations between the parties. As with parents and children, participants in serious negotiations need not be, and often are not, of equal status. The lack of veto power does not render participation ungenuine. What is required is a framework that tries to provide that all the participants are represented and moves toward a resolution, which all parties can hopefully accept. As in any negotiated outcome, tradeoffs are made by participants between individual wants or needs and overall resolution.

Briefly, this diplomatic, negotiated approach is sketched, using as a frame of reference a child with cancer whose disease has recurred and for whom cure is unlikely. At the time of recurrence, parents would be told that there is be a family meeting to explore what options are available. A physician/investigator explains what will be covered in the meeting (eg, disease status, risks and benefits of what will be offered, and prognosis) and ascertains what the parents would be comfortable having said with the child present. For example, parents might indicate a willingness to have a discussion about the various options, even their potential risks and benefits, in front of or with their child, but not the child's prognosis.

It is extraordinarily important as well as beneficial for physicians to pursue with parents why they do not want particular information shared with a child, not just because of what is involved in terms of talking to the child. Such discussions provide physicians with an opportunity not only to explain what they think a child needs to know but also with an opportunity to explore from a different vantage point what is of concern to the parents regarding their child's condition and available options for care and treatment. In talking with parents about what they do not want a child to know, physicians can become aware of misunderstandings about various care and treatment options and even the prognosis as well as other issues in a family that may be effecting the choice parents are making. Physicians may also learn of other problems that the parents may be experiencing (eg, financial difficulties, siblings acting out, or marital problems).[15]

Physicians should open a dialog by acknowledging to parents that they understand where the parents are coming from. In the course of conversation, a physician might note that from experience that the child knows the likely outcome. To reinforce this point, a physician might give some examples of the ways that children indicate their desire to know more from their parents as well as cues that children give that indicate what they know and their desire for more information. The physician might ask the parents what are they most afraid would happen if, for example, the disease's incurability came up. A physician might suggest that perhaps further discussion with the child, with the parents present or with the physician alone, would be helpful for all of them, if not now then perhaps in the future.

Parents may continue to refuse to have discussions with the child present or to have a physician engage in discussions with the child that would include the child's prognosis, side effects, or efficacy, for example. The groundwork has been laid, however, for further discussions, and insights have been gained that will serve the physician well in other situations as they arise with these parents and their child.

After meeting with the parents, the physician should meet with the child. Although especially with older children it is helpful to meet a child alone, not all children are comfortable meeting with a physician alone. In these situations, discussions should be conducted in such a way that parents remain in the background. The focus is on the child with questions, responses, and remarks directed to the child.

Whether or not a parent is present, cues should be taken from the child. Physicians need to listen and to explore what a child knows and is worried about. Weithorn[68] advises professionals to "carefully assess and explore the child's behavior, level of interest and preferences rather than making any assumptions and drawing conclusions without consulting them." Sometimes, there is less discussion and more quiet time as the child is allowed to lead and share with what might at first appear to be random thoughts or actions or with direct expressions or more metaphorical musings.

Physicians also must make clear in the meetings alone with a child and in meetings with the parents and child present that although the child will be listened to by the parents and physician, and the child's wishes taken into account, the decision is not be the child's alone to make. This is a collaborative process. Not insignificantly, this also relieves children of a burden they should not have.[44] Children are involved in the process but do not themselves determine the outcome.

This does not mean that a child cannot disagree with parents. A child can but needs to know just how dissent will be taken into account, because from a legal standpoint, if a child is a minor, the ultimate decision is with the parents.

In this shuttle diplomacy framework, there is room for dissent and there is room for negotiation. If that negotiation fails to bring about a satisfying result, the child has been included in a meaningful way, not set up for something that he or she cannot have.[34,35]

A child's inability to control the process has not kept the child from being an active player. And the fact that a child has been told that he or she is not the final decision maker may also relieve second thoughts for everyone later on, because, tragically, the parents will survive the child.

The approach and framework outlined in this article have a great deal of flexibility and adaptability and can be tailored to meet the abilities, vulnerabilities, capacities, competencies, needs, and styles of individual patients and families on different issues at different points in the illness trajectory. They are well suited to a wide range of children and adolescents because they acknowledge individual children's or adolescents' understanding, take them from where they are, and remain open ended. Joffe and colleagues[26] point out their usefulness in working with adolescents over age 15 who, as others have suggested, are no less competent than adults[36,69] and can easily become cynical when their desires are solicited but then not acted on.

The reality is that decisions are made with which children do not agree. The guidelines and regulations concerning involving children in the decision-making process must recognize this from the outset. If children do not agree with a decision, the best that can be hoped for is that they accept the process by which it was made. To secure this, the other participants, especially physicians, must be honest with children about the process and how it works.

In conclusion, although the approach outlined in this article needs further development and is undergoing further research, the authors suggest that it is the right place to begin a dialog on how to approach involving children in decision making about their care and treatment because it addresses not only the more vexing ethical issues but also the social realities where decision-making takes place as ensuring a meaningful role for children is sought.

REFERENCES

1. Chambers L, Dood W, McCulloch R, et al. A guide to the development of children's palliative services. Bristol (UK): ACT (Association for Children's Palliative Care); April 2009. Report written by a working party of ACT.
2. Field MJ, Behrman RE, editors. When children die: improving palliative and end-of-life care for children and their families/committee on palliative and end-of-life care and their families, board on health sciences policy. Washington, DC: The Institute of Medicine of The National Academies Press; 2003.
3. Alderson P, Sutcliffe K, Curtis K. Children's competence to consent to medical treatment. Hastings Cent Rep 2006;36(6):25–34.
4. American Academy of Pediatrics Committee on Bioethics. Informed consent, parental permission, and assent in pediatric practice. Pediatrics 1995;95(2): 314–7.
5. American Medical Association. Confidential care for minors. Available at: http://www.ama-assn.org/ama1/pub/upload/mm/code-medical-ethics/5055a.pdf. Accessed August 26, 2009.
6. General Medical Council. Consent: patients and doctors making decisions together. 2008. p. 25 [Paragraphs 54–6]. Available at: http://www.gmc-uk.org. Accessed July 19, 2009.
7. Medical Research Council of Canada, Natural Sciences and Engineering Research Council of Canada and Social Sciences and Humanities Research Council of Canada: Tri-Council Policy Statement. Ottawa (Canada): Ontario Public Works and Government; 1998. Article 2.7. p. 40. Available at: http://pre.ethics.gc.ca/english/policystatement/policystatement.cfm. Accessed August 16, 2009.

8. Society for Adolescent Medicine. Access to health care for adolescents and young adults: position paper of the society for adolescent medicine. J Adolesc Health 2004;35:342–4.

9. Society for Adolescent Medicine. Confidential health care for adolescents: position paper of the society for adolescent medicine. J Adolesc Health 2004;35(1):1–8.

10. Smith DH, Veatch RM. Guidelines on the termination of life-sustaining treatment and the care of the dying: a report by the Hastings Center. Bloomington (IN): Indiana University Press; 1987. p. 33–4.

11. World Medical Association Declaration of Ottawa on the Rights of the Child to Health Care. Adopted by the 50th World Assembly Ottawa, Canada, 1998. Available at: http://www.wma.net/e/policy/c4.htm. Accessed August 19, 2009.

12. Bluebond-Langner M. In the shadow of illness: parents and siblings of the chronically ill child. Princeton (NJ): Princeton University Press; 1996.

13. Bluebond-Langner M, DeCicco A, Belasco JB. Involving children with life-shortening illnesses in decisions about participation in clinical research: a proposal for shuttle diplomacy and negotiation. In: Kodish E, editor. Ethics and research with children: a case based approach. Oxford: Oxford University Press; 2005. p. 323–43.

14. Bluebond-Langner M, Belasco JB, Goldman A, et al. Understanding parents' approaches to care and treatment of children with cancer when standard therapy has failed. J Clin Oncol 2007;25(17):2414–9.

15. Bluebond-Langner M, Belasco JB, Goldman A. On going review and analysis of findings and data collected as part of a study conducted from 2001 through 2005, "Decision making for children with cancer when cure is not likely: implications for end-of-life and palliative care." [Work in progress].

16. Leiken S. Minors' assent, consent, or dissent to medical research. IRB 1983; 15(2):1–7.

17. Kripalani S, Bengtzen R, Henderson LE, et al. Clinical research in low-literacy populations: using tech-back to assess comprehension of informed consent & privacy information. IRB 2008;30(2):13–9.

18. Hazen RA, Drotar D, Kodish E. The role of the consent document in informed consent for pediatric leukemia trials. Contemp Clin Trials 2007;28:401–40.

19. Hinds PS, Drew D, Oakes LL, et al. End-of-life care preferences of pediatric patients with cancer. J Clin Oncol 2005;23(36):9146–54.

20. Miller VA, Drotar D, Kodish E. Children's competence for assent and consent: a review of empirical findings. Ethics Behav 2004;14(3):255–95.

21. Dorn LD, Susman EJ, Fletcher JC. Informed consent in children and adolescents: age, maturation and psychological state. J Adolesc Health 1995;16(3):185–90, 186.

22. Bluebond-Langner M. The private worlds of dying children. Princeton (NJ): Princeton University Press; 1978.

23. Bluebond-Langner M, Perkel D, Goertzel T, et al. Children's knowledge of cancer and its treatment: impact of an oncology camp experience. J Pediatr 1990; 116(2):207–13.

24. Bluebond-Langner M, Perkel D, Goertzel T. Pediatric cancer patients' peer relationships: impact of an oconology camp experience. J Psychosoc Oncol 1991;9(2):67–79.

25. Gibson F, Twycross A. Children's participation in research. Paediatr Nurs 2007; 19(4):14–7.

26. Joffe S, Fernandez CV, Pentz RD, et al. Involving children with cancer in decision-making about research participation. J Pediatr 2006;149(6):862–8.

27. Kuther TL, Posada M. Children and adolescents' capacity to provide informed consent for participation in research. Adv Psychol Res 2004;32:163–73.

28. Martenson EK, Fagerskiold AM. A review of children's decision-making competence in health care. J Clin Nurs 2007;17:3131–41.
29. Weir RF, Peters C. Affirming the decisions adolescents make about life and death. Hastings Cent Rep 1997;27:29–40.
30. Crisp J, Ungerer JA, Goodnow JJ. The impact of experience on children's understanding of illness. J Pediatr Psychol 1996;21(1):57–72.
31. Britto M, Cote M, Horning R, et al. Do adolescents with chronic illnesses want to make decisions about their treatment? J Adolesc Health 2004;34(2):120.
32. Broome ME, Richards DJ. The influence of relationships on children's and adolescents' participation in research. Nurse Res 2003;52(3):191–7.
33. Knopf JM, Hornung RW, Slap GB, et al. Views of treatment decision making from adolescents with chronic illnesses and their parents: a pilot study. Health Expect 2008;11:343–54.
34. Kon AA. Assent in pediatric research. Pediatrics 2005;117(5):1806–10.
35. Kon AA. Assent in pediatric research: in reply. Pediatrics 2006;118(4):1801.
36. Kuther TL. Medical decision-making and minors: issues of consent and assent. Adolescence 2003;38(150):343–58.
37. Olechnowicz JQ, Eder M, Simon C, et al. Assent observed: children's involvement in leukemia treatment and research decisions. Pediatrics 2002;109:843.
38. Stegenga K, Ward-Smith P. On receiving the diagnosis of cancer: the adolescent perspective. J Pediatr Oncol Nurs 2009;26:75–80.
39. Broome M, Richards D, Hall J. Children in research: the experience of ill children and adolescents. J Fam Nurs 2001;7(1):32–49.
40. Bluebond-Langner M, Belasco J, Goldman A. Decision making for children with cancer when cure is not likely: implications for end-of-life and palliative care. Atlanta (GA): Children's Oncology Group Meetings; 2003.
41. Unguru Y, Sill AM, Kamani N. The experiences of children enrolled in pediatric oncology research: implications for assent. Pediatrics 2010;125(4):e876–83.
42. Glaser BG, Strauss AL. Awareness of dying. Chicago: Aldine Publishing Company; 1965.
43. Zwaanswijk M, Tates K, van Dulmen S, et al. Young patients', parents', and survivors' communication preferences in paediatric oncology: results of online focus groups. BMC Pediatr 2007;7:35–45.
44. Kunin H. Ethical issues in pediatric life-threatening illness: dilemmas of consent, assent, and communication. Ethics Behav 1997;7(1):43–57.
45. Erlen JA. The child's choice: an essential component in treatment decisions. Child Health Care 1987;15(3):156–60.
46. Mohrmann M. Whose interests are they, anyway? J Relig Ethics 2006;34(1):141–50.
47. Young B, Dixon-Woods M, Heney D. Identity and role in parenting a child with cancer. Pediatr Rehabil 2002;5(4):209–14.
48. Dixon-Woods M, Young B, Heney D. Rethinking experiences of childhood cancer: a multidisciplinary approach to chronic childhood illness. London: Open University Press; 2005.
49. Dunsmore J, Quine S. Information, support, and decision-making needs and preferences of adolescents with cancer: implications for health professionals. J Psychosoc Oncol 1995;13(4):39–56.
50. Britto M, Slap GB, DeVillis RF, et al. Specialists' understanding of health care preferences of chronically ill adolescents. J Adolesc Health 2007;40(4):334–41.
51. Scherer DG. The capacity of minors to exercise voluntarism in medical treatment decisions. Law Hum Behav 1991;15:431–49.

52. Susman EJ, Dorn LD, Fletcher JC. Participation in biomedical research: the consent process as viewed by children, adolescents, young adults, and physicians. J Pediatr 1992;121(4):547–52.
53. Bartholome WG. A new understanding of consent in pediatric practice: consent, parental permission and child assent. Pediatr Ann 1989;18(4):262–5.
54. Wendler D, Shah S. Should children decide whether they are enrolled in non-beneficial research? Am J Bioeth 2003;3(4):1–7.
55. Twycross A, Gibson F, Coad J. Guidance on seeking agreement to participate in research from young children. Paediatr Nurs 2008;20(6):14–8.
56. Ashcroft R, Goodenough T, Williamson E, et al. Children's consent to research participation: social context and personal experience invalidate fixed cutoff rules. Am J Bioeth 2003;3(4):16.
57. Baylis F, Downie J, Kenny N. Children and decision making in health research. IRB 1999;21(4):5–10.
58. Fernandez CV. Context in shaping the ability of a child to assent to research. Am J Bioeth 2003;3(4):24–30.
59. Fisher C. Goodness of fit ethic for child assent to non-beneficial research. Am J Bioeth 2003;3(4):27–8.
60. Ladd RE. Child assent revisited. Am J Bioeth 2003;3(4):37–8.
61. Murphy TF. Assent and dissent in 407 research with children. Am J Bioeth 2003; 3(4):1–4.
62. Nelson RM, Reynolds WW. We should reject passive resignation in favor of requiring the assent of younger children for participation in nonbeneficial research. Am J Bioeth 2003;3(4):11–3.
63. Parekh SA. Child consent and the law: an insight and discussion into the law relating to consent and competence. Child Care Health Dev 2006;33(1):78–82.
64. Taylor HA. Children under age 14 deserve more. Am J Bioeth 2003;3(4):33–4.
65. Toner K, Schwartz R. Why a teenager over age 14 should be able to consent, rather than merely assent, to participation as a human subject of research. Am J Bioeth 2003;3(4):38–40.
66. Wendler D, Shah SA. A response to commentators on "should children decide whether they are enrolled in nonbeneficial research?" Am J Bioeth 2003;3(4): W37–8.
67. Moeller CJ. Moral responsiveness in pediatric research ethics. Am J Bioeth 2003; 3(4):W1–3.
68. Weithorn LA. Involving children in decisions affecting their own welfare: guidelines for professionals. In: Melton GB, Koocher GP, Saks MJ, editors. Children's competence to consent. New York: Plenum Press; 1983. p. 75–91.
69. Grisso T, Vierling L. Minors' consent to treatment: a developmental perspective. Prof Psychol 1978;78:412–27.

Clinical Decision Making in Palliative Care and End of Life Care

Margaret M. Mahon, PhD, RN

KEYWORDS

• Palliative care • Decision making • Ethics • Nurses • End of life

Nurses often care for patients and their families who are in turmoil because of a new diagnosis or an exacerbation of a long-term diagnosis. This turmoil can be exacerbated by the decisions that must be made following a diagnosis or other newly disclosed information. The purpose of this article is to describe processes of clinical decision making, to identify a range of factors that affect decision making, and to explore three landmark cases that led to decision-making guidelines being accepted in the twenty-first century. Finally, nurses' responsibilities and opportunities in decision making are examined.

COMPONENTS OF DECISION MAKING
Decisions in the Clinical Arena

Most decisions about a patient's care are based simply on clinical data; for example, a specific disease or symptom X is best treated with medication Y. Other clinical decisions are made by considering specific dimensions of an individual patient's situation. For example, it may be important to minimize a patient's pill burden. In this case, one medication may be chosen out of several appropriate medications because it is administered once or twice a day rather than three or four times. A broad consideration, then, of the content and processes of decision making allows providers to identify and integrate the full range of factors necessary for the best decision for an individual patient.

Jonsen and colleagues[1] have developed a model to guide the integration of ethics into clinical decision making. Although the model was developed for the integration of ethical thinking into clinical decisions, its global and multidimensional considerations make it immediately applicable to any situation in which health care providers, patients, and families must come to a consensus.

Palliative Care and Ethics, School of Nursing, George Mason University, 4400 University Drive, Mail Stop 3C4, Fairfax, VA 22030, USA
E-mail address: mmahon@gmu.edu

Nurs Clin N Am 45 (2010) 345–362
doi:10.1016/j.cnur.2010.03.002   nursing.theclinics.com
0029-6465/10/$ – see front matter © 2010 Elsevier Inc. All rights reserved.

Jonsen and colleagues[1] described four dimensions of decision making: medical indications, patient preferences, quality of life, and contextual features. The diagnosis and medically indicated treatments circumscribe the choices available to patient and family and even to the health care team. The physician and other members of the health care team bring to the discussion the facts, the raw information that patients and families need to make decisions; these medical indications frame the rest of the discussion. The patient and family add the meaning and value of the choices, and the meaning and value of the consequences informed by the considerations of the other dimensions of the decision.

Medical indications

Medical indications dictate the therapeutic choices available to patients and families. For example, immunizations are given to prevent future disease. A fracture is treated with specific types of immobilization and sometimes surgery. Patients with lung disease, heart disease, and many other chronic illnesses are treated with medications and interventions that allow them to live as well as possible with a specific disease. In each of these cases, the diagnosis or risk of future disease determines the treatment. Specifics of the disease or comorbidities or even facts about insurance may further limit options. Regardless, in every case, the patient's medical condition is the first consideration in treatment options.

Patient preferences

Health care providers have come to recognize the importance of considering patient preferences in clinical decision making. "[D]ecisions regarding the treatment of patients should be anchored in terms of each patient's own values, preferences, and goals of care, as best understood, which determine what is best for each patient."[2] Patient preferences are just that: What does the patient want in the context of the medical indications? This is much more complex than it might initially seem. How the questions are asked is at least as important as what is asked. Open-ended, noncontextual questions, such as "What do you want us to do?" are rarely helpful and often engender a sense of confusion in patient and family. Before posing any questions, before considering any options, it is important that the patient understands the disease, injuries, or other pathophysiologic considerations.

Patient preferences, then, are based on accurate understanding from a clear list of options. It is the responsibility of the clinician to construct the clinical options and often to make recommendations. Making the choice also means considering the burdens and the benefits of each option. Health care providers are often very good about describing the benefits of a particular therapy but not as forthcoming about the burdens. Withholding information about the burdens or limitations of a specific therapy is not done out of any bad intention. Rather, when a provider espouses the benefits of a particular treatment, it is done out of a firm belief that *this* is what is best for the patients. The reality is that there is no treatment without risks and no therapy without cost.

A patient newly diagnosed with cancer is often told that the next step is chemotherapy. Before deciding whether a patient should have chemotherapy (or any other treatment) the goals of that treatment must be specified. The goals of treatment are very specific outcomes to be achieved with the therapy. What will chemotherapy do for this patient? Is the goal to cure the disease or to prolong the patient's life without eradicating the disease? If the goal is to prolong the patient's life, then by how much—weeks, months, or years? What goal is realistic, or what is the likelihood of achieving the goal? Finally, what are the burdens of this treatment? What will the patient's quality of life be if she receives the chemotherapy or if she does not? Understanding what each treatment is meant to accomplish allows providers, patients, and families to enter treatment with a shared understanding. For most patients with cancer, chemotherapy or some other form of treatment is the best option. The same questions can and should be asked about preference for treatments for heart disease, lung disease, major trauma, or infectious diseases.

Quality of life

The quality-of-life dimension addresses not only what quality of life is acceptable to the patient, but first what quality of life is realistic with the proposed therapies. Quality-of-life decisions are based on an accurate understanding of the clinical realities of the disease or injury. For example, for a patient on chronic dialysis, quality of life is compromised; a tremendous commitment of time and energy is inherent in the therapy. Patients often do not feel well even after dialysis. Can a patient make a truly informed decision about whether to start dialysis without understanding the experience of dialysis? It may be helpful for a patient to observe dialysis and to speak with a patient on dialysis. Quality of life is not only about whether the patient survives but also about how the patient lives. Dialysis is an excellent therapy for many patients. The decision about whether to start can often be better informed than it is for many patients.

Contextual features

Understanding the context of a clinical situation is essential for optimal decision making.[3] Jonsen and colleagues[1] described contextual factors as including family and other social relationships, as well as factors about the institution, and financial and legal factors. The consideration of contextual factors has to do with identifying elements that affect the ability to implement any particular decision. If a hospital has three continuous venovenous hemodialysis (CVVHD) machines that are all in use and a fourth person needs hemodialysis, what should be done? Does one patient have to come off of dialysis? Do those patients already on CVVHD have priority? Can another treatment be substituted? Consideration of contextual factors may compound the difficulty of the decision-making process. In other cases, contextual factors actually limit certain options. For example, a patient's insurance might dictate the hospitals where she can receive care. If the physician chosen by the patient does not have staff privileges at that hospital, options may be narrowed. The patient can have either the hospital or the physician but not both. Clarification of the contextual factors affects how and whether the decision can be implemented as planned.

Factors Affecting Decision Making

In the late twentieth century, inclusive decision making (medical decision making with participation of patients, families, and a variety of health care providers; sometimes called shared decision making) was brought into sharp focus by three landmark cases. The common element in these cases is the challenge of integrating new technology into traditional clinical decision making. These cases were breakthroughs because they highlight the limitations of clinical decision making at the time. Up to the time of the case of Karen Ann Quinlan, new medical technology had been considered as an inevitable good to be utilized at every opportunity. Any new technology, despite its potential promise, brings with it the responsibility to consider not only when it should be used, but also whether there are any circumstances under which it should not be used. This latter consideration, whether not to use a technology, almost inevitably occurs much later than the considerations of how a technology should be used.

This tendency to rush to use a new treatment in health care applies to more than machines. Prescribers are likely to use newer medications, even if there are extant medications with proven and perhaps better efficacy for the patient's specific condition.[4,5] Pressure to use newer (usually more expensive) medications is compounded because patients often demand them. Direct-to-consumer advertising contributes to these demands, as patients often request medication for which they have seen or heard advertisements.[6] These advertisements rarely appeal primarily to medical indications. Instead, advertisements almost universally include an emotional appeal (95%) and often portray the medication as a medical breakthrough (58%) that will lead to social approval (78%).[7]

Pharmaceutical companies spend billions of dollars a year to urge prescribers to use their new, more expensive medications. Many of these medications fill a void, but many do not. Billions more dollars are spent on direct-to-consumer advertising, and prescribers then feel even greater pressure to prescribe the new medication. As a result, patients not uncommonly receive medications that may not provide the optimal benefit, or that they do not need.

As much as this is true for medications, so too is it true for other technologies also. Because the medication exists, we feel compelled to prescribe it. Because the technology exists, we feel compelled to use it. Mathematician John von Neumann wrote, "Technological possibilities are irresistible to man."[8] Victor Fuchs[9] described physicians' desire to use new technologies as what came to be called the "technological imperative". Callahan[10] wrote, "Nothing so characterizes and defines contemporary healthcare as the pursuit of scientific knowledge and technological applications." This perceived imperative to use technology has shaped much of health care in the late twentieth and early twenty-first centuries. Because a technology exists, health care providers feel compelled to use it. Further, because a technology exists, patients and families often expect it will (and should) invariably be used. In US society, and in some other western societies that are wealthy enough to have a plethora of technologies available, the dimension of decision making about when *not* to use a technology is still not widely understood.

There are certain patients, about a dozen, whose cases became public and then landmark, usually through the courts. The publicity of these cases has provided a forum for discussion among both lay and professional audiences. Such landmark cases embody the evolution of thought, of understanding, and of optimal processes for decision making. Understanding three such cases provides greater understanding of questions to be asked in the process of good decision making, and the influence of technology on this process.

Landmark Cases

Karen Ann Quinlan
The case Karen Ann Quinlan was born on March 29, 1954. She was the oldest of the 3 children of Joseph and Julia Quinlan. At 21 years of age, she moved into a house with friends in Cranberry Lake, New Jersey. Quinlan had recently been dieting. On April 14, 1975, while at a bar celebrating a friend's birthday, she mixed alcohol with other drugs. When she complained that she was not feeling well, she was taken home by friends and put to bed. When the friends checked on her a short time later, they found she was not breathing. Friends called for emergency assistance and attempted resuscitation.[11] Quinlan arrived at the hospital with "pupils unreactive...[she was] unresponsive even to deep pain. Legs: Rigid, curled up. Impression: Overdose, unknown substance, with decorticate brain activity."[11(pp15)]

Quinlan was in the intensive care unit on a ventilator, diagnosed as being in a coma.[12] Shortly thereafter, a tracheostomy was inserted; a nasogastric tube was used for feedings. Although comatose, family and friends were struck by her restless, thrashing behaviors.[11(pp16,18)]

She was eventually diagnosed as being in the recently described persistent vegetative state (PVS). Quinlan's parents came to recognize that she would never recover. Several factors affected their subsequent decisions. First, Julia Quinlan remembered that her daughter had commented on the dying of 2 people she knew from cancers. Karen Quinlan had said that she would not want to be "kept alive like that."[11(pp18,34)] Joseph and Julia Quinlan each consulted their parish priest. They were reminded that for centuries the Roman Catholic Church had not required its members to accept extraordinary means. The Quinlans acted based on the medical facts, their acceptance of the reality of her condition, and the reassurance that their decision was not incompatible with their faith. On July 31, 1975, they requested that the physician "discontinue all extraordinary measures, including the use of a [ventilator] for our daughter Karen Quinlan."[11(pp19)]

Neurologist Robert Morse, Karen Quinlan's physician, denied the Quinlans' request. His response reflected the understanding of both medical science and the law at the time; Dr Morse believed that discontinuation of the ventilator would be homicide.[11(pp21)] On September 12, 1975, a motion was filed with the New Jersey Superior Court; Mr Quinlan sought guardianship of his daughter with the intention of seeking permission to have the ventilator discontinued.

The case gained traction in the media; across the country and around the world different views of the case were starkly demarcated. The assertion by some was that, given that Karen Quinlan did not meet Harvard Brain Death Criteria,[13] withdrawing the ventilator was murder. Conversely, given that PVS was a permanent, neurologically devastating condition that precluded Quinlan's abilities to perceive or interact with the environment, it would be disrespectful not to discontinue ventilatory support.

Judge Robert Muir Jr denied the Quinlans' request, dismissing the claims offered by their attorney Paul Armstrong for relief on the grounds of privacy, religion, and freedom from cruel and unusual punishment. Muir wrote that Karen Quinlan's views, expressed through her mother, lacked the strength of a real understanding, and that her father's emotional involvement precluded him from the objectivity needed to be her guardian.[11(pp43)] Ultimately, the physicians' wishes were followed; the judge's statements allowed discontinuation of life-prolonging treatments to be equated with homicide.

In January 1976, the New Jersey Supreme Court heard the case that had been appealed by Armstrong. In their decision, the Justices focused primarily on who should make decisions about Quinlan's care. On March 31, 1976, the Court decided that Joseph Quinlan could make decisions on his daughter's behalf, including the decision to discontinue artificial ventilation.

Although the decision was made at the end of March, and the Quinlans requested that it be implemented immediately, throughout April Dr Morse and others did not implement the decision. They continued artificial ventilation and told the family to "be patient." Rather than withdraw the ventilator as Mr Quinlan had requested and the New Jersey Supreme Court had allowed, the staff at St Clare's hospital weaned Karen Quinlan over a period of 3 weeks. Thus, although still in a PVS, she no longer required ventilatory support. She was transferred to a long-term care facility. Quinlan died nine years later, on June 11, 1985, from a pneumonia that was not treated with antibiotics.

Significance Lessons from the dying of Karen Ann Quinlan are related primarily to the interrelationship of technology and the diagnosis of PVS, as well as to the evolution of the content and processes of decision making. PVS was first described in 1972 by Jennett and Plum[14] as "a syndrome in search of a name." Since that time, understanding of the condition has been slow to emerge; as a result, how to care for patients with PVS has been slower yet to be understood and implemented. PVS was first defined as "a form of eyes-open permanent unconsciousness in which the patient has periods of wakefulness and physiologic sleep/wake cycles, but at no time is the patient aware of himself or his environment. Neurologically being awake, but unaware is the result of a functioning brainstem, and the total loss of cerebral cortical functioning."[15] PVS cannot be diagnosed until 3 months after a nontraumatic injury and 6 months after a traumatic injury.[16]

Perhaps the greatest challenge of PVS is that although PVS is (mis)understood as related to coma, in fact the patients appear very different. It seems incongruous that someone who can awaken, who can move spontaneously, and whose eyes are open actually has no capacity to perceive stimuli from the environment. To this day, the condition is widely misunderstood.

The case of Karen Ann Quinlan brought national attention to the problem of the artificial prolongation of life, a clinical question with ethical dimensions. Quinlan's case also initiated the first step toward consideration of the right to refuse treatments. Quinlan's parents sought to refuse treatment for a therapy that could not cure their daughter, or in any way contribute to an improved quality of life for her. Prior to this case, there existed no formal mechanism for refusing a treatment. Health care providers did not know whether to stop or how to discontinue the use of technologies, especially ventilators.

In the New Jersey Supreme Court case *in re Quinlan,* because the patient's wishes were not known, and could never be known, her parents' wishes of what they believed she would want were accepted.[12] (Although they had specific statements about what she would want, the court concluded that her statements were too remote from her own situation to represent a real understanding.) This *substituted judgment* standard meant that a decision could be based on what a patient *would have wanted* under these circumstances.

In 1976, the California Natural Death Act was passed. This was the first law in the United States that specified the right to refuse life-prolonging therapies. The law also protected physicians from being sued for failing to provide treatments at the end of a patient's life. Over the next 5 years, 15 states passed legislation that allowed patients to designate preferences for the care at the end of their lives.[17] Although many of the documents, especially living wills, were replete with problems, they also did a great deal to open the discussion about when to stop certain therapies at the end of life.

Nancy Cruzan

The case On January 11, 1983, 25-year-old Nancy Davis (later to be known to the public by her maiden name, Nancy Cruzan) was driving to her rural Missouri home when she took a curve in the road too quickly. Her car overturned, landing 35 feet away from the road. Davis was thrown from the car; she was found face down and unresponsive. Although the police at the scene believed she had died, paramedics eventually restored Davis's heartbeat.[18] She was likely anoxic for about 20 minutes.

Davis was taken to the operating room to repair liver damage and extensive facial wounds. While she was in the operating room, nurses twice came out to give a report to her husband, parents, sister, and other family members. All present were relieved when the second nurse reporting from the operating room said, "I think she's going to be fine."[18(pp14)]

Although Davis initially required ventilatory support, by the end of the month, she was breathing on her own.[18(pp19)] Because Davis was unresponsive and unable to participate in decision making, "the staff generally turned to Paul, as Nancy's husband, for necessary decisions."[18(pp21)] Although Nancy Davis had no formal document indicating that her husband should represent her wishes in decision making, as her husband, Paul Davis was the presumed decision maker. When Paul Davis was unavailable, health care providers turned to Nancy Davis's father, Joe Cruzan, to sign the necessary forms. Joe Cruzan signed the form for the insertion of his daughter's gastrostomy tube on February 7, 1983.

In January 1984, one year after the car crash, it was clear to many in the family, her husband and parents among them, that Nancy Davis would never recover. At that time, her parents, Joe and Joyce Cruzan, went to court seeking guardianship of their daughter because her husband had been increasingly absent. Guardianship was granted, allowing them to make decisions for Nancy, though those decisions had to be in her best interest. Six months later the Cruzans went to court again, seeking a divorce between Nancy and Paul Davis. Paul Davis did not oppose the request. Nancy Davis became Nancy Beth Cruzan again.

Because they recognized that she was not improving, and would not improve, in 1987, Nancy Cruzan's parents eventually chose to request that the hospital stop their daughter's tube feedings. The hospital, Missouri Rehabilitation Center, sought a court order to prevent the removal of the feeding tube. The state trial court affirmed the right to refuse treatment. The Missouri State Supreme Court reversed this decision, asserting that the State had an interest in "the preservation of life."[19] The State Supreme Court also ruled that the parents did not have a right to decide *for* their daughter. Rather, they ruled that under Missouri law there had to be "clear and convincing" evidence of what Nancy Cruzan would want. The court wanted to be sure that *her* wishes were clearly represented. The Missouri court thus decided that substituted judgment was not adequate for so crucial a decision. The Court decided that it was not enough to know what the patient would likely have wanted; rather, explicit patient preferences had to be clear. The case was appealed to the US Supreme Court.

The US Supreme Court supported the right of competent patients to refuse treatment, even if that decision resulted in the patient's death. The Court also decided that discontinuation of a feeding tube is no different from refusing any other medical treatment. This rendered some state laws unconstitutional. Finally, the Supreme Court decided that states could, as Missouri had done, apply a "clear and convincing evidence standard in proceedings where a guardian seeks to discontinue nutrition and hydration of a person diagnosed to be in a persistent vegetative state."[19] That is, it was not enough to base a decision on what those closest to Cruzan were convinced she would want. Rather, the court demanded proof (clear and convincing evidence) that the request represented Cruzan's own wishes. The US Supreme Court left it to the states to establish mechanisms "for protecting an incompetent individual's liberty interest in refusing medical treatment."[19] (O'Connor concurring).

The case was then remanded, or sent back to the Missouri court, who were to render a decision in light of the US Supreme Court's decision. The case was covered widely in the media, including pictures of Cruzan before the crash. Cruzan had been married twice; her first husband's name was Hayes. Two women who had known Nancy Hayes came forward to testify in the new Missouri hearing. They described conversations they had had with Hayes (née Cruzan) in which she specifically said she would not want to live "like a vegetable." In addition, another friend came forward to tell of Cruzan's statements about the Quinlan case, stating that she "wouldn't want to live like that." These statements of Nancy Cruzan met the "clear and convincing" evidence standard; the Court allowed the tube to be removed. "Within minutes of receiving the final trial court ruling, Nancy Cruzan's feeding tube was removed, the gastrostomy hole in her stomach was taped over with white athletic tape, and Nancy was moved to the hospice wing of the state hospital,"[20(pp286)] where she later died.

Significance As in Quinlan's case, the facts in Cruzan's case centered on a young woman in a PVS. The question that arose for Cruzan also involved the discontinuation of a technology, in this case a tube inserted for the purpose of providing nutrition and hydration. Nancy Cruzan's family knew of no statements, oral or written, about her preferences for end-of-life care. At the center of their decision making was the question, "What would Nancy want?"[19(pp41)] Her parents and sister were united in their belief that Nancy Cruzan would not want to be kept alive in a PVS. The medical indications, the facts about PVS, framed the options for clinical care. In this case, the question was not about what could prolong patient life, but whether the feeding tube could provide a benefit that Cruzan could appreciate. Her parents petitioned the lower court in Missouri to be allowed to remove the feeding tube and to allow a "natural death." When the state Supreme Court did allow for the removal of the tube, the case was appealed, because the state believed it had to protect Cruzan. As a result, unlike Quinlan's case, Cruzan's case went to the US Supreme Court.

The US Supreme Court did not rule specifically on the right not to continue a therapy for which the patient could not recognize a benefit. The Supreme Court did, however, assume a right to refuse unwanted treatment as a protected civil liberty. The court also agreed that states could set a standard about the strength of evidence necessary for a patient's decision. In Cruzan's case, the standard that had been applied by Missouri was a "clear and convincing evidence" standard. Decisions about whether to continue or discontinue a life-prolonging therapy should be based on the patient's stated preference, even if the patient is no longer able to reiterate previously made statements.

Another important dimension of Cruzan's case was that the therapy to be discontinued was artificial nutrition and hydration (ANH). Based on the patient's eventually discovered stated preferences, a decision to implement the patient's refusal of treatment was allowed. ANH is not the same as food; the technology is invasive and often causes discomfort.[21-23] The right to refuse treatment, then, extends to the right to refuse ANH.

There is an extensive body of literature on cases in which patients cannot recognize a benefit of ANH. Regardless, still many people, including providers, consider ANH equivalent to naturally ingested food and fluids. Although health care providers might consider it a minor procedure, for patients it is not minor. Although ANH is beneficial for many patients, the medical indications, including the ability to appreciate the benefit, are not present in people with PVS, dementia, and other diseases.

The other major implication of Cruzan's case was the genesis of advance directives. After Karen Ann Quinlan's death, there was increasing recognition of the need to establish a mechanism of decision making for people who had lost capacity. Since the late 1960s, there had been sporadic efforts by physicians and legislators to get people to express their wishes for end-of-life care.[24] These efforts all lacked significant impact. While the issues around decision making gained traction with Quinlan's case, the most significant legislative effort did not occur until Cruzan's case.

The Patient Self-Determination Act (PSDA)[25] was passed in 1990 and went into effect in 1991. The PSDA mandates that all institutions participating in Medicare or Medicaid are required to provide specific information to patients. This information includes that patients have the right to be involved in medical decision making;

patients have the right not only to informed consent but also to refuse treatments, even if that refusal means that the patient will die. In both Quinlan and Cruzan, the decision was to refuse all therapies that could not benefit the patient.

The PSDA also requires that patients receive information about advance directives. Advance directives are a mechanism to accomplish 2 things: they allow patients to designate a surrogate, and they allow the patient to specify preferences for medical therapies in the context of certain disease states. *Surrogate* comes from the Latin *surrogatus*, meaning "to put in the place of" or sometimes translated as "to stand in the shoes of." Advance directives provide a means for patients to designate who can represent their decisions if they are unable or choose not to participate in health care decision making. The focus of a surrogate decision maker should be to represent the patient's wishes in decision making. In both Quinlan and Cruzan, the parents were acting as surrogates, standing in to voice not their opinions, but those of their daughters.

Commonly known types of advance directives are Living Wills and Durable Powers of Attorney for Health Care. Each of these types of document allows both identification of a surrogate and indication of preferences for decision making. Living wills are often more difficult to implement, because they have statements that are sharply delimited. For example, a typical living will or some durable powers of attorney will have statements such as, "I ___ do / ___ do not want artificial nutrition." Any document that conveys the message, "I never want this therapy" or "I always want this therapy" is likely to be unhelpful in clinical decision making. Understanding the context of any decision is extremely important, but many advance directives preclude this. When patients or family members make such absolute pronouncements, they usually have specific beliefs about the context of the statement. One patient might mean, "If I am dying, I do not want artificial nutrition." The same patient might intend, "If it will help me recover, I do want artificial nutrition." The medical indications frame preferences, but many advance directives do not allow for this specification.

The patient preference, then, is often a manifestation of the patient's understanding of the goals of care. That is, is this therapy a bridge to a quality of life that would be acceptable to the patient? Or, conversely, will this therapy merely prolong the patient's dying? Although simple, analyzing a therapy as either a bridge to a better living or a prescription for how the patient will spend the end of his life can be helpful in discussions with the family, as well as with other health care providers.

Advance directives are still a mystery to many today. It was specified in the PSDA that hospitals should help patients and families to complete and presumably to understand advance directives. There remain, however, multiple problems with advance directives. A majority of adults do not have advance directives. If a patient does have an advance directive in which a surrogate has been designated, often that surrogate is not aware that she has been designated as the surrogate decision maker. If a surrogate has been designated, *and* if the surrogate is aware that she is the surrogate, it is still unlikely that a discussion about the patient's preferences has occurred.[26] Finally, *if* a surrogate has been appointed, and *if* the surrogate has been informed that she is the surrogate, and *if* the discussion about the patient's preferences has occurred, the surrogate is still likely to be incorrect in about one-third of the cases.[26]

People who are married are most likely to appoint their spouse as surrogate. Moorman and Carr[27] studied spouses' ability to predict preferences for end-of-life care for people with dementia or severe pain. Spouses were accurate only 77% of the time in the situation of cognitive impairment and only 62% of time in the case of severe pain. Given these rates of inaccuracies, the responsibility of health care providers is increased. Specifically, health care providers can focus on patient preferences *with the patient* while the patient is healthy and able to consider and articulate preferences. In cases in which decision making is done with a surrogate, it is essential to keep the focus of decision making on the patient. That is, the question should be, "If your mother were able to sit at the table with us, what would she tell us?" rather than, "What do you want us to do?"

Terri Schiavo

The case[a] Theresa Marie Schindler was born on December 3, 1963, 1 of the 3 children of Mary and Robert Schindler.[28] As an adolescent, Terri Schindler struggled with her weight and likely had an eating disorder. In 1984, Terri Schindler married Michael Schiavo. In 1986, the couple moved to Florida, where Mrs Schiavo's parents then lived.

On February 25, 1990, Terri Schiavo had a cardiac arrest, possibly due to hypokalemia resulting from her eating disorder. After the arrest, she had prolonged anoxia leading to brain damage; Schiavo was eventually diagnosed as being in a PVS. (Two medical malpractice cases led to more than $1 million for Mrs Schiavo's care as well as money for Michael Schiavo.) In June 1990, Michael Schiavo was appointed his wife's guardian. For three years after the initial cardiac arrest, Michael Schiavo and the Schindlers were united in their pursuit of cure for Terri Schiavo. Her care included experimental therapies, speech therapy, occupational therapy, rehabilitation, and more.

In July 1993, the Schindlers went to court to have Michael Schiavo removed as guardian. This Court, and several others uniformly found that Michael Schiavo was acting in his wife's best interest. This began a 12-year battle about decisions for how Terri Schiavo would live and how she would die.

In May 1998, Michael Schiavo sought permission from the court to have his wife's percutaneous endoscopic gastrostomy (PEG) tube removed. He based this request on statements his wife had made that would be applicable in the context of a diagnosis of PVS. The Schindlers were adamantly opposed. The ensuing protracted legal battle was extremely acrimonious, and very public. Legal proceedings involved more than 100 petitions, motions, and hearings before the Pinellas County Circuit Court, the Second District Court of Appeals, and the Florida Supreme Court, District Courts, and even the US Supreme Court (though they refused to hear the case).

Finally, on April 24, 2001, the Pinellas County Circuit Court and the Second District Court of Appeals ordered Terri Schiavo's PEG tube removed. On April 26, 2001, a Circuit Court judge ordered the tube reinserted.

More legal efforts and attempted mediation ensued. Most of these efforts addressed Michael Schiavo's efforts to implement his wife's wishes to have the PEG tube removed, and the Schindlers' efforts to have the PEG tube reinserted.

On October 15, 2003, Mrs Schiavo's PEG tube was removed for the second time. At this point, governmental involvement began. This eventually included intervention attempts by Florida Governor Jeb Bush, the Florida House of Representatives, and the Florida Senate, seeking to have the PEG tube reinserted. These efforts, intended only to apply to Terri Schiavo, became known as Terri's Law. Despite Michael Schiavo's legal efforts to prevent the implementation of these laws, on October 21, 2003, the PEG tube was reinserted.

---

[a] Many of the facts in this section are from the work of Cerminara and Goodman.[28] They compiled an extensive report of the unprecedented decision making in the case of Schiavo. Every court appearance, legislative effort, and other interventions are described in almost day-by-day coverage.

At this point, President George W. Bush publicly praised the efforts of his brother, Governor Jeb Bush, on behalf of Terri Schiavo. Michael Schiavo sought to have Terri's Law declared unconstitutional. Throughout the rest of 2003 and all of 2004, there were multiple legal and legislative efforts by Michael Schiavo, the Schindlers, multiple judges, and various branches of government. Much of the debate focused on the legality of Terri's Law.

In March 2004, Pope John Paul II[29] broadened the religious dimension of the debate by making statements that seemed to indicate that Roman Catholics would be required to accept ANH, even in the case of PVS. His comments included.

I should like particularly to underline how the administration of water and food, even when provided by artificial means, always represents a natural means of preserving life, not a medical act. Its use, furthermore, should be considered, in principle, ordinary and proportionate, and as such morally obligatory, insofar as and until it is seen to have attained its proper finality, which in the present case consists in providing nourishment to the patient and alleviation of his suffering.[29(pp12)]

Many in the Roman Catholic Church continue to struggle with this issue to this day. Many Roman Catholic scholars recognize ANH as a medical treatment that can be refused when the patient can appreciate no benefit.

In September 2004, the Florida Supreme Court unanimously declared Terri's Law unconstitutional. In January 2005, the US Supreme Court refused to review the Florida Decision on Terri's Law. There were ongoing and simultaneous efforts to have Schiavo's PEG tube removed, countered by others to have the PEG tube remain in place.

In March 2005, additional legislative efforts in Florida, as well as by the US House of Representatives sought to mandate the prolongation of Terri Schiavo's life. Regardless, removal of the PEG tube was again scheduled. Despite round the clock and national efforts, Terri Schiavo's PEG tube was removed for the third time on March 18, 2005. During March 19–20, the US Senate and the US House passed a federal version of Terri's law, signed by President Bush at 1:11 AM on March 21, 2005. Legal and legislative efforts continued unabated. Terri Schiavo died on March 31, 2005.

Significance In clinical decision making, the facts about the patient's condition shape decisions to be made. Medical indications are the data that frame the clinical options. These options allow for the integration of patient preferences, quality of life, and contextual factors.

In Terri Schiavo's case, this was largely set aside. The Schindlers wanted to save their daughter's life at any cost. Her husband wanted to implement a decision based on respecting her wishes. The Schindlers truly believed their daughter could be saved, cured, or at least to some degree healed. Michael Schiavo was looking for his wife and she was not there; Mrs Schindler was looking for her baby and she was very much there (Charles Harrison, MD, Columbia, MD, personal communication, 12 November 2009).

In one of their final appeals to the Eleventh Circuit Court, days before her death, the Schindlers contended they heard their daughter say, "I want to live."[28] (25 March, 2005) The Florida medical examiner's autopsy report provided the final data on the impossibility of this act; examination of her brain confirmed extensive cortical atrophy. John Thogmartin, MD, went on to say, "No amount of therapy or treatment would have regenerated the massive loss of neurons."[28] (15 June, 2005).

The Schindlers' beliefs are understandable. They were getting information from multiple sources that their daughter could recover. None of this advice, however, was from people with a true understanding of the condition. Regardless, the Governor, Senate Majority Leader Bill Frist (a heart surgeon who, upon observing videotapes, stated that Schiavo was not in a PVS), the President, Jesse Jackson, and countless others made public statements that failed to consider the objective, physical, clinical reality of Schiavo's brain injuries.

Unlike the cases of Quinlan and Cruzan in which medical indications ultimately shaped clinical decision making, in Schiavo's case, ignorance of the medical facts led to poor overall decision making. Further, nonlegal questions and answers about patient preferences, with the notable exception of Michael Schiavo, did not focus on Terri Schiavo's preferences, but rather on the preferences and beliefs of others. There is a distinction between killing and letting die that rests in the understanding of the current and future state of the disease. This has to be integrated into decision making. No one wanted Terri Schiavo to die; however, her death was deemed less burdensome and more respectful than continued living in a condition that she would never be able to appreciate.

IMPLICATIONS FOR NURSES' INVOLVEMENT IN DECISION MAKING

Patients face decisions across the course of an illness. Whether the patient will recover completely from a disease, whether the patient will live for years with a chronic illness, or whether a disease is likely to cause the patient's death in a relatively short period of time, the prognosis has little effect on the inevitability of health care decision making. Decisions may address small questions ("At what time should I take this medication?") or questions with great import ("I've been diagnosed with Alzheimers. How do I plan for the rest of my life?"[30]).

Although the landmark cases presented have to do with patients in a PVS, the principles of decision making remain the same: clinical realities shape options for decision making. Knowledge of the facts of *this* patient's illness or injuries at *this* time, often in the context of comorbidities, developmental stage, and other factors, is the first stage of decision making. Physiologic realities frame clinical options.

Many factors affect patients' and families' decisions. These include their understanding of the disease (accurate or inaccurate), experiences, hopes and goals, the desire to please health care providers, family support, beliefs about quality of life, beliefs of family or friends, fears, religious or spiritual beliefs, practicalities of daily living, and other factors.[31-34] Barriers to optimal decision making include lack of accurate information, inadequate disclosure of pertinent information, lack of time, perceived legal influences, an emphasis on family (rather than patient) preferences, lack of decision-making process skills, attitudes, bias, lack of belief in the process, and others.[34-36]

"The patient's right to make his or her own medical decisions is one-half of the working basis of the physician-patient relationship, regardless of the patient's current capacity to make choices."[37(pp213)] This notion of partnership and reciprocal responsibility extends to the entire health care team working collaboratively. It is extremely unlikely that health care providers will be aware of all the pertinent facts affecting a patient's or family's decision-making processes. The patient or family might not even be aware of why they are afraid, reticent, angry, or unsure. The role of the health care team in decision making is first to know and present the medical facts. Based on these facts, options are constructed from which a choices will be made. Sometimes the options are few. (A bacterial infection or arrhythmia or other disease is treated with specific medications determined by evidence-based standards.) Sometimes several options exist. Options still depend on the physical realities of the condition. Medical indications shape clinical options. The questions that follow, then, are who should make the decision and what the decision will be.

Respect for autonomy leads to processes that preserve the patient as the decision maker. Patients may be too ill to participate in decision making or may choose not to participate in decision making, especially if they are comfortable about the decision making that would occur even without their involvement.[38] Even if the patient is not participating in decision making, the patient's preferences still guide decision making. This places a clear responsibility on providers to structure questions in such a way as to elicit patient preferences. Patients may be asked, "given what we have discussed…" establishes that what follows is based on what came before. "Given what we have discussed, how would you like to proceed?" This statement may be followed by a restatement of the options. "Do you want to try X, or is Y right for you at this time?"

Open-ended questions may afford patients latitude, but failure to place the questions in the context of medical indications and structured options leaves families adrift and confused. Similarly, options presented to family members are ideally structured in a way to keep the focus on the patient's preferences, not on what the surrogate wants or hopes. "Did you ever speak with your husband about what he would want in these circumstances?" Often these discussions have not occurred. In this case, questions should be structured to elicit patient's likely preferences. "Did he ever know someone in circumstances like this?" "Did he ever see anything on television like this? What did he say about it?" Such questions not only provide a good view of the patient preferences but also can reassure the family member that the decision is respecting what the patient would want. Proper guidance by providers can unburden family members from feeling that they made a decision that caused harm; it can reassure them that they were doing what was medically indicated and respecting patient preferences.

In some circumstances, the surrogate not only does not know the patient's preferences but also is unable to extrapolate from similar circumstances. In such cases, it is helpful to ask, "What is most important to her in her daily living?" Structuring subsequent discussions on the likelihood of the patient ever being able to enjoy these activities or interactions again establishes quality of life as a further dimension of patient preferences in decision making.

Discussion about medical indications and patient decision making are most often and appropriately led by a physician. One of the hallmarks of palliative care is involvement of an interdisciplinary team. The nurse is a member of that team; that is the standard of care. Nurses are often described as the professionals with the most patient contact; as such, nurses are often positioned to have an important role in decision making.[39] Their role in decision making is often affected by knowledge, experiences, organizational structures, and personal beliefs and attitudes.[39] Unfortunately, nurses often misunderstand the role of palliative care, thereby limiting options for patients and families.[40] Consultation with the palliative care team can help optimize the role of each person involved in the patient's care.

Patients and families often need additional information to make decisions; they may be unclear about information they have already been given. Patients and families often turn to the nurse for clarification. Nurses often feel very willing to assist patients and families in decision making. Sulmasy and colleagues[41] found that nurses were more comfortable than house officers and attending physicians in discussions with patients and families about do not resuscitate orders. Although sometimes nurses are in a position to be involved in decision making, whether they have an official or formal role in decision making is often unclear. It is essential for nurses to know the policies and practices within their institutions.

In addition to knowing about procedural factors affecting decision making, it is important to consider whether the nurse is qualified to provide factual input or formal teaching about the topic under consideration. Some nurses are qualified, but many are not. In Nancy Cruzan's case, the well-intentioned but uninformed statement of a nurse who said "I think she's going to be fine" may have temporarily reassured the family, but it was wrong, perhaps based more on a desire to reassure than to provide accurate information. There is no benefit to false reassurance. It is essential that nurses are willing to say, "I don't know," if they do not have the necessary information. They must then, however, get the information and provide it to the patient, or to the family when appropriate.

A related consideration is whether institutional policies allow the nurse to assess what the patient knows. Some physicians, institutions, and nurses are not comfortable with the nurse asking, "What do you understand about your condition?" These questions sometimes elicit important information about the patient's concerns about the illness, its treatment, and the prognosis. If the nurse has concerns about whether the patient has accurate information to make a decision, they should be shared with the primary team. The team can then collaborate to help the patient receive the information necessary for decision making.

In palliative care and in end-of-life care, decision making often has to do with the appropriate use of technology or other medical interventions. Focusing on the goals of care for the therapy under consideration (eg, a ventilator, surgery, antibiotics, a feeding tube, etc) should be specified. Does this therapy allow the overall goals of care for this patient to be achieved? "The test is what a technology will do for the overall life and welfare of the patient, not what it will do to forestall a coming death or to sustain organ systems."[10(pp248)] Most patients do not want to be kept alive with technology if they are not likely to lead a "meaningful life".[42]

Consideration of benefits of the therapy is relatively straightforward. Less often explicated, especially with the same degree of specificity, are the burdens of the therapy. Decision making absent considerations of the benefits *and* the burdens is, by definition, incomplete.

Decision making about technology and other treatments involves decisions not only about when to use a therapy but also, of equal importance, about when not to use or when to discontinue specific therapies. Therapies may be started at times when serious injury or sudden changes in the patient's condition necessitate emergent intervention. Therapies are started with the hope of achieving a specific goal. If it becomes apparent that the goal of that therapy (cure or achievement of a quality of life acceptable to the patient) is not possible, the goals of therapy should change. Treatments that cannot benefit the patient, that cannot achieve the desired goal should not be started. If it becomes clear that a treatment the patient is already receiving cannot achieve the stated goals, that treatment should be discontinued. Several similar guidelines can help in an ongoing integration of goals of therapy and benefit/burden considerations (**Box 1**).

Palliative care often involves the care of terminally ill patients. Still too often, a patient's death is viewed as a failure. "One of our human ends, not unimportant, is to be allowed to die when nothing more of any serious value can be done for us."[10(pp249)] Decision making sometimes involves consideration of what the end of life will be like, as well as what can be done to alleviate suffering with excellent symptom management and continued support in decision making. It is not uncommon to hear providers and family members suggest that information not be completely forthcoming, with the explanation, "I don't want to take away hope." That statement reflects an incomplete understanding of hope. Hope is not a static concept. Hope

---

Box 1
Principles of withdrawing and withholding life-prolonging therapies

1. There is no difference between withdrawing and withholding a life-prolonging therapy.

2. Providers should never start a therapy that they are not willing to discontinue.

3. The goals of care both for a specific therapy and for the patient overall care should be specified.

4. Medical indications should be considered first when determining clinical options.

5. If the efficacy of a particular therapy is unknown, a trial of that therapy is often reasonable.

6. Though specific therapies may be withdrawn, the patient care should be uninterrupted, often with aggressive attention to symptom management.

7. There is a tremendous difference between allowing a death and causing a death.

From Mahon MM. Withdrawing and withholding life-prolonging therapies in children. In: Ravitsky V, Fiester A, Caplan AL, editors. The Penn Center guide to bioethics. New York: Springer; 2009. p. 485; with permission.

---

evolves over the course of serious illness. People who are dying do have hope! For most it is not hope for a cure. Rather, while still recognizing hope as important, people who are facing the end of their lives express clear home to live well or "to the fullest", for a death without suffering, for good lives for their family members, and more.[43] The participants in Duggleby and Wright's study[43] described hope as a choice.

Hope is dynamic; it is real even for patients at the end of life. Health care providers have an important role in fostering hope while simultaneously being honest.[44] These roles are not mutually exclusive but rather are 2 sides of the same coin. To take this proactive role, however, providers have to be aware of the complex and dynamic nature of hope. Recognizing the patient as a multidimensional person and affirming the worth of the patient, including through dying, can support the patient's maintenance of hope in the context of dying.[45]

Decision making can be complex and difficult. The decisions confronted in palliative care and end-of-life care often have multiple facets with significant implications. The nurse's role in these decisions may be unclear. A nurse at one institution may be considered a valuable source of information, a conduit with the patients, and a member of the team providing information to patients and families, clarifying what the medical team has said, and working with the team, including the patient and family as the decision is made and implemented. In another institution, the nurse may not be allowed to gather, share, or clarify information. The actual physical care provided by these two nurses may be identical. The interactions with the patient and family around this care may be affected not only by the nurse's knowledge and skills, but also by the contextual factors of formal institutional policies and informal unit or team rules.

In any case, the nurse should never feel alone in nursing practice. It is important to identify resources that can help with decision making. The Hospice and Palliative Nurses Association (HPNA) has several position statements that can provide help in analyzing and understanding specific cases. HPNA position statements address the use of opioids,[46] pain management,[47] and withholding or withdrawing life-sustaining therapies[48] and ANH.[23] The American Academy of Hospice and Palliative Medicine also has position statements that can be helpful; these include ANH at the end of life[49] and the use of clinical practice guidelines in palliative care.[50] The palliative care team of a hospital can be a very helpful resource, as can an institution's ethics committee. Of greatest importance are resources for support and education within one's unit and organization.

SUMMARY

Many aspects of clinical decision making have evolved because of the 3 cases described herein. The lessons are important and should be more widely understood than they are. Of equal importance, though, is that these lessons apply to patients across diagnoses and independent of goals of care. It is essential to identify goals of care, both for the patient overall and for each intervention. Answering these questions and explicating the medical indications are the foundations of good decision making. Good decisions also include knowing how and when to provide and when to discontinue certain therapies to achieve the goals of care. The Jonsen, Siegler, and Winslade model[1] provides nurses with a useful framework to approach clinical decision making. The model applies to a variety of clinical situations encountered by nurses in day-to-day practice. Although widely used for decisions faced by seriously ill and injured patients, the model's comprehensive nature lends to its application across the clinical spectrum.

REFERENCES

1. Jonsen AR, Siegler M, Winslade WJ. Clinical ethics: a practical approach to ethical decisions in clinical medicine. 6th edition. New York: McGraw-Hill; 2006.
2. Bacon D, Williams MA, Gordon J. Position statement on laws and regulations concerning life-sustaining treatment, including artificial nutrition and hydration, for patients lacking decision-making capacity. Neurology 2007;68:1097.
3. Gunnerson BM, Stomberg MW. Factors influencing decision making among ambulance nurses in emergency care situations. Int Emerg Nurs 2009;17:83–9.
4. Dai C, Stafford RS, Alexander C. National trends in cyclooxygenase-2 inhibitor use since market release. Arch Intern Med 2005;165:171–7.
5. Jeske AH. Selecting new drugs for pain control. J Am Dent Assoc 2002;133: 1052–6.
6. Law MR, Majumdar SR, Soumerai SB. Effect of illicit direct to consumer advertising on use of etanercept, mometasone, and tegaserod in Canada: controlled longitudinal study. Br Med J 2008;337:a1055.
7. Frosch DL, Krueger PM, Hornik RC, et al. Creating demand for prescription drugs: a content analysis of television direct-to-consumer advertising. Ann Fam Med 2007;5:6–13.
8. Mumford L. The pentagon of power: the myth of the machine. New York: Harcourt Brace Jovanovich; 1970. p. 185–6.
9. Fuchs VR. Health care and the United States economic system. An essay in abnormal physiology. Milbank Mem Fund Q 1972;50:211–44.
10. Callahan D. What kind of life? The limits of medical progress. Washington, DC: Georgetown University Press; 1995. p. 162. Available at: http://www.flipkart.com/kind-life-daniel-callahan-limits/0878405739-c9w3fu6faf#previewbook. Accessed September 17, 2009.
11. Filene PG. In the arms of others: a cultural history of the right-to-die in America. Chicago: Ivan R. Dee; 1998.
12. In re Quinlan. Supreme Court of New Jersey, 355 A.2nd 647 (NJ 1976).

13. A definition of irreversible coma: report of the Ad Hoc Committee of the Harvard Medical School to examine the definition of brain death. JAMA 1968;205:337–40.

14. Jennett B, Plum F. Persistent vegetative state after brain damage. A syndrome in search of a name. Lancet 1972;1:734–7.

15. American Academy of Neurology. Position statement of the American Academy of Neurology on certain aspects of the care and management of the persistent vegetative state patient. Neurology 1989;39:125–6 125.

16. Practice parameters: assessment and management of patients in the persistent vegetative state. Report of the Quality Standards Subcommittee of the American Academy of Neurology. Neurology 1995;45:1015–8.

17. Menikoff J. Law and bioethics. An introduction. Washington, DC: Georgetown University Press; 2001.

18. Colby WH. Long goodbye: the deaths of Nancy Cruzan. Carlsbad (CA): Hay House; 2002.

19. Cruzan v Director, Missouri Department of Health. Supreme Court of the United States, 497 US 261 (1990).

20. Colby WH. From Quinlan to Cruzan to Schiavo: what have we learned? Loyola Univ Chicago Law J 2006;37:289–96.

21. Casarett D, Kapo J, Caplan A. Appropriate use of artificial nutrition and hydration – fundamental principles and recommendations. N Engl J Med 2005;353:2607–14.

22. Ganzini L. Artificial nutrition and hydration at the end of life: ethics and evidence. Palliat Support Care 2006;4:135–43.

23. Hospice & Palliative Nurses Association. HPNA position statement. Artificial nutrition and hydration in end-of-life care. Available at: http://www.hpna.org/pdf/Artifical_Nutrition_and_Hydration_PDF.pdf; 2003. Accessed October 21, 2009.

24. Jones CJ. Say what? How the patient self-determination act leaves the elderly with limited English out in the cold. Elder Law J 2005;13:489–93.

25. Patient Self Determination Act: Omnibus Budget Reconciliation Act of 1990, Pub. L. No. 101–508, § 4206 and 4751, codified as U.S.C. 1395cc (a) (1) (q), 1395 mm (c) (8), 1395 cc (f), 1396a (57), (58), 1396a (w).

26. Shalowitz DI, Garrett-Mayer E, Wendler D. The accuracy of surrogate decision makers. A systematic review. Arch Intern Med 2006;166:493–7.

27. Moorman SM, Carr D. Spouses' effectiveness as end-of-life health care surrogates: accuracy, uncertainty, and errors of overtreatment or undertreatment. Gerontologist 2008;48:811–9.

28. Cerminara KL, Goodman KW. Key events in the case of Theresa Marie Schiavo. University of Miami Ethics Program; 2005. Available at: http://www.miami.edu/ethics2/schiavo/timeline.htm. Accessed August 19, 2009.

29. John Paul Pope II. Address of John Paul II to the participants in the international congress on "life-sustaining treatments and vegetative state: Scientific advances and ethical dilemmas. Saturday, 20 March, 2004. Available at: http://www.vatican.va/holy_father/john_paul_ii/speeches/2004/march/documents/hf_jp-ii_spe_20040320_congress-fiamc_en.html. 2004. Accessed November 19, 2009.

30. Mahon MM, Sorrell JM. Palliative care for people with Alzheimer's disease. Nurs Philos 2008;9:110–20.

31. Christopoulou I. Factors affecting the decision of cancer patients to be cared for at home or in hospital. Eur J Cancer Care 1993;2:157–60. DOI: 10.1111/j.1365-2354.1993.tb00189.

32. Hawley ST, Griggs JJ, Hamilton AS, et al. Decision involvement and receipt of mastectomy among racially and ethnically diverse breast cancer patients. J Natl Cancer Inst 2009;101:1337–47.

33. Koeda M, Shibata T, Asai K, et al. Care policy for patients with dementia: family's decision and its impact. BioMedical Engineering and Informatics 2008;2:843–7. DOI: http://doi.ieeecomputersociety.org/10.1109/BMEI.2008.355.

34. Shepherd HL, Tattersall MH, Butow PN. Physician-identified factors affecting patient participation in reaching treatment decisions. J Clin Oncol 2008;26:1724–31.

35. Aita K, Takahashis M, Miyata H, et al. Physicians attitudes about artificial feeding in older patients with severe cognitive impairment in Japan: a qualitative study. BMC Geriatr 2007;7:22. DOI: 10.1186/1471-2318-7-22.

36. Légaré F, Ratté S, Gravel K, et al. Barriers and facilitators to implementing shared decision-making in clinical practice: update of a systematic review of health professionals' perception. Patient Educ Couns 2008;73:526–35.

37. King NMP. Making sense of advance directives. (revised edition). Washington, DC: Georgetown University Press; 1996. p. 213.

38. Clover A, Browne J, McErlain P, et al. Patient approaches to clinical conversations in the palliative care setting. J Adv Nurs 2004;48:333–41.

39. Barthow C, Moss C, McKinlay E, et al. To be involved or not: factors that influence nurses' involvement in providing treatment decisional support in advanced cancer. Eur J Oncol Nurs 2009;13:22–8.

40. Mahon MM, McAuley WJ. Oncology nurses' personal understandings about palliative care. Oncol Nurs Forum, in press.

41. Sulmasy D, He MK, McAuley R, et al. Beliefs and attitudes of nurses and physicians about do not resuscitate orders and who should speak to patients and families about them. Crit Care Med 2008;36:1817–22.

42. Heyland DK, Dodek P, Rocker G, et al, for the Canadian Researchers, End-of-Life Network (CARENET) what matters the most in end-of-life care: perceptions of seriously ill patients and their family members. Can Med Assoc J 2006;174: 627–33.

43. Duggleby W, Wright K. Elderly palliative care cancer patients' descriptions of hope-fostering strategies. Int J Palliat Nurs 2004;10:352–9.

44. Clayton JM, Butow PN, Arnold RM, et al. Fostering coping and nurturing hope when discussing the future with terminally ill cancer patients and their caregivers. Cancer 2005;103:1965–75.

45. Kylmä J, Duggleby W, Cooper D, et al. Hope in palliative care: an integrative review. Palliat Support Care 2009;7:365–77.

46. Hospice & Palliative Nurses Association. HPNA position statement. The ethics of opiate use within palliative care. Available at: http://hpna.org/DisplayPage.aspx?Title=Position%20Statements. 2003. Accessed October 21, 2009.

47. Hospice & Palliative Nurses Association. HPNA position statement. Pain management. Available at: http://hpna.org/DisplayPage.aspx?Title=Position%20Statements. 2008. Accessed October 21, 2009.

48. Hospice & Palliative Nurses Association. HPNA position statement. Withholding and/or withdrawing life sustaining therapies. Available at: http://hpna.org/DisplayPage.aspx?Title=Position%20Statements. 2008. Accessed October 21, 2009.

49. American Academy of Hospice and Palliative Medicine. Statement on artificial nutrition and hydration near the end of life. Available at: http://www.aahpm.org/positions/nutrition.html. 2006. Accessed October 21, 2009.

50. American Academy of Hospice and Palliative Medicine. Statement on clinical practice guidelines for quality palliative care. Available at: http://www.aahpm.org/positions/quality.html. 2006. Accessed October 21, 2009.

Assessing Respiratory Distress When the Patient Cannot Report Dyspnea

Margaret L. Campbell, PhD, RN[a,b,]*

KEYWORDS

- Dyspnea • Assessment • Cognitive impairment
- Dying • Distress

Ensuring patient comfort begins with a comprehensive assessment for symptom distress. The dying patient poses unique challenges for assessment because of the high prevalence of declining and impaired cognition that typifies this population. The focus of this paper is on the practical clinical question: How can we recognize respiratory distress when the patient cannot provide a report about dyspnea?

DEFINITIONS

Symptoms are subjective phenomena that can be perceived and verified only by the person experiencing them. An expert panel representing the American Thoracic Society defined dyspnea as: a subjective experience of breathing discomfort that consists of qualitatively distinct sensations that vary in intensity.[1] Symptom distress has been conceptualized as the need to alter actions in response to a symptom; and the physical or mental anguish and suffering that results from the symptom.[2] A sign is any abnormality indicating disease that is detectable by the individual or by others. Respiratory distress has been conceptualized as an observable corollary to dyspnea relying on signs that indicate the likely presence of dyspnea.[3] Respiratory distress, for the purpose of this paper, is the physical and/or emotional suffering that results from the experience of dyspnea and is characterized by behaviors that can be observed and measured.

PREVALENCE OF DYSPNEA AND COGNITIVE IMPAIRMENT AT THE END OF LIFE

A systematic review of symptom prevalence studies was done to determine the extent to which patients with chronic progressive diseases have similar symptom profiles.[4]

---

a Center for Health Research, College of Nursing, Wayne State University, 5557 Cass Avenue, Detroit, MI 48202, USA
b Nursing Research, Detroit Receiving Hospital, 4201 St Antoine, Detroit, MI 48201, USA
* Nursing Research, Detroit Receiving Hospital, 4201 St Antoine, Detroit, MI 48201.

Nurs Clin N Am 45 (2010) 363–373
doi:10.1016/j.cnur.2010.03.001
0029-6465/10/$ – see front matter © 2010 Elsevier Inc. All rights reserved.

The prevalence of dyspnea and confusion across the 5 common conditions is illustrated in **Table 1**.

Heart disease is the leading cause of death in the United States, with chronic pulmonary diseases ranked fourth. Pneumonia is the fifth leading cause for persons older than 65 years.[5] The World Health Organization predicts that by 2020 chronic obstructive pulmonary disease (COPD) will increase from the twelfth most prevalent disease worldwide to the fifth and from the sixth most common cause of death to the third.[6] As expected, the prevalence of dyspnea is highest among people with COPD and heart disease.

Declining or impaired cognition is also highly prevalent among terminally ill patients, particularly those who are elderly or referred from long-term care.[7,8] Likewise, hypoxemia temporarily impairs cognition, particularly if the Pao_2 is less than 50 mm Hg;[9] hypercarbia produces a narcotic effect at $Paco_2$ levels greater than 70 mm Hg.[10,11] Patients with COPD who experience chronic blood gas alterations are likely to have mild, chronic, cognitive impairment even when their oxygenation is stable with declines from baseline occurring when they are hypoxemic.[12–15]

Patients with declining or impaired cognition are vulnerable to under recognition and over or under treatment of their distress because clinicians may lack the ability to identify signs associated with the autonomic and emotional responses. A retrospective audit of 185 charts from 5 long-term care facilities in Canada found that half of the residents who died were cognitively impaired; dyspnea was the most common symptom (62%) but only 23% of residents with dyspnea had it treated.[7] A corresponding result was found in a large mortality follow-back survey of family members of patients who died in an institutional setting. Families reported that 22% of patients with dyspnea did not receive any or enough treatment.[16] More than half the terminally ill hospitalized patients (54%) in a prospective study were unable to provide even a simple yes or no response to the query "Are you short of breath?" Inability to self-report was associated with unconsciousness, impaired cognition, and nearness to death.[17]

Theoretically, the same physiologic changes that induce dyspnea in the patient with intact cognition will produce respiratory distress when the patient is experiencing declining cognition. The only difference in the 2 patient cohorts is in their ability to reliably report their distress. The prevalence of respiratory distress at the end of life is not known because patients unable to report have been largely excluded from prevalence estimates.

COMMON SELF-REPORT TOOLS FOR ASSESSING DYSPNEA

The simplest form of assessment for dyspnea is to ask the patient: "are you short of breath?" The yes or no response does not provide any qualitative information and

Table 1						
Prevalence of dyspnea and confusion across conditions						
Conditions	Dyspnea Prevalence (%)	Number of Studies	N	Confusion Prevalence (%)	Number of Studies	N
Cancer	10–70	21	10,029	6–93	19	9154
AIDS	11–62	2	504	30–65	2	
Heart disease	60–88	6	948	18–32	3	343
COPD	90–95	4	372	18–33	2	309

Data from Solano JP, Gomes B, Higginson IJ. A comparison of symptom prevalence in far advanced cancer, AIDS, heart disease, chronic obstructive pulmonary disease and renal disease. J Pain Symptom Manage 2006;31(1):58–69.

cannot be used to measure the intensity of the patient's experience, but it does give the examiner initial information. In the case of a cognitively impaired patient the simple yes or no response may be all the patient can provide.

More informative but unidimensional tools include a numeric rating scale (NRS) and a visual analog scale (VAS). The VAS is typically a 100-mm line anchored at either end with descriptors such as "no breathlessness" to "greatest breathlessness."[18] The patient marks a point on the line to represent the intensity of breathlessness, which is thus converted to a numerical value by measuring the millimeters in length expressed. Horizontal and vertical versions of the VAS have high correlation ($r = 0.97$) and have demonstrated construct and discriminate validity and responsiveness in therapeutic trials.[18] The NRS is a 0 to 10 integer scale that may be anchored with descriptors such as 0 = "no shortness of breath" and 10 = "shortness of breath as bad as can be." The NRS has shown concurrent validity to VAS ($r = 0.56$) and construct validity for incident or short time frame dyspnea assessments.[19]

Patient report is considered the gold standard for measuring symptom distress. Consciousness is necessary for cognition and cognitive functions are necessary to generate and report a symptom or symptom distress. The patient must be able to interpret sensory stimuli, pay attention to instructions and concentrate to form a report, be able to communicate in some fashion, and be able to recall the previous report if trending is requested. When cognition is impaired, reliance on proxy assessments may occur. Concordance with the family's perspective about the patient's behavior and level of comfort can be sought. However, proxy reports about respiratory distress when the patient is unable to provide a self-report may be less reliable than reliance on behavioral cues.[20]

BEHAVIORAL ASSESSMENT

As we evolved from water-dwelling to air-breathing organisms the dyspnea response to asphyxiation began and has persisted over millions of years.[21] This primal ancient response produces compensatory behaviors and induces basic aversive emotions, including fear.

The following theoretical model of respiratory distress (**Fig. 1**) was derived from a synthesis of animal and human studies of biobehavioral responses to an asphyxial threat. The model relies on subcortical neurologic systems in the emotional and autonomic domains that are rapidly triggered in response to a threat of asphyxia.[22] These evolutionary ancient reactions produce compensatory responses oriented to survival.[21] Conditions that produce dyspnea (inspiratory effort, hypercarbia, and hypoxemia) trigger a near immediate autonomic and primal fear reaction that produces an array of observable behaviors.

ASPHYXIAL THREAT

An asphyxial threat is produced when pulmonary pathology produces 1 or more of inspiratory effort, hypoxemia, or hypercarbia. A sense of inspiratory effort is produced by conscious awareness of voluntary activation of skeletal muscles. Muscle receptors provide feedback about muscle force and tension and information from these chest wall receptors produce the conscious awareness of respiratory effort. The respiratory muscles also activate autonomic central respiratory motor centers (pons and medulla) that can contribute to the sense of effort; effort has been strongly correlated with breathlessness.[23]

Hypercarbia and hypoxemia have long been known to produce an involuntary motor response mediated in the brainstem to increase ventilation through increased rate and

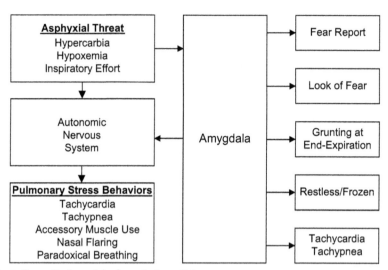

Fig. 1. A theoretical model of respiratory distress.

volume of breathing. Hypercarbia and hypoxemia also make independent contributions to the sensation of distress.[24] Generally, hypercarbia will produce dyspnea and its associated physiologic and emotional reactions when the partial pressure of carbon dioxide (Pco_2) increases by 5–10 mm Hg from the patient's baseline level.[25] Severe hypercarbia (Pco_2 >80 mm Hg) produces a narcotic effect and at very high levels suppresses the brainstem respiratory center causing death.[10] Pathologic conditions that produce respiratory distress do so by more than 1 mechanism. Sense of effort, hypoxemia, and hypercarbia, however, are common to the pathologic conditions that produce respiratory distress particularly during severe exacerbations and respiratory failure.[26]

AUTONOMIC NERVOUS SYSTEM ACTIVATION

Respiratory sensors consist of central (medulla, pons, and cerebellum) and peripheral chemoreceptors (aortic and carotid bodies) and peripheral sensory receptors found in the chest wall, airways, and lungs. Stimulation of the respiratory center elicits an increased respiratory and cardiac response through activation of the parabrachial complex in the pons,[27,28] sympathetic nervous system, and activation of the adrenal medullary catecholamines (epinephrine and norepinephrine). Increased cardiac and pulmonary performance from central respiratory control and the sympathetic nervous system produce compensatory responses including accelerations in heart and respiratory rates and increased lung volumes through recruitment of thoracic and abdominal accessory muscles.[29] These well-understood cardiorespiratory responses and pulmonary stress behaviors are intended to restore respiratory homeostasis and preserve life.

FEAR ACTIVATION

Emotions are short-lived psychophysiologic phenomena representing adaptation to changing environmental demands. The emotion system is a set of interconnected structures including the anterior thalamus, hypothalamus, septum, amygdala, hippocampus, cingulate cortex, and the bed of the stria terminalis.[30,31] These primitive subcortical brain areas evolved after the brainstem but before the neocortex.[32]

An eliciting stimulus, such as an asphyxial threat, leads to a subcortical appraisal. An important function of any emotion is the coordination of an optimal physiologic environment to support the behavior that is called forth. Recruitment of responses from the central and autonomic nervous systems provides for capacity to adapt and survive. Some emotion systems, such as fear, are so primitive that conscious awareness of their activation is not necessary for response recruitment given the predominance for survival over deliberation.[33]

Fear is the primal emotion most often associated with respiratory disability.[34–36] The amygdala is closely associated with the ability to identify threats, and in turn activates a fear response array. The amygdala receives input via 2 pathways: cortical (conscious) and subcortical (unconscious). Threat stimuli are communicated by both pathways. The most rapid communication is from the sensory thalamus to the amygdala with no conscious perception; this produces, in animals or humans, a rapid response to the threat that precedes conscious awareness. A slower pathway traverses the sensory thalamus to the sensory cortex to the amygdala providing conscious appraisal of the threat stimulus.[37] Thus, patients with brain lesions that contribute to declining or impaired cognition may have a distorted or absent conscious appraisal of threats but retain fear responses and behaviors because threat stimuli are communicated via the rapid thalamic pathway.

The amygdala projects to multiple brain regions controlling endocrine, autonomic, and motor activity.[38] A threat elicits an amygdaloid response that controls brainstem nuclei underlying facial expression, startle excitability, freezing behavior, and respiratory and cardiovascular changes.[39–42] Fear is an aversive state triggered in people and animals when survival is threatened. It is an evolutionarily old brain response that controls behaviors necessary for survival of the individual and ultimately survival of the species.

FEAR ACTIVATION BY AN ASPHYXIAL THREAT

The mechanisms that produce the sensation of uncomfortable breathing also produce the strongly correlated negative emotional responses through activation of the amygdala and other central nervous system processes. Investigators using brain imaging techniques revealed elevated and robust activation of the amygdala and other subcortical structures when air hunger was induced in healthy human subjects.[43–49] Asphyxia may induce a primal, innate, unconditioned, autonomic array of pulmonary stress and fear behaviors because the threat to survival cannot be controlled.

BEHAVIORS ASSOCIATED WITH RESPIRATORY DISTRESS

This theoretical model is composed of behaviors activated simultaneously from the autonomic nervous system and the amygdala. The autonomic pulmonary stress behaviors include the recruitment of accessory muscles (sternocleidomastoid, intercostals, abdominal) that are displayed as elevation of the clavicles and/or paradoxic breathing, which is an inward movement of the abdomen on inspiration[50–52] tachycardia and tachypnea,[53] and an outward flaring of the distal external nares.[54,55]

Subcortical elicitation of fear produces an organized response array of facial, vocal, motor, and physiologic responses that can be observed as measurable behaviors. Fear in response to an asphyxial threat produces a characteristic look of fear.[56] The universal fearful facial expression is characterized by (1) the upper iris is visible, (2) the teeth are visible, (3) the teeth are not parted, (4) there are lines in the forehead, (5) the eyebrows are flat, (6) the eyebrows are raised, and (7) there are no wrinkles in the nose (**Fig. 2**).[57] Fear in response to asphyxia is also postulated to produce grunting at end expiration,[58] restlessness,[59–61] or freezing,[62] and fear-specific physiologic support through heightened activation of the autonomic nervous system, adrenal medulla, and ventromedial pons. These evolutionarily ancient brain areas react to the threat of asphyxiation and produce compensatory responses oriented to the survival of the individual and ultimately of the species. Fear has been strongly correlated with dyspnea in studies of patients with respiratory disease.[51,63–66]

FEAR AND PULMONARY STRESS BEHAVIORS TO AN ASPHYXIAL THREAT ACROSS COGNITIVE STATES

An exploratory study was conducted to test the aforementioned biobehavioral theoretical model of responses to an asphyxial threat. Patients undergoing a ventilator weaning trial ($n = 12$) were assessed and observed at baseline and during weaning with a capnograph/oximeter and video camera. Cognitive state (intact, mild, or moderately or severely impaired) was categorized at baseline, and an emotion report was elicited after the weaning trial. Pulmonary stress and fear behaviors were similar across cognitive states and included in order of descending frequency: tachycardia/tachypnea, accessory muscle use, fearful facial expression, paradoxic breathing, and nasal flaring. Hypercarbia predicted activation of fear behaviors. Gender differences characterized emotion reporting; men did not report fear. An asphyxial threat induced an innate array of behaviors that were not volitionally controlled and had the same appearance across cognitive states (intact, mild, or moderately impaired).[66]

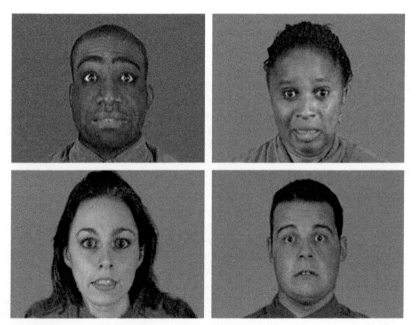

Fig. 2. Characteristic facial expression denoting fear. (*Courtesy of* Ursula Hess, Professor of Psychology, University of Quebec at Montreal.)

DEVELOPMENT AND TESTING OF A RESPIRATORY DISTRESS OBSERVATION SCALE

A Respiratory Distress Observation Scale (RDOS) was developed from the aforementioned biobehavioral models (see Appendix) and was subsequently tested for reliability and convergent and discriminant validity.[67] Patient reports about dyspnea were compared with displayed respiratory distress behaviors in 3 groups of 70 patients or volunteers ($n = 210$). In the first group, pulmonary rehabilitation patients were assessed with the RDOS after controlled exercise that induced hypoxemia as measured by oximetry. The individuals were subsequently asked to report current dyspnea on a dyspnea visual analog scale (DVAS). In the second group, patients with postoperative orthopedic pain were evaluated with the RDOS and asked to report current pain (pain numeric report) and dyspnea. In the third group, healthy volunteers were assessed with the RDOS at rest and asked to report current dyspnea. The internal consistency (alpha) of the RDOS was 0.78 ($N = 210$). A positive correlation between the RDOS and DVAS ($P<.01$) and an inverse correlation between RDOS and peripheral oxygen saturation (Spo_2; $P<.01$) were found, indicating convergent validity. Significant mean differences were found when RDOS and DVAS scores from dyspneic patients were compared with RDOS from patients with pain ($P<.01$) and with healthy volunteers ($P<.01$) indicating discriminant validity. Of necessity, the RDOS was tested with study participants who were cognitively intact and able to provide a dyspnea self-report because there is no gold standard respiratory distress observation tool with which to test convergent validity.[67] The instrument has subsequently been revised and has undergone additional reliability and validity testing with terminally ill patients dying from 1 or more of the following diagnoses: pneumonia, heart failure, COPD, and lung cancer.[67] Additional testing was needed with terminally ill patients unable to self-report.

An observational design was used with 89 consecutive patients referred for inpatient palliative care consultation and at risk for dyspnea who had 1 or more of lung cancer, COPD, heart failure, or pneumonia. Patients were observed and the RDOS scored once each day for up to 3 days after the initial consultation. Other measures included dyspnea self-report, neurologic diagnoses, opioid or benzodiazepine use, peripheral oxygen saturation, end-tidal carbon dioxide level, consciousness, cognitive state, nearness to death, and patient demographics. Perfect interrater reliability across data collectors was achieved. No differences in RDOS scoring were found by patient demographics. RDOS was associated with the use of oxygen ($P<.01$), oxygen saturation ($P<.01$), and nearness to death ($P<.01$). A significant decrease in RDOS was found between the initial palliative care consultation and day 2 that corresponded with treatment ($P<.01$) and with a significant increase in opioid administration ($P<.01$). The reliability of this 8-item scale is sufficient ($\alpha = 0.64$).[68]

Declining consciousness and/or cognition are expected when patients are near death. The RDOS performed well when tested with terminally ill patients who were at risk for respiratory distress, most of whom could not self-report dyspnea. The tool was sensitive to detect changes over time and measure response to treatment. The RDOS is simple to use; scoring takes less than 5 minutes. The RDOS has clinical and research usefulness to measure and trend respiratory distress and response to treatment.

SUMMARY

Standard measures of dyspnea, such as a numeric report or VAS, rely on the patient's self-report. Declining consciousness and/or cognitive function and nearness to death may interfere with dyspnea reporting making the patient vulnerable to under or over treatment. The ability to give even the simplest self-report (yes or no) about dyspnea is lost in the near death phase of terminal illness, yet the ability to experience distress may persist and may be overlooked and under or over treated. Other methods for symptom assessment are needed in this context.

REFERENCES

1. American Thoracic Society Dyspnea. Mechanisms, assessment, and management: a consensus statement. American Thoracic Society. Am J Respir Crit Care Med 1999;159(1):321–40.
2. Rhodes VA, Watson PM. Symptom distress–the concept. Semin Oncol Nurs 1987; 3(4):242–7.
3. Campbell ML. Terminal dyspnea and respiratory distress. Crit Care Clin 2004; 20(3):403–17.
4. Solano JP, Gomes B, Higginson IJ. A comparison of symptom prevalence in far advanced cancer, AIDS, heart disease, chronic obstructive pulmonary disease and renal disease. J Pain Symptom Manage 2006;31(1):58–69.
5. Centers for Disease Control. Hyattsville (MD): National Center for Health Statistics; 2007.
6. Lopez AD, Murray CC. The global burden of disease, 1990–2020. Nat Med 1998; 4:1241–3.
7. Hall P, Schroder C, Weaver L. The last 48 hours of life in long-term care: a focused chart audit. J Am Geriatr Soc 2002;50:501–6.
8. Brandt HE, Deliens L, Ooms ME, et al. Symptoms, signs, problems, and diseases of terminally ill nursing home patients. Arch Intern Med 2005;165:314–20.
9. Moosavi SH, Golestanian E, Binks AP, et al. Hypoxic and hypercapnic drives to breathe generate equivalent levels of air hunger in humans. J Appl Phys 2003; 94:141–54.
10. Dean JB, Mulkey DK, Garcia AJ, et al. Neuronal sensitivity to hyperoxia, hypercapnia, and inert gases at hyperbaric pressures. J Appl Phys 2003;95:883–909.
11. Taxen DV. Permissive hypercapnea. In: Tobin MJ, editor. Principles and practices of mechanical ventilation. New York: McGraw-Hill; 1994.
12. Kozora E, Filley CM, Julian LJ, et al. Cognitive functioning in patients with chronic obstructive pulmonary disease and mild hypoxemia compared with patients with mild Alzheimer disease and normal controls. Neuropsychiatry Neuropsychol Behav Neurol 1999;12(3):178–83.
13. Incalzi RA, Marra C, Giordano A, et al. Cognitive impairment in chronic obstructive pulmonary disease: a neuropsychological and spect study. J Neurol 2003; 250:325–32.
14. Liesker JJ, Postma DS, Beukema RJ, et al. Cognitive performance in patients with COPD. Respir Med 2004;98(4):351–6.
15. Hung WW, Wisnivesky JP, Siu AL, et al. Cognitive decline among patients with chronic obstructive pulmonary disease. Am J Respir Crit Care Med 2009; 180(2):134–7.
16. Teno JM, Clarridge BR, Casey V, et al. Family perspectives on end-of-life care at the last place of care. JAMA 2004;291(1):88–93.
17. Campbell ML, Templin T, Walch J. Patients who are near death are frequently unable to self-report dyspnea. J Palliat Med 2009;12:881–4.
18. Gift AG. Clinical measurement of dyspnea. Dimens Crit Care Nurs 1989;8(4): 210–6.

19. Gift AG, Narsavage G. Validity of the numeric rating scale as a measure of dyspnea. Am J Crit Care 1998;7:200–4.
20. Radbruch L, Sabatowski R, Loick G, et al. Cognitive impairment and its influence on pain and symptom assessment in a palliative care unit: development of a Minimal Documentation System. Palliat Med 2000;14:266–76.
21. Gooden BA. The evolution of asphyxial defense. Integr Physiol Behav Sci 1993; 28:317–30.
22. Campbell ML. Respiratory distress: a model of responses and behaviors to an asphyxial threat for patients who are unable to self-report. Heart Lung 2008; 37(1):54–60.
23. El-Manshawi A, Killian KJ, Summers E, et al. Breathlessness during exercise with and without resistive loading. J Appl Physiol 1986;61(3):896–905.
24. Manning HL, Schwartzstein RM. Mechanisms of dyspnea. In: Mahler DA, editor. Dyspnea. New York: Marcel Decker; 1998. p. 63–95.
25. Banzett RB, Lansing RW, Evans KC, et al. Stimulus-response characteristics of CO_2-induced air hunger in normal subjects. Respir Physiol 1996;103:19–31.
26. Beach D, Schwartzstein RM. The genesis of breathlessness: what do we understand? In: Booth S, Dudgeon DJ, editors. Dyspnoea in advanced disease. New York: Oxford University Press; 2006. p. 1–18.
27. Harper RM, Gozal D, Bandler R, et al. Regional brain activation in humans during respiratory and blood pressure challenges. Clin Exp Pharmacol Physiol 1998;25: 483–6.
28. Chamberlin NL, Saper CB. A brainstem network mediating apneic reflexes in the rat. J Neurosci 1998;18:6048–56.
29. West JB. Respiratory physiology: the essentials. Philadelphia (PA): Lippincott, Williams and Wilkins; 1999.
30. Carlson NR. Physiology of behavior. Boston: Allyn and Bacon; 2001.
31. Maddock RJ. The retrosplenial cortex and emotion: new insights from functional neuroimaging of the human brain. Trends Neurosci 1999;22:310–6.
32. MacLean PD. The triune brain in evolution: role in paleocerebral functions. New York: Plenum Press; 1990.
33. Levenson RW. Human emotion: a functional view. In: Ekman P, Davidson RJ, editors. The nature of emotion: fundamental questions. New York: Oxford University Press; 1994. p. 123–6.
34. Chiu T, Hu W, Lue B, et al. Dyspnea and its correlates in Taiwanese patients with terminal cancer. J Pain Symptom Manage 2004;28(2):123–32.
35. Heinzer MMV, Bish C, Detwiler R. Acute dyspnea as perceived by patients with chronic obstructive pulmonary disease. Clin Nurs Res 2003;12(1): 85–101.
36. Kessler R, Stahl E, Vogelmeier C, et al. Patient understanding, detection, and experience of COPD exacerbations: an observational, interview-based study. Chest 2006;130(1):133–42.
37. LeDoux J. The emotional brain, fear, and the amygdala. Cell Mol Neurobiol 2003; 23:727–38.
38. Davis M, Whalen PJ. The amygdala: vigilance and emotion. Mol Psychiatry 2001; 6:13–34.
39. Applegate CD, Kapp BS, Underwood MD, et al. Autonomic and somatosensor effects of amydala central N. stimulation in awake rabbits. Physiol Behav 1983; 31(3):353–60.
40. Davis M, Hitchcock JM, Rosen JB. Anxiety and the amygdala: pharmacological and anatomical analysis of the fear-potentiated startle paradigm. In: Bower G,

editor. The psychology of learning and motivation. New York: Academic Press; 1987. p. 263–305.

41. Harper RM, Frysinger RC, Trelease RB, et al. State-dependent alteration in respiratory cycle timing by stimulation of the central nucleus of the amygdala. Brain Res 1984;306(1–2):1–8.

42. Takayama K, Okada J, Miura M. Evidence that neurons of the central amygdaloid nucleus directly project to the site concerned with circulatory and respiratory regulation in the ventrolateral nucleus of the cat: a WGA-HRP study. Neurosci Lett 1990;109(3):241–6.

43. Banzett RB, Mulnier HE, Murphy K, et al. Breathlessness in humans activates insular cortex. Neuroreport 2000;11(10):2117–20.

44. Corfield DR, Fink GR, Ramsay SC, et al. Evidence for limbic system activation during CO_2-stimulated breathing in man. J Physiol 1995;488:77–84.

45. Brannan S, Liotti M, Egan G, et al. Neuroimaging of cerebral activations and deactivations associated with hypercapnia and hunger for air. Proc Natl Acad Sci U S A 2001;98(4):2029–34.

46. Evans KC, Banzett RB, Adams L, et al. Bold fMRI identifies limbic, paralimbic, and cerebellar activation during air hunger. J Neurophysiol 2002;88:1500–11.

47. Liotti M, Brannan S, Egan G, et al. Brain responses associated with consciousness of breathlessness (air hunger). Proc Natl Acad Sci U S A 2001;98:2035–40.

48. Parsons LM, Egan G, Liotti M, et al. Neuroimaging evidence implicating cerebellum in the experience of hypercapnia and hunger for air. Proc Natl Acad Sci U S A 2001;98:2041–6.

49. Peiffer C, Poline JB, Thivard L, et al. Neural substrates for the perception of acutely induced dyspnea. Am J Respir Crit Care Med 2001;163:951–7.

50. Breslin EH, Garoutte BC, Kohlman-Carrieri V, et al. Correlations between dyspnea, diaphragm and sternomastoid recruitment during inspiratory resistance breathing in normal subjects. Chest 1990;98(2):298–302.

51. Gift AG, Cahill CA. Psychophysiologic aspects of dyspnea in chronic obstructive pulmonary disease: a pilot study. Heart Lung 1990;19(3):252–7.

52. Gosselink R. Controlled breathing and dyspnea in patients with chronic obstructive pulmonary disease. J Rehabil Res Dev 2003;40(5):25–34.

53. Campbell ML, Bizek KS, Thill M. Patient responses during rapid terminal weaning from mechanical ventilation: a prospective study. Crit Care Med 1999;27(1):73–7.

54. Strohl KP, O'Cain CF, Slutsky AS. Alae nasi activation and nasal resistance in healthy subjects. J Appl Phys 1982;52(6):1432–7.

55. Gold AR, Smith PL, Schwartz AR. Effect of alae nasi activation on maximal nasal inspiratory airflow in humans. J Appl Phys 1998;84:2115–22.

56. Tarzian A. Caring for dying patients who have air hunger. J Nurs Scholarsh 2000; 32(2):137–43.

57. Benson PJ. A means of measuring facial expressions and a method for predicting emotion categories in clinical disorders of affect. J Affect Disord 1999;55(2-3): 179–85.

58. Demers AM, Morency P, Myberyo-Yaah F, et al. Risk factors for mortality among children hospitalized because of acute respiratory infections in Bangui, Central African Republic. Pediatr Infect Dis J 2000;19(5):424–32.

59. Hirose S. Restlessness of respiration as a manifestation of akathisia: five case reports of akathisia. J Clin Psychiatry 2000;61(10):737–41.

60. Goodlin SJ, Winzelberg GS, Teno JM, et al. Death in the hospital. Arch Intern Med 1998;158(14):1570–2.

61. Lichter I, Hunt E. The last 48 hours of life. J Palliat Care 1990;6(4):7–15.

62. Mongeluzi DL, Rosellini RA, Ley R, et al. The conditioning of dyspneic suffocation fear: effects of carbon dioxide concentration on behavioral freezing and analgesia. Behav Modif 2003;27:620–36.
63. DeVito AJ. Dyspnea during hospitalization for acute phase of illness as recalled by patients with chronic obstructive pulmonary disease. Heart Lung 1990;19:186–91.
64. Kellner R, Samet J, Pathak D. Dyspnea, anxiety, and depression in chronic respiratory impairment. Gen Hosp Psychiatry 1992;14:20–8.
65. Brenes GA. Anxiety and chronic obstructive pulmonary disease: prevalence, impact, and treatment. Psychosom Med 2003;65:963–70.
66. Campbell ML. Fear and pulmonary stress behaviors to an asphyxial threat across cognitive states. Res Nurs Health 2007;30(6):572–83.
67. Campbell ML. Psychometric testing of a respiratory distress observation scale. J Palliat Med 2008;11(1):44–50.
68. Campbell ML, Templin T, Walch J. Psychometric testing of a revised respiratory distress observation scale. J Palliat Med 2010;13:285–90.

APPENDIX: RESPIRATORY DISTRESS OBSERVATION SCALE (RDOS)

Variable	0 Points	1 Point	2 Points	Total
Heart rate (beats per minute)	<90	90–109	≥110	
Respiratory rate (breaths per minute)	≤18	19–30	>30	
Restlessness: nonpurposeful movements	None	Occasional slight movements	Frequent movements	
Paradoxic breathing pattern: abdomen moves in on inspiration	None		Present	
Accessory muscle use: rise in clavicle during inspiration	None	Slight rise	Pronounced rise	
Grunting at end expiration: guttural sound	None		Present	
Nasal flaring: involuntary movement of nares	None		Present	
Look of fear			Eyes wide open, facial muscles tense, brow furrowed, mouth open, teeth together	
Total				

Instruction for use:

1. RDOS is not a substitute for patient self-report if able.
2. RDOS is an adult assessment tool.
3. RDOS cannot be used when the patient is paralyzed with a neuromuscular blocking agent.
4. Count respiratory and heart rates for 1 minute; auscultate if necessary.
5. Grunting may be audible with intubated patients on auscultation.
6. Fearful facial expressions.

Sickle Cell Disease: An Opportunity for Palliative Care Across the Life Span

Diana J. Wilkie, PhD, RN[a,b,]*, Bonnye Johnson, MS, RN[c],
A. Kyle Mack, MD[d], Richard Labotka, MD[c],
Robert E. Molokie, MD[e,f]

KEYWORDS

- Sickle cell • Pain • Symptoms • Advance care planning
- Grief • Bereavement • Palliative care

People living with sickle cell disease (SCD) face many types of morbidity and early mortality. SCD is an inherited hemoglobin disorder characterized by chronic hemolytic anemia, increased susceptibility to infections, end-organ damage, and intermittent episodes of vascular occlusion that result in acute and chronic pain.[1] In some African countries, nearly all babies born with SCD die in early childhood. In the United States,

This publication was made possible by Grant Numbers 1R01 HL078536 and U54 HL090513 from the National Institutes of Health, National Heart Lung and Blood Institute, and P30 NR010680 from the National Institute of Nursing Research. Its contents are solely the responsibility of the authors and do not necessarily represent the official views of the National Heart Lung and Blood Institute or the National Institute of Nursing Research. The final peer-reviewed manuscript is subject to the National Institutes of Health Public Access Policy.
[a] Department of Biobehavioral Health Science (MC 802), Center for End-of-Life Transition Research, University of Illinois at Chicago, 845 South Damen Avenue, Room 660, Chicago, IL 60612-7350, USA
[b] Comprehensive Sickle Cell Center, University of Illinois at Chicago, 820 South Wood Street, Suite 172 (MC 712), Chicago, IL 60612-7350, USA
[c] Department of Medicine, College of Medicine and Comprehensive Sickle Cell Center, 820 South Wood Street, Suite 172 (MC 712), Chicago, IL 60612-7350, USA
[d] Division of Pediatric Hematology/Oncology/Stem Cell Transplantation, Children's Memorial Hospital, Northwestern University-Feinberg School of Medicine, 2300 Children's Plaza, PO Box 30, Chicago, IL 60614, USA
[e] Department of Medicine, College of Medicine, Department of Biopharmaceutical Sciences, College of Pharmacy, and Comprehensive Sickle Cell Center, 820 South Wood Street, Suite 172 (MC 712), Chicago, IL 60612-7350, USA
[f] Jesse Brown VA Medical Center, 820 South Damen Avenue, Chicago, IL 60612-3728, USA
* Corresponding author. Department of Biobehavioral Health Science (MC 802), Center for End-of-Life Transition Research, University of Illinois at Chicago, 845 South Damen Avenue, Room 660, Chicago, IL 60612-7350.
E-mail address: diwilkie@uic.edu

newborn screening, prophylactic penicillin treatment in childhood, and other aggressive treatments for pain and disease complications have increased the average life expectancy for the 100,000 people with SCD to age 42 years for men and 48 years for women.[2] Recent advances in the treatment of SCD, such as hydroxyurea, prolong and improve the quality of life for many people, with some living into their 80s. People with SCD live with many threats to the quality of life for them and their families. Palliative care offers the hope of reducing these threats. The purpose of this article is to profile the many opportunities for implementation of palliative care concepts across the life span, toward the goal of further improving the quality of life for infants, children, adolescents, adults, and older adults who inherited SCD, and for their families. Specifically, the article discusses an ecological model of palliative care that is patient centered and family focused, as a way to improve awareness and communication about SCD, understand the challenges of SCD, manage pain and other symptoms during a lifetime, and cope with loss, grief, and bereavement.

ECOLOGICAL MODEL OF CARE FOR PEOPLE WITH SCD
Patient-centered and Family-focused Care for People with SCD and their Families

A health ecological model is useful for planning comprehensive care of people with SCD because it can be a means to improve quality of life with a special focus on patient-centered and family-focused care (**Fig. 1**). Within a health ecological model, it is important to consider personal and environmental factors as they influence palliative care needs. Focus should include awareness of the disease, advance care planning, symptom experiences throughout the life span, and bereavement. Based on the human response model,[3,4] a health ecological model allows incorporation of the essential components of palliative care for individuals and families across the life span.[5–10] A health ecological model is also consistent with the National Quality Forum's priorities for high-quality palliative care.[10] It is important for the

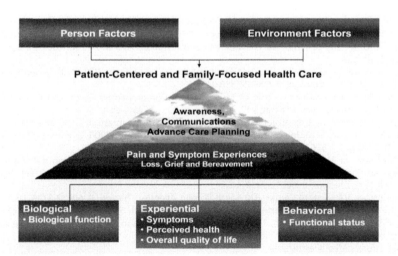

Fig. 1. Ecological framework for palliative care of people with SCD. (*Modified from* University of Illinois College of Nursing, Center for End-of-Life Transition Research, © 2007; with permission.)

comprehensive care of people living with SCD that clinicians recognize the palliative care needs and life-threatening nature of this disease.

As shown in **Fig. 1**, palliative care for the person with SCD requires that clinicians have biologic expertise to better manage symptoms and to maintain or improve functional status. Similarly, clinicians with behavioral and community expertise are needed to deal with (1) personal (individual) factors, such as awareness of the genetic transmission of the disease and effective communication; and (2) external (environmental) factors, such as cultural norms that contribute to behavior, advance care planning or adherence to prescribed analgesic therapies. Attention to salient personal and environmental factors is important for implementing interventions at the personal or community level, thereby maximizing patient-centered and family-focused palliative care of people with SCD.

Model Components

Personal factors and environmental factors are keys to understanding the constellation of factors that contribute to palliative care. Personal factors are either fixed characteristics or modifiable dimensions,[7] such as age and ethnicity (fixed characteristics) and physical symptoms, and a sense of purpose and meaning (modifiable dimensions). Environmental factors include home, community, and health care system factors that exist outside the person to influence health care outcomes.[7] Palliative care is directed toward assessing and changing personal (individual) vulnerability or resilience factors that are modifiable, and it is directed toward manipulating or helping individuals to manipulate environmental factors that constitute risks or resources, with the goal of improving the quality of life. Care system interventions exist on several levels: the family, the larger social group (communities), and health care institutions, including health care providers, to facilitate awareness about the challenges of SCD and the life-threatening nature of the disease.

As shown in **Fig. 1**, awareness of SCD transmission and disease trajectory and effective communication are central to advance care planning to allow the individual or the parents of a child to plan in advance of a critical event the type of care preferred. Ideally, advance care planning occurs before the patient and family are facing death. It also recognizes that individuals' previous experiences with end-of-life experiences can influence subsequent advance care planning. Advance care planning indicates the type of care desired when one approaches death, be it aggressive medical treatment (eg, mechanical ventilation, tube feeding, and cardiopulmonary resuscitation in persons with SCD) or be it solely aggressive palliative care to promote symptom control and maintain function. Providing comfort to the dying individual is important for managing the pain and symptom experience and to reducing complications during the bereavement process. Bereavement refers to having experienced the loss of someone significant through death.[11] Although bereavement is viewed as a normal life event, and most bereaved people go through the grieving process without any outside intervention, various personal and environmental factors can make certain individuals vulnerable to negative physical and mental health outcomes.[12] For example, the death of a child, even one with SCD, is often seen as an unnatural event that can place a parent at risk for a negative health outcome, such as major depression. Offering support groups for bereaved parents, siblings, and friends or schoolmates or for raising awareness of and coping with SCD is a palliative care-oriented intervention, which is typically offered by communities (eg, faith communities, organizations) or comprehensive SCD centers.

Within the health ecological framework and in the context of palliative care, nurses and other health care providers focus on related components, including biologic function, symptoms, perceived health, quality of life, and functional status. These components represent realms that can be measured physiologically, experientially (personally reported), or behaviorally (observed). Awareness about the transmission of SCD and communication issues that occur across the life span is vital to understanding the importance of assessing these components and providing palliative care as appropriate to the life stage.

Awareness and Communication Issues

Inherited genetic disease

SCD results from the inheritance of a gene for abnormal hemoglobin (sickle hemoglobin or hemoglobin S [Hb S]), which, on deoxygenation, forms an intracellular polymer that transforms the red blood cell to a dense and rigid sickle cell. The sickle cells have difficulty flowing through small blood vessels and can block effective blood flow, which results in tissue damage and death. Several closely related genetic conditions can each lead to a form of SCD, with more than 400 hemoglobin variants in the United States. In each case, the patient inherits a gene for Hb S from 1 parent, and a second abnormal hemoglobin gene from the other parent. The commonest (and generally the most severe) form of SCD is homozygous hemoglobin S (Hb SS). Other common variants include sickle hemoglobin C disease (Hb SC) and sickle β thalassemia (Hb Sβ thal). SCD is most common in people descendant from Africa, the Mediterranean area, the Middle East, and India.

Because SCD is a recessive genetic disease, both parents must be carriers (sometimes referred to as having the trait) of an abnormal hemoglobin (at least 1 being Hb S) and/or have the disease (Hb SS) to produce offspring with SCD. In the United States, SCD primarily affects African Americans (AA). The incidence is 1 in 500 births, and 10% (1 in 10) of AAs are carriers of the trait. If both parents are carriers of an abnormal hemoglobin gene, then with each pregnancy there is a 25% chance that the offspring will be born with SCD. There is also a 25% chance that the offspring will be born with normal hemoglobin, and a 50% chance that the offspring will be born with the trait that was carried by the parent(s).[13] This inheritance pattern is illustrated in **Fig. 2**. Gallo and colleagues,[14] however, found that many parents are unaware of their potential to transmit SCD to their children.

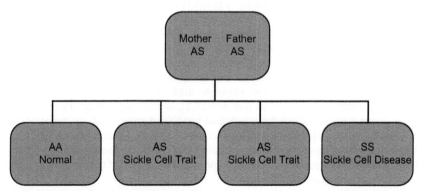

Fig. 2. Inheritance pattern of parents with heterozygous hemoglobin variant S. A normal hemoglobin gene; S abnormal hemoglobin gene.

Awareness of SCD transmission

The Comprehensive Sickle Cell Center at the University of Illinois at Chicago (UIC), in partnership with board members of the Have A Heart For Sickle Cell Anemia Foundation, a not-for-profit community sickle cell advocate program, conducted an informal survey about sickle cell awareness. Most people surveyed were not aware of the possibility of screening for SCD or of whether they were carriers of sickle cell trait (SCT) or of other hemoglobin variants (B Johnson, J Bilder, R Molokie [Community-University partnership for sickle cell screening], unpublished raw data, University of Illinois at Chicago Medical Center, Chicago, Illinois, 2009). Widespread community education and screening events are crucially needed to increase awareness in people at risk for SCT. In addition, discussions with individuals with SCD and SCT should address several topics, for example: (1) disease burdens and consequences for the affected individual as well as the caregiver; (2) the genetic transmission of SCD; and (3) the reproductive risks of having an affected child, as well as reproductive options that will allow for informed reproductive decisions and the practice of appropriate reproductive health behaviors.[15] This lack of awareness of the genetic transmission of the disease and lack of awareness of one's own trait carrier status are major areas requiring improved communication within families, communities, and the public health and health care systems.

There remains a lack of awareness of SCD transmission and care needs not only among the general population but also (disturbingly) among health care providers and those who are affected by this devastating disease. Griffin[16] reported to the SCD Association of America-Dallas Chapter's newborn screening program that challenges for proper SCD care included "a pervasive lack of awareness of sickle cell risk among the target population; a lack of effective parental notification and referral mechanisms to ensure family access to required testing, education, counseling and support services; inadequate parental health knowledge and health supervision to improve outcomes for children affected by SCD; and inadequate medical homes limiting children's access to care that is accessible, family centered, culturally competent, compassionate, comprehensive and continuous."[16(pp1)] Awareness of the key facts, decisions, and practices related to SCD transmission is an important area for a public health approach to palliative care that has been advocated by the International Workgroup on Death, Dying and Bereavement.[17]

Care communication issues

When parents give birth to a child with SCD, several communication issues become critically important for a palliative care approach to SCD. SCD is characterized by chronic hemolytic anemia, increased susceptibility to infections, end-organ damage, and intermittent episodes of vascular occlusion that result in acute and chronic pain.[1] All of these complications compromise the quality of life for the person with SCD, as well as for the family. Helping each patient to attain optimal quality of life is the goal of palliative care,[18] and this occurs through open and effective communication.[19] Effective communication among the health care professional team, patient, and family is essential for positive patient outcomes, well-being, and satisfaction. Poor communication often occurs between patients and health care professionals, which results in suspicion and mistrust.[20] Patients perceive themselves as labeled as drug seekers (although occasionally they are), and they think that the medical community is merely tolerant of them. These patients believe they are confronted by an unsympathetic system and hence respond to health care professionals in a hostile fashion. The result is often an adversarial relationship between the 2 groups. Use of good communication skills by health care professionals is vital to good health practice and healthy patient-provider relationships.[20]

Advance care planning

Ethical decision making is another core value of integrated palliative care that should be integrated into the care of patients with SCD. For example, not only must SC patients make decisions on reproductive choices but also they should make decisions regarding advance care planning. Advance care planning includes informed consent, surrogate decision making, advance directives and do-not-resuscitate (DNR) orders. Progress has been made in the management of SCD, especially among the pediatric population; however, these patients' life expectancy is significantly lower than that of the general population.[2] Integrated palliative care facilitates advance care planning discussions across the life span.

Individuals with decision-making capacity have a legal and ethical right to participate in health care decision making. Ethical guidelines require 5 elements in order for informed consent to occur: (1) the person must have the capacity to make decisions; (2) all relevant facts must be disclosed; (3) the person must understand what has been disclosed; (4) the decision must be voluntary; and (5) the person must give consent.[21] For the person lacking capacity for decision making, there are basic standards for surrogate decision making that ensure that the person's previously stated wishes are honored. Two examples are substituted judgment standard and best interest standard. Substituted judgment standard is doing what the patient would have chosen if he or she were able to choose. Written evidence such as advance directives, verbal evidence (such as conversations with family, friends, or professionals regarding their wishes), and relational evidence (personal knowledge of an individual) are acceptable forms of evidence for the substituted judgment standard. The best interest standard applies if there is no available information of what a person would have wanted; then surrogates are obliged to do what is in the patient's best interest.[21]

Advance directives are a way that individuals can make their wishes for end-of-life treatment known before losing their decision-making capacity. Advance directives usually take the form of written evidence of a person's wishes. There are 2 basic types of advance directive: one that stipulates one's treatment preferences (eg, living wills); and the other that stipulates who will be the surrogate decision makers (eg, a durable power of attorney for health care). Typically, advance directives are completed more frequently by white, middle- to upper-class individuals than by individuals of ethnic and minority populations. Generally, some groups in the United States fear that they may be denied treatment at the end of life and they are therefore unlikely to complete an advance directive. A DNR order serves as written evidence that informed consent discussion has occurred between the health care professional and the patient or his/her legal surrogate.[21]

Similar to adults, children with SCD must have advance care planning as well. Decision making needs to occur, and parents are considered to be the best surrogate decision makers for a minor child. Because children do not have a history of prior choices, parents are held to the best interest standard. The model for informed parental consent includes parental informed permission combined with the assent of the child. The purpose of an assent is to gain the child's cooperation and agreement as much as possible. Also, assent considers the developmental capabilities of the child and assesses the child's knowledge and response to tests and treatments.[21] Advance care planning is needed early in the life of individuals with SCD and throughout their lives as they encounter the many challenges of SCD. Living one's entire life with the realities and burdens of SCD provides experience that leaves each patient with SCD able to contribute realistically to discussions about clinical decisions.

CHALLENGES OF SCD

Since SCD was first described in the Western literature a century ago,[22] understanding of the disease mechanisms and sequelae has been important to guide care of people with the disease. SCD was considered primarily a pediatric condition because of extremely high childhood morbidity and mortality. In the 1960s, only 50% of patients with SCD survived to age 20 years;[23] however, in the first decade of the twenty-first century, the probability of survival to adulthood had improved to nearly 95%,[24] with a parallel reduction in life-threatening complications. These improvements can be attributed to several medical advances, including the introduction of penicillin prophylaxis for prevention of pneumococcal infections,[25,26] conjugated *Haemophilus*,[27,28] and pneumococcal[29] vaccines in early childhood; universal newborn screening for hemoglobinopathies;[30,31] and prevention of primary strokes.[32,33]

Currently, newborn screening for hemoglobinopathies is practiced in all 50 states. Hence, in contrast to previous years, the parents of virtually all patients with SCD in the United States become aware of their child's condition shortly after birth. On being informed for the first time of the diagnosis of SCD in their newborn child, parents face a multitude of issues. Although most have heard of SCD, unless they or another family member also have the disease, parents are likely to have little understanding of the condition or its potential effect on the health and life expectancy of their children. Many new parents are surprised to learn that they were at risk of having a child with SCD, and were unaware that they and/or their partner were carriers of a genetic abnormality. In addition to feeling guilt for having passed on a genetic illness to their child, they may feel helpless or uncertain for the future.

From early in life and throughout their lives, people with SCD have great need for palliative care. Although a child with SCD is asymptomatic at birth (because of high levels of fetal hemoglobin), by 3 to 6 months of age the child is at risk for early complications of the disease. Frequently, dactylitis or hand-and-foot syndrome is the first clinical manifestation in an infant or toddler with SCD. Dactylitis is characterized by swelling of the dorsum of the hands or feet, or swelling of the fingers or toes. Progressive loss of splenic function begins in infancy and leads to a lifelong risk for potentially deadly bacterial infections, such as septicemia, pneumonia, meningitis, and osteomyelitis. Because of infection risk, young children with SCD are frequently hospitalized when they develop a fever. Infants or young children may develop potentially fatal splenic sequestration crises, caused by trapping of the blood by the dysfunctional spleen, or aplastic crises associated with common viral infections (eg, parvovirus). In these situations, red blood cell transfusions may be lifesaving. Parents may feel ambivalent or fearful of the risks of transfusions, or may have religious objections, lending further emotional trauma to such situations. Families find themselves needing to adapt their lifestyles to accommodate frequent visits to the doctor or hospital, daily medications, blood tests, and other medical procedures.

In addition to infections, the risk for certain complications of SCD begins early in life and continues throughout life. Examples[34] include painful vasoocclusive crises and acute chest syndrome (ACS), which is an acute illness characterized by fever and respiratory symptoms in a patient with SCD and accompanied by a new pulmonary infiltrate on a chest radiograph.[35] This syndrome of pulmonary infarction may arise from a variety of causes, including bacterial or viral pneumonitis, pulmonary infarction, fat embolus from marrow necrosis during vasoocclusive crisis, or acute respiratory compromise. Although more common in young children, the condition is more likely to be fatal in adults.[36]

School-aged children with SCD face additional challenges. Painful crises or hospitalizations may lead to frequent school absences, with difficulty in maintaining school performance and passing grades. Risk for debilitating strokes is high throughout the school years, with a peak incidence for cerebral infarction at about 7 years of age.[37] The vascular pathology leading to infarctive strokes in children with SCD is incompletely understood, but frequently involves the large cerebral arteries. In this case, inflammatory endothelial damage results from adherent sickle cells or the products of hemolysis in conjunction with high blood flow rates caused by anemia and vasoconstriction from nitric oxide depletion. Intimal hyperplasia ensues, the caliber of the affected vessels narrows, and a thrombus ultimately occludes the vessel.[38] A child having a stroke or found through screening to be at high risk for a stroke may start a chronic red blood cell transfusion program. This program involves transfusions approximately monthly; this is about 90% effective in reducing stroke risk.[32] Because discontinuing a program of regular transfusions is associated with return of high stroke risk,[39] chronic transfusion therapy may be maintained for many years. This therapy is not without risks. Chronic transfusion therapy leads to excessive iron accumulation in body organs (transfusional hemosiderosis), which results in liver, cardiac, or endocrine abnormalities, and potentially contributes to premature mortality.[40] In addition to overt strokes, a different lesion of the central nervous system known as silent infarction may be found in children with SCD.[41] These children may experience attention deficit, hyperactivity, or various learning disabilities. Silent infarcts, which can be diagnosed based on characteristic brain lesions seen on magnetic resonance imaging,[42,43] may progress to overt stroke.[44] Neuropsychiatric testing and development of an individualized education plan at school may help a child perform to his or her fullest potential.

Children and teens with SCD face additional physical and social challenges. The renal damage caused by SCD leads to loss of urinary-concentrating ability during childhood.[45] As a result, young people with SCD have a high incidence of primary enuresis, which may be embarrassing. Body image issues are common in adolescents and teens with SCD; these frequently include short stature and delayed puberty,[46] as well as chronic jaundice. Participation in sports and physical activities is frequently limited. Not only do chronic anemia and propensity to dehydration limit the exercise capacity of patients with SCD but also painful crises may be triggered by vigorous exercise or environmental extremes, including summer heat, swimming in cold water, or travel to high altitudes. Despite these limitations, physical activity may be beneficial in patients with SCD[47] and should be judiciously encouraged. Denial, or a desire to be like other teens, may induce a patient with SCD to engage in risky behaviors,[48] or to forgo his or her medications or medical treatments, sometimes with serious consequences.

As teens grow into adulthood, the transition to being an adult living with a chronic medical condition is difficult.[49] The young adult must leave the familiar setting of the pediatric physicians and nurses who have cared for the patient for his or her entire life, and establish a relationship with an unfamiliar medical care team. In addition, the responsibility for managing the patient's medical condition, taking medicines, making appointments, and so forth, is transferred from the parent to the patient. Medicaid or parental private insurance coverage terminates at the age of majority, and the patient must secure new medical coverage through an employer, Medicare, or Supplemental Security Income disability. If the pediatric sickle cell center has a transition program, that program may be a valuable resource in guiding the patient through this process.[50]

Certain medical complications of SCD become increasingly frequent in the teenage to young adult years. Because of sickle vasculopathy and poor wound healing, cutaneous leg ulcers may arise from apparently trivial injury, such as insect bites or minor abrasions.[51] Ulcers may become large and debilitating, sometimes lasting for years. Avascular necrosis of bones occurs, most frequently in the femoral head, leading to chronic hip disease.[52,53] The patient ultimately may need a hip replacement to relieve pain and restore function. Avascular necrosis also may occur in the humeral head, leading to shoulder dysfunction. Collapse of infarcted vertebral bodies may lead to chronic back pain. Vasculopathy also leads to sickle retinopathy,[54] which includes retinal hemorrhages, neovascularization, and retinal detachment, and may lead to blindness. This complication is particularly frequent in patients with hemoglobin SCD.[55] Frequent eye examinations are essential to identifying and treating retinal vascular lesions early.[56] Cholelithiasis is a frequent complication of SCD. If asymptomatic, no intervention is required; however, cholelithiasis may progress to symptomatic cholecystitis requiring cholecystectomy.[57]

Priapism, a painful, prolonged involuntary erection, is a potentially serious condition in teens and young men with SCD. It may occur repeatedly; recurrent priapism leads to lifelong impotence in many cases.[58] Priapism frequently begins at night, and prompt interventions that patients may try at home include voiding, ejaculation, warm baths, and analgesics.[59] However, the occurrence of a painful erection lasting more than 2 hours should be considered an emergency, and the patient should seek medical attention immediately, to reduce the risk for impotence. There is no universal approach to the medical management of priapism, but intervention may include oral vasoactive agents, transfusion, penile aspiration and injection with epinephrine or phenylephrine, and surgical shunting.[58]

Although many women with SCD can safely bear children, pregnancy is considered high risk[60] because of a high frequency of sickling complications, as well as spontaneous miscarriage, preeclampsia, premature delivery, and low birth weight infants. Teens and young adults should be counseled to use effective methods of birth control to avoid unintended pregnancies. When they become pregnant, women should initiate prenatal care promptly from an obstetrician experienced in the management of SCD. Teens and young adults with SCD should receive genetic counseling, to understand the risk of having children with SCD. Their partners should also be tested for a hemoglobinopathy; this testing should be by means of hemoglobin electrophoresis or high-performance liquid chromatography, and not merely a sickle preparation, as the latter misses other hemoglobinopathies such as hemoglobin C or β thalassemia.

As a result of chronic pain, physical disabilities, frequent acute pain episodes or other complications resulting in hospitalization, patients with SCD may be fired for excessive job absences, and may have difficulty in securing employment. Employed patients should be encouraged to file federal Family and Medical Leave Act papers with their employer, to protect their jobs whenever possible. Similarly, patients may experience difficulties with marital and other personal relationships.

Despite medical advances, SCD in adults is a debilitating disorder leading ultimately to premature mortality. The Cooperative Study of SCD (CSSCD), a national study of the natural history of SCD, found in 1994 that patients with persistently high levels of fetal hemoglobin (Hb F) had prolonged survival compared with those with low Hb F. The protective effect of Hb F has been observed for many years[61] and forms the basis for the treatment of patients with hydroxyurea,[62] a chemotherapy agent capable of inducing Hb F production in some patients with SCD. Long-term follow-up of patients who participated in a definitive trial of hydroxyurea therapy[63] has provided some preliminary evidence that use of this drug may prolong survival. Patients often succumb to chronic organ failure, dying from an illness that in other circumstances would not be fatal. Common causes of death include pulmonary hypertension, sudden death because of unknown causes, renal failure, ACS, or acute multiorgan failure, often in the context of hospitalization for painful crisis, sepsis, cardiac disease, thromboembolism, stroke, or iron overload.[64] Frequently, more than 1 of these conditions contributes to the death.

Despite the multitude of challenges facing persons living with SCD and their loved ones, many adults are able to lead successful careers and fulfilling family lives. Such patients' optimism has been eloquently expressed by the late Linda Collins, a beloved and respected Chicago sickle cell activist, UIC patient, and the founder of the Have a Heart for Sickle Cell Foundation, whose motto was "SCD is not who you are; it is what you have." With the focus on the person with SCD, effective management of the pain and other symptoms of the disease is important for patient-centered and family-focused care and central to high quality of life, as advocated by a palliative care approach to SCD management.

SCD PAIN AND SYMPTOM MANAGEMENT

Pain and SCD are so intertwined that ancient African tribal words for SCD are onomatopoeic for pain. The first patient reported with SCD in the Western literature was hospitalized for 62 days for "muscular rheumatism."[65] Whereas SCD has been associated with many groundbreaking discoveries, our understanding of pain syndromes associated with it, the pathophysiology of the pain, and its treatment have not advanced nearly to the same degree. Pain syndromes in those with SCD do not generally start until after the first few months of life, when the amount of fetal hemoglobin in the red blood cells decreases, and sickle hemoglobin increases, an observation first reported by Watson in 1948.[66] The importance of increased fetal hemoglobin in adults to decrease disease severity was first reported by Perrine, in 1972.[67] Both of these findings are the underpinning for the development of therapies that increase fetal hemoglobin production to ameliorate pain and other symptoms of the disease. The consequences of unrelieved pain in those with SCD are substantial.[68]

Many different pain syndromes are associated with the sickle hemoglobinopathies; however, the most common is the acute vasoocclusive crisis, which represents more than 90% of admissions to hospital for SCD.[34] Acute vasoocclusive crisis is a complicated physiologic event, involving endothelial red blood cell interaction, leukocyte adhesion, hemoglobin polymerization, and coagulation activation.[69] It has been described as having 4 phases. The first phase is prodromal, with symptoms of numbness, aches, and paresthesias that develop in areas subsequently affected by pain. This phase can last up to 2 days. The second phase, the initial infarct, shows increasing pain, which usually peaks by the second or third day. This phase is followed by the postinfarction phase, with persistent and severe pain associated with signs and symptoms of inflammation, followed by the resolution phase.[34] The pain may involve any part of the body, and its severity and time from development to resolution can vary greatly. Someone can be well, and a few minutes later in severe pain, needing admission to the hospital, whereas for others their pain can be easily controlled at home. Other causes of acute pain include ACS, hepatic crisis, cholecystitis, priapism, hand-and-foot syndrome, and splenic sequestration syndrome. Chronic pain can be associated with avascular necrosis of joints, skin ulcers, osteomyelitis, and chronic pain syndromes, including neuropathic pain.[34]

The CSSCD's prospective study of the natural history of pain in people with SCD is the largest prospective study of the natural history of pain in patients with SCD.[70] The study followed 3578 children and adults and documented 12,290 pain episodes in 18,356 patient years. A pain episode was defined as pain in the extremities, back, abdomen, chest, or head that lasted at least 2 hours, required a visit to the hospital, and could be explained only by SCD. Patients with Hb SS and those with Hb Sbeta; thal[0] had higher mean pain frequency (0.8 and 1.0 episodes/y) compared with patients with hemoglobin SCD or Hb Sbeta; thal[+] (0.4 episodes/y). These investigators also showed the wide variability in the frequency of these painful episodes within each phenotype. As defined for the study, 39% of patients had no pain episodes/y, whereas 1% of patients had 6 or more/y.

The CSSCD researchers also found significant differences in the frequency in pain episodes between age groups, with children 4 years of age or less having 0.4 episodes/y and those 25 to 29 years of age having 1.21 episodes/y.[70] A lower fetal hemoglobin and higher hemoglobin were independent risk factors for these pain events. Although there is little doubt as to the importance of the CSSCD pain study, it may not represent fully the pain experience of those with SCD. To be considered a painful event, the patient's pain needed to be severe enough for the patient to be seen by a health care provider, and if they had more than 1 event in a week, it was considered as 1 event. Therefore, the number of painful episodes may be underrepresented.

The pain experiences of those with SCD are more frequent and complex than the CSSCD study suggested. Nurse scientists have contributed substantially to understanding the sensory, emotional, cognitive, and temporal characteristics of acute pain in children with SCD by using the Adolescent Pediatric Pain Tool.[71–73] Dampier and colleagues[74] reported on 37 child and adolescent patients with SCD who completed pain diaries at home, for a total of 18,377 pain diary days. Only 2 patients did not report pain during the study, whereas the remaining 35 reported 518 pain episodes. Smith and colleagues[75] prospectively studied 232 adults with SCD for up to 6 months, using a daily self-reported pain diary. They found that patients reported pain on more than 50% of the days, and 30% experienced pain on more than 95% of the study days. Only 22% of days that the patients reported acute pain resulted in an admission.

Our group at UIC recently reported on the pain of 145 adults who used PAIN*Reportlt*,[76] an electronic version of the McGill Pain Questionnaire.[77] We found that the SCD pain at a usual clinic visit was more severe than pain severity reported for cancer pain or childbirth pain.[78] Furthermore, our findings[78] suggested that the pain experienced by adults with SCD may include a component that is neuropathic (pain arising as a direct consequence of a lesion or disease affecting the somatosensory system),[79] in addition to the nociceptive pain (pain from injury to somatic or visceral tissue) commonly associated with a vasoocclusive event.

Pain in people with SCD also has a significant effect on quality of life. Schwartz and colleagues[80] studied 40 adolescent patients with SCD and found that they missed 12% of the school year, and 35% missed at least 1 month of school. These investigators also reported that parent-reported pain frequency and attendance at clinic appointments were significantly associated with the school absenteeism.[80]

It is not clear why some people have more severe disease. Ballas,[81] however, first suggested that there were 2 distinct phenotypes of sickle cell: those with frequent

Table 1
Differences in grief responses by age, gender, and person

Age	Responses
Babies	May withdraw and stop eating, or be listless and fussing
Toddlerhood	Toddlers' sense of what they want guides how they see the situation around them. They believe that people can read their minds and that wishing for something will make it happen. Frequently, they blame themselves for what does happen, including the death of a family member. Toddlers may not distinguish between going away and death. They may show their distress in nonverbal ways as agitated behaviors, body language or in dreams. Sometimes in play situation, a toddler may cry 1 moment and run outside and play in the next moment
Preschool-kindergarten age	Children between the ages of 3 and 6 years begin to recognize their own behavior even although they may not be able to fully control their feelings and actions. By age 4 years, children may have a limited understanding of the word "death." They may think the dead come back to life. There is an interaction with the social environment. For example, if the mother died when the child was 2 years old and the father remarries, the child at the age of 4 years feels cared for by this second mother but still may want to visit the grave of his mother
Elementary school age	Children are on a continuum of development, and they learn quickly not only about relationships but also how to read and develop more resources for themselves. These children are able to separate their point of view from that of others. Elementary school age children realize that there is a connection between events, that their father being sick led to his death. They have concerns as to who will take their father's place. These children understand death as the cessation of functions. Death processes and funerals are on their minds. Older children know that death is universal. There can be emotional disturbances such as poor school performance, appetite changes, shortened attention span, depression, guilt, and fear. They may complain of stomachache and other somatic symptoms. They frequently do not bring up their concerns

Adolescence	This period of time is one of rapid cognitive, emotional, and physical development. They act more independently and are able to think abstractly, to also recognize their own feelings and point of view as well as others' feelings and points of view. Maintaining relationships and receiving approval from their peers are vitally important to them. When death occurs in the family, they begin to contain their feelings and are less likely to talk about them, whereas girls do. Questions about death are natural and an integral part of an attempt to reach a new understanding of life. Initial response to death may be shock, confusion, depression, anger, fear, blaming, lethargy, and guilt, which decrease with time. Acting out behavior such as driving fast or taking risks may be seen
Gender	
Feminine (conventional)	Sharing intense feelings with others, expressing feelings through crying, responding favorably to interventions that are traditional, affect-intensive strategies (eg, open sharing of feelings and group support)
Masculine	Remaining silent, engaging in solitary mourning, secret grief, taking physical or legal action, becoming immersed in activity, exhibiting addictive behavior, seeking companionship (in line of support), using humor or other ways of expressing feelings (but managing anger and aggression)
Other Factors	
Personal factors	Past experiences with loss and completion of grief work, when in the life cycle the loss occurred, relationship with deceased, how loss occurred (sudden, expected, unexpected, preventable), health history (physical health, mental health, suicide attempts, life crises)

Modified from Wilkie DJ, Brown MA, Corless I, et al. Toolkit for nursing excellence at end of life transition for nurse educators (TNEEL-NE). Version 1.0. Chicago: University of Illinois Chicago College of Nursing; 2001; with permission.

painful episodes and fewer leg ulcers, and those with fewer painful episodes, but more leg ulcers. Serjeant and others were also able to develop a twofold model with either predominantly painful crises or leg ulcer phenotypes in patients with SCD from Jamaica.[82] They also found that the painful crisis group had higher frequencies of dactylitis, meningitis, septicemia, ACS, and stroke.[82] More recently, others have found a hyperhemolysis phenotype to be more associated with increased blood pressure, priapism, leg ulcer, and pulmonary hypertension, whereas osteonecrosis and pain occurred less often in this group.[83] Some pain syndromes can be addressed with specific procedures, such as arthroplasty for severe avascular necrosis, and surgery for cholecystitis, but the management of the acute vasoocclusive event and chronic pain syndromes can be more difficult.

Opioids are the mainstay for management of severe vasoocclusive events; however, health care providers are often reluctant to provide adequate therapy. The reasons for inadequate medication use are complex.[84] A disturbing survey found that 53% of emergency department physicians and 23% of hematologists believed that more than 20% of those with SCD are addicts.[85] Using nonpain-related symptoms, however, Elander and colleagues[86] showed that only 2% met DSM-IV (Diagnostic and Statistical Manual of Mental Disorders, fourth edition) criteria for dependence, whereas others found an incidence of 0.2% to 2.0%.[87] Studies are needed in people with SCD to determine the effect of drugs commonly used for neuropathic pain, such as gabapentin, on the pain that they describe with neuropathic descriptors. A palliative care approach that includes attention to the complete pain experience of SCD may help to improve outcomes and quality of life for this vulnerable population.

When patients cannot control their pain at home and need to go to the emergency department for care, Tanabe and colleagues[88] found that the median time to administration of an initial analgesic was 90 minutes (25th to 75th interquartile range, 54–159 minutes). These investigators also found that 92% received the recommended dose, based on American Pain Association Guidelines, but only 55% received the drug by the recommended route (intravenously or subcutaneously).[88]

A major advance in the care of patients with SCD has been the acute care facility, or day hospital. In 1984, Grady Hospital in Atlanta opened a center, 24 hours a day, 7 days a week, for adult patients with SCD. In addition to providing outpatient care, this facility substituted for the emergency department for most of the adult patients with SCD who were having painful events that they could not control at home (obstetric cases were triaged to obstetrics, trauma cases to trauma). The admission rate for those who now use this facility is only 20%, with a reduced admission rate from 2.5 to 0.5 active subjects/y, and improved patient satisfaction (Alan Platt, Atlanta, GA, personal communication, 2009). In 2000, Benjamin and colleagues[89] reported on the Day Hospital of the Bronx Comprehensive Sickle Cell Center at the Montefiore Medical Center, Bronx, NY. During their first 5 years of operation, they, too, were able to discharge more than 80% of the patients to home, compared with the emergency department's 94% hospital admission rate.[89] Similar findings have been reported in the United Kingdom,[90] in Jamaica,[91] and for pediatric patients.[92] There are few such facilities in the United States.

Although it has been almost 100 years since SCD was first reported in the Western literature,[65] we are lacking in our understanding of the physiology and complicated nature of pain in SCD, as well as its effect on the quality of life for patients. Overall, the delivery of health care and adequate pain management for those with SCD is lacking. We now understand that pain is almost a daily experience in those with SCD, yet patients often have problems in obtaining appropriate care. Most find themselves in an adversarial relationship with many health care providers, who do not understand the severity of their pain. This breakdown in the patient-provider relationship undermines self-reliance and self-knowledge and reduces the capacity for self-management.[93] The palliative care philosophy of a partnership between patients and their health care providers, starting at the earliest of ages, may be the most effective health care model for those with SCD.[94] A palliative care focus is needed not only to foster adequate pain management but also to facilitate coping with the losses associated with SCD, as well as the grief and bereavement related to death in this vulnerable population.

COPING WITH LOSS, GRIEF, AND BEREAVEMENT

Individuals and families living with SCD face many kinds of loss, not only the possibility of death at a young age but also the multiple losses along the way as the person experiences the challenges of the disease. For example, the husband whose wife has SCD and has had multiple strokes will be faced with the loss of a partner who shared the household responsibilities, and he may need to take on the task of paying the bills, doing the gardening and grocery shopping, and more. Because he must assume the responsibilities that his wife once did for both of them, his grieving process starts long before her actual death. At the same time, as his wife's illness and disability worsen, she too grieves the loss of roles, activities, and experiences in which she is no longer able to participate. For example, her work as a bank vice-president was a key part of her identity, but her health challenges associated with SCD force her to miss work, a big loss for her. Similarly, she grieves for not being able to continue her active support of her teenage daughter's involvement in competitive gymnastics. As patients and families focus on the challenges of the illness, they experience multiple losses.

The spectrum of losses includes those that often come to mind, as well as those rarely considered (**Box 1**). Grief is a normal response to loss. People of all ages have grief responses, but the responses differ by age, gender, and other factors (**Table 1**). Some grief responses persist and interfere with the individual's health and functioning to the extent that the person is considered to have complicated grief. Uncomplicated grief is managed by the person and his/her communities (eg, work, faith, neighbors) without need for professional help. In contrast, people with complicated grief often require counseling support from health professionals.

Many health professionals commonly express feelings of inadequacy at helping patients with SCD and their families cope with loss, grief, and bereavement. Two simple strategies can be implemented to help patients, families, and health professionals cope with the loss, grief, and bereavement that are common in the face of SCD. One strategy is to recognize the importance of rituals to assist in coping with loss and grief. Rituals are embedded within our cultures and offer comfort, especially at the time of a death. Some health care professionals intentionally attend funerals of their patients as a means of offering support to the bereaved but also to help them cope with their sense of loss. It is also helpful for health professionals in clinics or inpatient units to participate in an annual remembrance of patients who died during the year with a recognition event.

Another strategy that many health professionals might find helpful is to write condolence letters or notes to their patients who have experienced a loss (eg, stroke) or to a bereaved family after a death. Often, however, health professionals lack confidence in their ability to say the right thing, and they fear that their words will cause more distress to a patient with a loss or the family after a death. **Table 2** shows a basic structure for a condolence letter or note with example language suggested by grief

---

Box 1
The spectrum of losses in people living with SCD

Loss of a significant loved or valued person through death

1. Self (imminent or future)

2. Spouse, partner, children (including through abortion, miscarriage, stillbirth), siblings

3. Other relatives, close friends, pets

4. Fellow workers, business associates, colleagues, acquaintances

5. Celebrities, well-known personalities (eg, presidents, leaders [Martin Luther King], entertainment figures [Elvis Presley, John Lennon, Michael Jackson])

6. Strangers (in random violence and in disasters)

    geographically close or distant

    people with whom we can and cannot easily identify

Loss of significant people through other means

1. Divorce, separation, desertion

2. Temporary or permanent removal of people from home or the community and placement in:

    Institutions (eg, hospitals, nursing homes, mental hospitals, prisons, the armed forces) or

    Substitute living arrangements (eg, adoptive home or foster homes)

3. Illness (eg, strokes), accidents, or the consequences of aging (which can potentially result in such profound changes in significant persons that they are no longer the same persons we once knew and are literally gone from our lives)

4. Geographic moves (eg, because of the military, different jobs, travel)

Loss of a part of self

Physical loss

1. Structural losses: through amputation (eg, mastectomy, colostomy, hysterectomy, heart and kidney transplant) and through disfigurement caused by congenital deformation, accidents, burns, and so forth

2. Functional losses: through loss of mobility caused by paralysis, stroke, spinal cord injury; loss of 1 or more of the 5 senses; loss of elimination control; loss of sexual functioning; loss of health, and so forth

Psychological loss

1. Loss of mental processes and mental acuity (eg, loss of memory, loss of feeling, loss of mental control)

2. Loss of dignity, self-esteem, self-concept, sense of adequacy

Social loss

1. Economic loss: loss of work or income and its related loss of status, prestige, self-concept, workplace-generated losses

2. Loss of social roles (eg, role of parent, spouse, student, leader)

3. Loss of home, country, or culture, through immigration or refugee status

4. Losses resulting from addictions (of all kinds) and losses caused by surrendering such addictions

Loss of external material objects

Loss of all kinds of possessions: those with economic, practical, or convenience value and those with sentimental, emotional value can elicit grieving responses.

Developmental losses

All growing involves relinquishing (ie, losing certain ways of functioning to gain new skills, patterns and modes of functioning). These losses occur across the entire life span, from birth and infancy through older age.

Modified from Wilkie DJ, Brown MA, Corless I, et al. Toolkit for nursing excellence at end of life transition for nurse educators (TNEEL-NE). Version 1.0. Chicago: University of Illinois Chicago College of Nursing; 2001; with permission.

Table 2
Zunin's and Zunin's[95] elements of a letter of condolence or condolence note

Element	Example Language
Salutation	Dear John,
Acknowledge the loss	I was saddened when Troy called this evening to tell me the news of Bobbie's death. Even though I had been expecting it, the final word was still difficult.
Express your sympathy	Words are so inadequate, but with this letter comes my deep sympathy on the loss of your beloved wife. I, too, cared deeply for her.
Note special qualities of the deceased	Bobbie was a vibrant, talented, caring, and funny woman. Everyone cherished her, but for me, she was even more. She was a rare and treasured friend.
Recount a memory about the deceased	As I write, I recall the precious memories of the day when Bobbie and I were driving to the lake for what we thought would be a lazy afternoon of fishing. Instead, our car broke down and the 2 of us had quite a time trying to fix it. We were covered in grease and laughing like little girls, but we fixed it! And we made it to the lake just in time to catch the biggest fish either of us ever caught.
Note special qualities of the bereaved	I know you will miss her so very much, but I also know that you will find strength remembering the beautiful years you shared. Bobbie loved you so and you were always a source of strength and courage to her. I recall her once saying that your love of life and enduring optimism gave her much peace. I hope that these same qualities will help support and guide you during this difficult time.
Offer assistance	Please know that you have my sympathy and my friendship. I would appreciate if you would turn to me for any help I might give. I'll call soon to see if there's anything I can do.
Close with a thoughtful word or phrase	My thoughts are with you, Or I send you my deepest sympathy, Or My prayers are with you,

Modified from Wilkie DJ, Brown MA, Corless I, et al. Toolkit for nursing excellence at end of life transition for nurse educators (TNEEL-NE). Version 1.0. Chicago: University of Illinois Chicago College of Nursing; 2001; with permission.

and bereavement experts.[95] Writing the letter or note is therapeutic for the health care professional, and receiving the letter or note is comforting to the family. Using a palliative care approach to care of people living with SCD and their families, health care professionals can incorporate condolence letters and notes into their routines. In addition, health care professionals should come to understand the benefits that a condolence letter or note has for themselves and the comfort it can bring to the bereaved.

SUMMARY

Patients with SCD often have painful episodes and other health challenges, but how they manage those issues can determine the quality of their lives, their successes and productivity. An ecological model of care that is patient centered and family focused may better equip a patient and his/her family and health care providers for success across the patient's life span. Personal factors, including improved communication and education, can benefit patients. In addition, environmental factors like support groups and advance care planning can help patients navigate the minefields of having a chronic, often debilitating disease. This palliative care approach can facilitate patient involvement and advocacy in their own care and ultimately help to improve the patient's quality of life and functional status.

Patients with SCD are at increased risk for morbidity and mortality. The life span of patients has improved over the years, which can be attributed to multiple factors; however, living with SCD still has numerous challenges. Patients must deal with having a chronic disease that often requires frequent hospital and outpatient visits. Patients with SCD live on average into their mid-40s and can have multiple physical and emotional struggles along the way, including leg ulcers, chronic hip pain, relationship challenges, marital discord, and difficulty maintaining insurance coverage. A person-centered and family-focused approach to care can help patients manage the multifaceted challenges of living with SCD.

Communication is important between the health care team and families with SCD. Often, parents with SCT may not be aware of the potential to transmit SCD to their offspring. Adolescents and young adults, therefore, must be aware of the potential of producing a child with SCD, who will have a decreased life span compared with his/her peers. Advance care planning, including informed consent, surrogate decision making, and the development of advance directives, can aid in improving the patient's quality of life, which is the ultimate goal of a palliative care approach.

Patients with SCD and pain crises make up most admissions to hospital. Although the exact genetic mutation that causes SCD has been known for years, there has been a lack of quality pain research. Researchers are just beginning to understand the broad effect of frequent admissions to hospital for pain, including routinely missing school and work. With the advent of recent research and establishment of day hospitals for managing patients' pain, admission rates can be significantly decreased.

Grief responses may differ for patients, depending on age and gender. Some patients lose their ability to provide for their families and fulfill their family roles. When grief responses interfere with an individual's ability to function, counseling from health care professionals may help. In addition, health care professionals may be better equipped to manage their patients' pain by improved communication and connection with their families.

The needs of the person with SCD and the family are amenable to intervention and support that is consistent with a simultaneous care plan that involves management of the SCD as well as palliative care. Such an approach could dramatically improve the experience of living with SCD.

ACKNOWLEDGMENTS

The investigators thank Kevin Grandfield for editorial assistance.

REFERENCES

1. Center TSCI. Sickle cell information–clinician summary. The Georgia Comprehensive Sickle Cell Center at Grady Health System. Available at: http://www.scinfo. org/prod05.htm. Accessed September 13, 2009.
2. Platt OS, Brambilla DJ, Rosse WF, et al. Mortality in sickle cell disease. Life expectancy and risk factors for early death. N Engl J Med 1994;330(23): 1639–44.
3. Heitkemper MM, Shaver JF. Nursing research opportunities in enteral nutrition. Nurs Clin North Am 1989;24(2):415–26.
4. Mitchell PH, Gallucci B, Fought SG. Perspectives on human response to health and illness. Nurs Outlook 1991;39(4):154–7.
5. Ruland CM, Moore SM. Theory construction based on standards of care: a proposed theory of the peaceful end of life. Nurs Outlook 1998;46: 169–75.
6. Widger KA, Wilkins K. What are the key components of quality perinatal and pediatric end-of-life care? A literature review. J Palliat Care 2004;20(2):105–12.
7. Emanuel EJ, Emanuel LL. The promise of a good death. Lancet 1998;351:sII21–9.
8. Field MJ, Cassel CK, editors. Approaching death: improving care at the end of life. Washington, DC: National Academy Press; 1997.
9. Field MJ, Behrman RE, editors. When children die: improving palliative and end-of-life care for children and their families. Washington, DC: The National Academies Press; 2003.
10. Forum NQ. A national framework and preferred practices for palliative and hospice care quality. Washington, DC: National Quality Forum; 2006.
11. Stroebe MS, Hansson RO, Stroebe W, et al. Introduction: concepts and issues in contemporary research on bereavement. In: Stroebe MS, Hansson RO, Stroebe W, et al, editors. Handbook of bereavement research. Washington, DC: American Psychological Association; 2001.
12. Schut H, Stroebe MS. Interventions to enhance adaptation to bereavement. J Palliat Med 2005;8(Suppl 1):S140–7.
13. Eckman JR, Platt AF. Problem oriented management of sickle syndromes; 1997. Available at: http://www.scinfo.org/prod04.htm. Accessed April 14, 2010.
14. Gallo AM, Knafl KA, Angst DB. Information management in families who have a child with a genetic condition. J Pediatr Nurs 2009;24(3):194–204.
15. Gallo AM, Wilkie DJ, Suarez ML, et al. Focus group findings about reproductive health decisions in people with sickle cell disease or trait. West J Nurs Res, in press.
16. Griffin MF. Improving sickle cell disease newborn notification and follow-up services in North Texas. Available at: http://www.sicklecelldisease.net/index. php?option=com_content&task=view&id=83&Itemid=54. Accessed April 14, 2010.
17. Becker C, Clark E, DeSpelder LA, et al. A call to action: an IWG charter for a public health approach to dying, death, and loss, in review.
18. Beider S. An ethical argument for integrated palliative care. Evid Based Complement Alternat Med 2005;2(2):227–31.
19. Anghelescu DL, Oakes L, Hinds PS. Palliative care and pediatrics. Anesthesiol Clin 2006;24(1):145–61, ix.

20. Thomas VJ, Cohn T. Communication skills and cultural awareness courses for healthcare professionals who care for patients with sickle cell disease. J Adv Nurs 2006;53(4):480–8.

21. Wilkie DJ, Brown MA, Corless I, et al. Toolkit for nursing excellence at end of life transition for nurse educators (TNEEL-NE). Version 1.0. Chicago: University of Illinois Chicago College of Nursing; 2001.

22. Herrick JB. Peculiar elongated and sickle-shaped red blood corpuscles in a case of severe anemia. Arch Intern Med 1910;6:517–21.

23. Scott RB. Health care priority and sickle cell anemia. JAMA 1970;214(4): 731–4.

24. Quinn CT, Rogers ZR, Buchanan GR. Survival of children with sickle cell disease. Blood 2004;103(11):4023–7.

25. Falletta JM, Woods GM, Verter JI, et al. Discontinuing penicillin prophylaxis in children with sickle cell anemia. Prophylactic Penicillin Study II. J Pediatr 1995; 127(5):685–90.

26. Gaston MH, Verter JI, Woods G, et al. Prophylaxis with oral penicillin in children with sickle cell anemia. A randomized trial. N Engl J Med 1986; 314(25):1593–9.

27. Marcinak JF, Frank AL, Labotka RL, et al. Immunogenicity of *Haemophilus influenzae* type b polysaccharide-diphtheria toxoid conjugate vaccine in 3- to 17-month-old infants with sickle cell diseases. J Pediatr 1991;118(1):69–71.

28. Schoendorf KC, Adams WG, Kiely JL, et al. National trends in *Haemophilus influenzae* meningitis mortality and hospitalization among children, 1980 through 1991. Pediatrics 1994;93(4):663–8.

29. Halasa NB, Shankar SM, Talbot TR, et al. Incidence of invasive pneumococcal disease among individuals with sickle cell disease before and after the introduction of the pneumococcal conjugate vaccine. Clin Infect Dis 2007;44(11):1428–33.

30. Cunningham G. Mortality among children with sickle cell disease identified by newborn screening during 1990–1994–California, Illinois and New York. MMWR Morb Mortal Wkly Rep 1998;47(9):169–72.

31. Yanni E, Grosse SD, Yang Q, et al. Trends in pediatric sickle cell disease-related mortality in the United States, 1983–2002. J Pediatr 2009;154(4):541–5.

32. Adams RJ, McKie VC, Hsu L, et al. Prevention of a first stroke by transfusions in children with sickle cell anemia and abnormal results on transcranial Doppler ultrasonography. N Engl J Med 1998;339(1):5–11.

33. Fullerton HJ, Adams RJ, Zhao S, et al. Declining stroke rates in Californian children with sickle cell disease. Blood 2004;104(2):336–9.

34. Ballas SK. Pain management of sickle cell disease. Hematol Oncol Clin North Am 2005;19(5):785–802, v.

35. Vichinsky EP, Neumayr LD, Earles AN, et al. Causes and outcomes of the acute chest syndrome in sickle cell disease. National Acute Chest Syndrome Study Group. N Engl J Med 2000;342(25):1855–65.

36. The management of sickle cell disease. NIH publication no. 02–2117; 2002. Available at: http://www.nhlbi.nih.gov/health/prof/blood/sickle/sc_mngt.pdf. Accessed April 14, 2010.

37. Ohene-Frempong K, Weiner SJ, Sleeper LA, et al. Cerebrovascular accidents in sickle cell disease: rates and risk factors. Blood 1998;91(1):288–94.

38. Switzer JA, Hess DC, Nichols FT, et al. Pathophysiology and treatment of stroke in sickle-cell disease: present and future. Lancet Neurol 2006;5(6):501–12.

39. Adams RJ, Brambilla D. Discontinuing prophylactic transfusions used to prevent stroke in sickle cell disease. N Engl J Med 2005;353(26):2769–78.

40. Kushner JP, Porter JP, Olivieri NF. Secondary iron overload. Hematology Am Soc Hematol Educ Program 2001:47–61.
41. Hindmarsh PC, Brozovic M, Brook CG, et al. Incidence of overt and covert neurological damage in children with sickle cell disease. Postgrad Med J 1987; 63(743):751–3.
42. Moser FG, Miller ST, Bello JA, et al. The spectrum of brain MR abnormalities in sickle-cell disease: a report from the Cooperative Study of Sickle Cell Disease. AJNR Am J Neuroradiol 1996;17(5):965–72.
43. Steen RG, Emudianughe T, Hankins GM, et al. Brain imaging findings in pediatric patients with sickle cell disease. Radiology 2003;228(1):216–25.
44. Miller ST, Macklin EA, Pegelow CH, et al. Silent infarction as a risk factor for overt stroke in children with sickle cell anemia: a report from the Cooperative Study of Sickle Cell Disease. J Pediatr 2001;139(3):385–90.
45. Allon M. Renal abnormalities in sickle cell disease. Arch Intern Med 1990;150(3): 501–4.
46. Platt OS, Rosenstock W, Espeland MA. Influence of sickle hemoglobinopathies on growth and development. N Engl J Med 1984;311(1):7–12.
47. Al-Rimawi H, Jallad S. Sport participation in adolescents with sickle cell disease. Pediatr Endocrinol Rev 2008;6(Suppl 1):214–6.
48. Britto MT, Garrett JM, Dugliss MA, et al. Risky behavior in teens with cystic fibrosis or sickle cell disease: a multicenter study. Pediatrics 1998;101(2): 250–6.
49. Kinney TR, Ware RE. The adolescent with sickle cell anemia. Hematol Oncol Clin North Am 1996;10(6):1255–64.
50. Bryant R, Walsh T. Transition of the chronically ill youth with hemoglobinopathy to adult health care: an integrative review of the literature. J Pediatr Health Care 2009;23(1):37–48.
51. Eckman JR. Leg ulcers in sickle cell disease. Hematol Oncol Clin North Am 1996; 10(6):1333–44.
52. Aguilar C, Vichinsky E, Neumayr L. Bone and joint disease in sickle cell disease. Hematol Oncol Clin North Am 2005;19(5):929–41, viii.
53. Smith JA. Bone disorders in sickle cell disease. Hematol Oncol Clin North Am 1996;10(6):1345–56.
54. Charache S. Eye disease in sickling disorders. Hematol Oncol Clin North Am 1996;10(6):1357–62.
55. Downes SM, Hambleton IR, Chuang EL, et al. Incidence and natural history of proliferative sickle cell retinopathy: observations from a cohort study. Ophthalmology 2005;112(11):1869–75.
56. Emerson GG, Lutty GA. Effects of sickle cell disease on the eye: clinical features and treatment. Hematol Oncol Clin North Am 2005;19(5):957–73, ix.
57. Williams CI, Shaffer EA. Gallstone disease: current therapeutic practice. Curr Treat Options Gastroenterol 2008;11(2):71–7.
58. Rogers ZR. Priapism in sickle cell disease. Hematol Oncol Clin North Am 2005; 19(5):917–28, viii.
59. Fowler JE Jr, Koshy M, Strub M, et al. Priapism associated with the sickle cell hemoglobinopathies: prevalence, natural history and sequelae. J Urol 1991; 145(1):65–8.
60. Hassell K. Pregnancy and sickle cell disease. Hematol Oncol Clin North Am 2005;19(5):903–16, vii,viii.
61. Sunshine HR, Hofrichter J, Eaton WA. Requirement for therapeutic inhibition of sickle haemoglobin gelation. Nature 1978;275(5677):238–40.

62. Charache S, Terrin ML, Moore RD, et al. Effect of hydroxyurea on the frequency of painful crises in sickle cell anemia. Investigators of the Multicenter Study of Hydroxyurea in Sickle Cell Anemia. N Engl J Med 1995;332(20):1317–22.

63. Steinberg MH, Barton F, Castro O, et al. Effect of hydroxyurea on mortality and morbidity in adult sickle cell anemia: risks and benefits up to 9 years of treatment. JAMA 2003;289(13):1645–51.

64. Darbari DS, Kple-Faget P, Kwagyan J, et al. Circumstances of death in adult sickle cell disease patients. Am J Hematol 2006;81(11):858–63.

65. Herrick JB. Peculiar elongated and sickle-shaped red blood corpuscles in a case of severe anemia. 1910. Yale J Biol Med 2001;74(3):179–84.

66. Watson J. The significance of the paucity of sickle cells in newborn Negro infants. Am J Med Sci 1948;215(4):419–23.

67. Brown MJ, Weatherall DJ, Clegg JB, et al. Benign sickle-cell anaemia. Br J Haematol 1972;22(5):635.

68. Benjamin L. Pain management in sickle cell disease: palliative care begins at birth? Hematology Am Soc Hematol Educ Program 2008466–74.

69. Morris CR. Mechanisms of vasculopathy in sickle cell disease and thalassemia. Hematology Am Soc Hematol Educ Program 2008:177–85.

70. Platt OS, Thorington BD, Brambilla DJ, et al. Pain in sickle cell disease. Rates and risk factors. N Engl J Med 1991;325(1):11–6.

71. Franck LS, Treadwell M, Jacob E, et al. Assessment of sickle cell pain in children and young adults using the Adolescent Pediatric Pain Tool. J Pain Symptom Manage 2002;23(2):114–20.

72. Jacob E, Beyer JE, Miaskowski C, et al. Are there phases to the vaso-occlusive painful episode in sickle cell disease? J Pain Symptom Manage 2005;29(4): 392–400.

73. Jacob E, Hesselgrave J, Sambuco G, et al. Variations in pain, sleep, and activity during hospitalization in children with cancer. J Pediatr Oncol Nurs 2007;24(4): 208–19.

74. Dampier C, Ely B, Brodecki D, et al. Characteristics of pain managed at home in children and adolescents with sickle cell disease by using diary self-reports. J Pain 2002;3(6):461–70.

75. Smith WR, Penberthy LT, Bovbjerg VE, et al. Daily assessment of pain in adults with sickle cell disease. Ann Intern Med 2008;148(2):94–101.

76. Wilkie DJ, Judge MK, Berry DL, et al. Usability of a computerized PAINReportIt in the general public with pain and people with cancer pain. J Pain Symptom Manage 2003;25(3):213–24.

77. Melzack R. The McGill pain questionnaire: major properties and scoring methods. Pain 1975;1:277–99.

78. Wilkie DJ, Molokie R, Boyd-Seal D, et al. Patient-reported outcomes: nociceptive and neuropathic pain and pain barriers in adult outpatients with sickle cell disease. J Natl Med Assoc 2010;102(1):18–27.

79. Treede RD, Jensen TS, Campbell JN, et al. Neuropathic pain: redefinition and a grading system for clinical and research purposes. Neurology 2008;70(18):1630–5.

80. Schwartz LA, Radcliffe J, Barakat LP. Associates of school absenteeism in adolescents with sickle cell disease. Pediatr Blood Cancer 2009;52(1):92–6.

81. Ballas SK. Sickle cell anemia with few painful crises is characterized by decreased red cell deformability and increased number of dense cells. Am J Hematol 1991;36(2):122–30.

82. Alexander N, Higgs D, Dover G, et al. Are there clinical phenotypes of homozygous sickle cell disease? Br J Haematol 2004;126(4):606–11.

83. Taylor JG, Nolan VG, Mendelsohn L, et al. Chronic hyper-hemolysis in sickle cell anemia: association of vascular complications and mortality with less frequent vasoocclusive pain. PLoS One 2008;3(5):e2095.

84. Pack-Mabien A, Labbe E, Herbert D, et al. Nurses' attitudes and practices in sickle cell pain management. Appl Nurs Res 2001;14(4):187–92.

85. Shapiro BS, Benjamin LJ, Payne R, et al. Sickle cell-related pain: perceptions of medical practitioners. J Pain Symptom Manage 1997;14(3):168–74.

86. Elander J, Lusher J, Bevan D, et al. Pain management and symptoms of substance dependence among patients with sickle cell disease. Soc Sci Med 2003;57(9):1683–96.

87. Martin JJ, Moore GP. Pearls, pitfalls, and updates for pain management. Emerg Med Clin North Am 1997;15(2):399–415.

88. Tanabe P, Myers R, Zosel A, et al. Emergency department management of acute pain episodes in sickle cell disease. Acad Emerg Med 2007;14(5):419–25.

89. Benjamin LJ, Swinson GI, Nagel RL. Sickle cell anemia day hospital: an approach for the management of uncomplicated painful crises. Blood 2000;95(4):1130–6.

90. Wright J, Bareford D, Wright C, et al. Day case management of sickle pain: 3 years experience in a UK sickle cell unit. Br J Haematol 2004;126(6):878–80.

91. Ware MA, Hambleton I, Ochaya I, et al. Day-care management of sickle cell painful crisis in Jamaica: a model applicable elsewhere? Br J Haematol 1999;104(1):93–6.

92. Raphael JL, Kamdar A, Beavers MB, et al. Treatment of uncomplicated vasoocclusive crises in children with sickle cell disease in a day hospital. Pediatr Blood Cancer 2008;51(1):82–5.

93. Wright K, Adeosum O. Barriers to effective pain management in sickle cell disease. Br J Nurs 2009;18(3):158–61.

94. McClain BC, Kain ZN. Pediatric palliative care: a novel approach to children with sickle cell disease. Pediatrics 2007;119(3):612–4.

95. Zunin LM, Zunin HS. The art of condolence. New York: Harper Collins; 1991.

Barriers to Effective Palliative Care for Low-Income Patients in Late Stages of Cancer: Report of a Study and Strategies for Defining and Conquering the Barriers

Laurie J. Lyckholm, MD[a],*, Patrick J. Coyne, MSN, APRN[b],
Kathleen O. Kreutzer, MEd[c], Viswanathan Ramakrishnan, PhD[d],
Thomas J. Smith, MD[a]

KEYWORDS

• Palliative • Poverty • Disparity • Minority • Barriers

The improvement of medicine would eventually prolong human life, but improvement of social conditions could achieve this result now more rapidly and more successfully.

–Rudolf Karl von Virchow, 1847

The discipline of palliative care is growing rapidly in the United States,[1] but multiple barriers exist to providing such care to low-income patients with end-stage cancer and other diseases.[2–6] Reports vary with regard to definition and scope of these and other barriers. This report briefly describes a pilot study of barriers to palliative

This work was supported by a grant from the Project on Death in America.
[a] Division of Hematology/Oncology and Palliative Care, Massey Cancer Center, Virginia Commonwealth University School of Medicine, PO Box 980230, Richmond, VA 23298-0230, USA
[b] Palliative Care Services, Massey Cancer Center, Medical College of Virginia Hospitals, Virginia Commonwealth University, PO Box 980007, Richmond, VA 23298, USA
[c] Curriculum Office, Virginia Commonwealth University School of Medicine, PO Box 980565, Richmond, VA 23298-0565, USA
[d] Department of Biostatistics, Massey Cancer Center, Virginia Commonwealth University School of Medicine, 730 East Broad Street, Richmond, VA 23298, USA
* Corresponding author.
E-mail address: lyckholm@vcu.edu

care and related issues in an urban cancer clinic, reviews the current literature regarding several important barriers, and suggests ways to overcome such barriers in low-income patients in late stages of cancer.

BARRIERS STUDY

In this pilot study, the authors sought to better identify barriers to good end-of-life care in low-income patients with late stages of cancer attending a hematology/oncology clinic in an urban medical center in a midsize city. Patients and their caregivers were surveyed as well as the health care providers caring for them as a population.

Methods

The survey instruments included demographics and Likert scale–based questions assessing perceived potential barriers to cancer and end-of-life care.

The barriers studied were identified from the clinical experience and observations of 2 of the investigators (LJL and PJC). Although not exhaustive, they were consistent with current literature about disparities in care of low-income patients.

Three versions of a Likert scale survey were designed, one each for patients, caregivers, and health care providers. The surveys were distributed to a convenience sample in the hematology/oncology clinic. The sample comprised 29 patients, 15 unmatched caregivers, and 34 health care providers (**Tables 1** and **2**) working in the hematology/oncology clinic and inpatient unit.

All patients had terminal cancer, with an estimated prognosis of less than 6 months. Treatment was funded by state-supported insurance, Medicaid, or Medicare Part A only. Prisoners were excluded. Surveys were completed by subjects or administered verbally by study staff according to subject preference. Informed consent was obtained under institutional review board guidelines.

Two other questions were asked: whether or not the patient had an advance directive, and if the patient or caregiver felt they were living a good quality of life, despite the patient having a life-limiting illness.

The study was conducted between 2001 and 2003; 3 of the investigators (LJL, PJC, and TJS) were funded faculty scholars of the Project on Death in America.

Results and Discussion of the Study

In general, the viewpoints of the patients and caregivers were similar regarding barriers. Beliefs of patients and families varied widely in many instances from the perspective of the providers. Providers believed there were more significant barriers than perceived by patients and caregivers. Caregivers and providers thought hospice was discussed more often than did patients (>90% of caregivers and providers vs 57% of patients). Forty-eight percent of patients said they had an advance directive.

Table 1 Characteristics of the respondents			
	Patients	**Unmatched Caregivers**	**Health Care Professionals**
Number	29	15	34
Median age	56	44	40
Average age	56	48	41
Race	African American 17 White 11 Asian American 1	African American 6 White 9	African American 5 White 28 No answer 1

Table 2	
Types of health care providers	
RN/LPN	14/2
Nursing assistant	2
Nurse practitioner	2
Social worker/social work intern	3/1
Physician	6
Occupational therapist/occupational therapy student	1/1
Pharmacist	1
Other	1

Abbreviations: LPN, licensed practical nurse; RN, registered nurse.

Finally, 72% of patients said they enjoyed life most or all of the time, and only 1 patient reported no enjoyment at all.

In this study, patients and caregivers differed considerably from health care providers in their perceptions of barriers to good care. Overall, health care providers overestimated the barriers perceived by patients and caregivers. The particular issues identified by medical personnel as barriers included transportation, insurance, unsafe neighborhood for hospice nurse visits, and reluctance to discuss health issues with health care providers. None of these was perceived as barriers by the patients or their caregivers.

The major constraints of the study included its size, limitation to 1 center, and the uncoupling of surveys of patients from those of their caregivers. The list of barriers was limited, and respondents were not given an opportunity to report other obstacles. There may be more and possibly more important barriers to palliative care of low-income patients with cancer than were considered and studied.

The research team concluded that the perceptions of barriers to good palliative and end-of-life care differed between the 3 groups, although patients and caregivers were more alike. Even experienced health care providers cannot predict the barriers to better care perceived by patients and caregivers. Thus, it is imperative to ask each patient and his or her caregivers specifically about perceived barriers to adequate cancer and palliative care. In addition, providers should observe and listen carefully for clues to other obstacles that may impede access to care.

BARRIERS TO PALLIATIVE CARE IN LOW-INCOME PATIENTS WITH LATE STAGES OF CANCER

Poverty is a significant barrier to health care in general. Barriers to cancer care in patients with low socioeconomic status have been well described and are often related to various issues involved with access to care.[7–9] Barriers to palliative care, specifically, in the same population, have recently come under more scrutiny.[6,10–16] Good palliative care of patients with late stages of cancer is focused on 3 primary domains: symptom management; communication among patients, their families, and health care providers; and promotion of patients' values and goals concerning decision making at the end of life.

The word, *poverty*, encompasses more than lack of financial resources; it also includes consideration of educational attainment, health literacy, and access to medical care. The literature regarding health care disparities is based on socioeconomic status and on race and ethnic background. Although minority status and socioeconomic status do not intersect at all times, and many white groups are significantly medically underserved,[8] ethnic minorities in general, especially African Americans, Hispanics and Latino populations, and American Indians and Alaskan Natives have a much higher rate of poverty in the United States.[9] Thus, in this review, minorities and those patients traditionally labeled "medically underserved" (without reference to racial background) are considered when examining barriers to low-income patients with cancer.

Poverty compounds suffering in people with cancer due to lack of resources as basic as food, shelter, and safety. Financial resources necessary for good palliative care include prescription copayments and full costs of over-the-counter medications, transportation, and indirect resources, such as lost patient and caregiver wages. Poverty thus directly affects symptom management. Out-of-pocket spending on health care creates a substantial burden for this population despite access to various government-sponsored insurance benefits.[17]

Multiple poverty-related concerns may limit access to medical care. These include factors as varied as lack of knowledge or education and distrust or fear of intimidation by health care providers. Personal health care may be compromised when there is no assistance with elder care or child care. Fear of leaving one's house due to neighborhood security issues may lead to missed appointments. Homelessness may be especially challenging for patients and providers alike, with attendant difficulties with continuity after treatment plans and maintaining contact with providers.

Some immigrants may confront such barriers as inability to communicate in English, follow treatment plans, or seek appropriate treatment. These barriers may be compounded by the fear of being discovered as an undocumented immigrant.

Poverty also affects health care providers. A study of Medicare data linked with physician surveys has suggested that low socioeconomic areas tend to have less well-educated health care providers, such as fewer board-certified physicians.[18] There may be less knowledge of palliative care, current symptom management techniques, and appropriate prognostication and referral to hospice. Physicians practicing in poor communities were also more likely than those in communities with more resources to report that they were unable to provide high-quality care, such as timely and appropriate imaging and consultations, to all their patients (27.8% vs 19.3%, $P =$ .005). The physicians treating African American patients reported facing greater difficulties in successfully referring their patients to high-quality subspecialists, which could include pain and palliative care specialists. They are also less likely to be reimbursed appropriately for services rendered, which may affect the quality of service offered to patients.

Access to Pain Control

Two of the greatest fears associated with dying are being a burden to family and being in pain. Obstacles to pain control in low-income populations are based on access as well as racial differences. There are 2 reports of pharmacies in low-income and minority areas that do not carry sufficient pain medicine to treat severe pain.[19,20]

Undertreatment of pain is widespread even in those patients who can self-report their pain.[21] Undertreatment is even more likely in those who cannot report pain. In a 1997 report of 281 minority outpatients with recurrent or metastatic cancer, 77% reported pain, and 65% received inadequate analgesic prescriptions compared with a previous study where 50% of patients from nonminority settings received inadequate pain prescriptions.[22] It was suggested by the investigators that reasons for inadequate prescribing for minority patients include concern about potential drug abuse, fewer resources with which to pay for analgesics, greater difficulty in accessing care and in filling analgesic prescriptions, and greater difficulty for health care providers in assessing pain in minority patients because of differences in language and cultural background.

Another reason for inadequate pain control is lack of expertise by the providers who treat these patients. This applies to more than minority or low-income patients: provider education in pain and symptom management is seriously lacking in all venues, rich and poor alike. As with many barriers to good care, knowledge and skill deficits may be accentuated in providers of low-income and minority patients.[22–25] The problems of medication theft and diversion are also a consideration.

Patient attitudes toward pain control can also impede good pain management. Patients may believe that pain is something to be endured or that suffering is an expected and necessary part of the dying process, as a result of lack of education or as part of a cultural, spiritual, or religious construct. Patients or their families may believe that using opioids means they are dying, that they will become addicted, or that it is a sign of weakness or giving up. It may be necessary to enlist the help of their clergy to understand their beliefs and feelings about pain management.

Access to Hospice

Researchers indicate that patients prefer to die at home, yet fewer than 29% of terminally ill patients enroll in hospice programs.[26] According to the National Hospice Foundation, 75% of Americans do not know that hospice care can be provided in the home, and 90% do not realize that hospice care can be fully covered through Medicare. Referrals to hospice and palliative care are often based on evidence of imminent death. As a result, mean survival after enrollment in hospice is 4 to 6 weeks (median 20 days), with between 20% and 35% of patients dying within 7 days.[27]

Underserved patients significantly underutilize hospice compared with other groups.[6,12,28–31] A recent review of Medicare beneficiaries revealed that minorities were more likely to die in hospitals and also had higher out-of-pocket expenditures than whites. Beneficiaries who resided in areas with lower average incomes and higher rates of poverty had higher end-of-life expenditures, likelihood of dying in the hospital, and lower rates of use of hospice.[32]

Lower-income and minority patients may be significantly more resistant to the idea of hospice. This may be due to distrust and to patients believing there is a difference in how health care professionals refer patients, with African American referred sooner because their providers are "giving up" on them sooner to reduce the cost of their care.[33]

Confusion exists among health care professionals about when it is appropriate to refer patients to hospice. This is not limited to providers caring for low-income patients, however; many providers are not aware of hospice and palliative care services available in their communities or time-appropriate ways to use these services.

Other barriers to hospice care for low-income patients are rooted in practicalities. For example, hospice workers are not able to go into certain communities or homes due to safety issues or to provide care in homeless shelters, halfway houses, or on the street. Although not a legal requirement, some hospices care for patients only if they have a caregiver living in the home with them. Some hospices do not provide care to immigrants or others who are uninsured or have no source of payment. Investigators have suggested, however, that some hospice agencies may provide some free care as an enticement to increase referrals from other health care entities.[34] It is, therefore, important for those caring for seriously ill patients to be familiar with and nurture community partnerships as a way to increase access for patients with limited access to hospice, palliative, and other types of care.

Barriers to Education and Health Literacy

The US Department of Health and Human Services has defined health literacy as "The degree to which individuals have the capacity to obtain, process, and understand basic health information and services needed to make appropriate health decisions."[35] Paasche-Orlow, and colleagues report: "Over 300 studies have demonstrated that most patient education materials, explanations of health services and benefits, and documents that purport to advance patients' rights are incomprehensible to a significant portion of the patients we serve."[36]

Functional health literacy is a measure of a patient's ability to perform basic reading and numerical tasks required to function in the health care environment. It is independently associated with poor self-rated health, poor understanding of one's condition and its management, and higher use of services.[37] Low functional health literacy, which may also include low numeracy, is a barrier to good palliative care. Low literacy or numeracy can impede obtaining financial assistance, access to providers, or even the ability to understand simple issues, such as date and location of an appointment. Low literacy or low numeracy can also interfere with understanding how to take medicines, in particular opioids and other medications, that may be ineffective and unsafe if taken improperly.

How does one screen for low literacy? Questions that may be helpful include, "Do you read very much?" or "Do you have any trouble seeing, or hearing, or reading?" Patients may be embarrassed but respond truthfully if asked kindly and confidentially. People who do not read well may not even look at written materials. They might offer excuses when asked to read written materials. Some identify medications by color/shape rather than name or by opening a bottle rather than reading the label.[38]

Ways to bridge the gaps presented by low literacy in patients needing palliative care include using materials with large print and simple language; planning to spend extra time and enlisting staff, caregivers, and pharmacists to assist in teaching and explaining; planning on more frequent visits and telephone calls; simplifying regimens; and using pill boxes. Perhaps of greatest importance is creating a shame-free environment so that patients feel comfortable and not afraid to disclose illiteracy.[38]

Issues in Communication and Understanding

Minority and low-income patients may have difficulty communicating goals and values to their health care providers. In a survey of white and African American patients who were eligible for hospice, 32% of African American patients felt they would receive better care if they were of a different race/ethnicity.[39] The majority of health care providers differ from these patients and their families in socioeconomic status and many in racial and ethnic status. Patients and providers often do not share the same cultural beliefs and traditions nor do they share spiritual beliefs. Patients may feel intimidated and even frightened of those who they believe live in such different worlds. End-of-life topics are especially challenging. Concepts related to death and dying are difficult enough to grasp and discuss without the constraints of language and cultural differences.

OVERCOMING THE BARRIERS

Barriers that hinder understanding and communication between patients and their health care providers may prevent patients and their caregivers from accessing available resources. Such barriers may also create and be created by suspicion of health care providers and the institution. As barriers are better identified, health care professionals may create strategies to overcome them. The magnitude and character of these challenges remain to be defined.

Although attempts are made to anticipate barriers to underserved patients, they may not be those identified as most important by the patients and their caregivers, or by the health care providers who interact most with them. This was demonstrated in the pilot study described in this article. To devise ways to overcome the most important barriers, they must first be correctly identified.

Ways to identify and overcome barriers include creative and humanistic ways of developing relationships between health care providers and patients. In order for providers to better understand the needs of patients and their families, "you gotta go to where they live."[14,40] Improved relationships lay the foundation for identifying and overcoming psychosocial barriers. As with any relationship, barriers are not overcome overnight. Continuity and truthfulness accompanied by the best care possible go far in development of a trusting, therapeutic relationship that transcends cultural and socioeconomic limitations.

Another recommendation is to train and collaborate with emergency department (ED) providers. Patients with advanced cancer come to an ED with a different context of care. Assisting ED personnel in development of skills in goal clarification and making them aware of options other than acute care admission for patients at the end of life may assist patients and their caregivers in overcoming knowledge and access barriers to result in better and more appropriate care.[41] Partnering with ED personnel toward these goals could allow more consistent implementation of end-of-life goals.

Empowering patients and families through education allows patients to gain control and to advocate for themselves, overcoming the obstacles identified as most important.[42] More timely referrals are necessary for patients and families to reap the full benefit of hospice and palliative care services. Thus, patients and loved ones and the professionals caring for them must be better educated about hospice and palliative care and other issues related to end-of-life care. Identifying widely used community resources and venues, such as churches, clinics, barbershops, and beauty salons, and trusted sources of information, such as clergy and teachers, is a way to better disseminate accurate information about these sensitive topics.

A simple but effective practice is for a health care provider to sit down with a patient and caregivers and complete a form inquiring about and documenting their perceptions of barriers to optimal health care, especially palliative care. The act of a provider, rather than an anonymous clerk, asking such questions, allows the patient, family, and provider to develop a relationship and the provider to understand better the actual rather than perceived barriers to palliative care of the patient. The patient may also identify barriers that are not named in the form but are important to the patient and family. Thus, the form in **Table 3** is useful as a method of needs assessment but also may be used as a way to better understand the patient and begin to develop a trusting, caring relationship.

Health policy must be implemented to effect change that will overcome obstacles to good palliative care in low-income patients. Still, each health care provider need not stand by helplessly but instead can act as a change agent by defining the particular barriers challenging each patient and institution and devising ways to tear them down, brick by ponderous brick.

Finally, health care providers must take a virtual walk in their patients' shoes. David Hilfiker, a physician and champion of care for the homeless, writes, "Most of us come from a different culture and do not understand, for instance, that the very poor are often so overwhelmed by the emotional, social and financial stresses in their lives that they simply cannot comply with our evaluation and treatment."[43]

Table 3
Risk assessment for barriers to palliative care

Patient Risk Factors	Yes	No
Uninsured?		
Underinsured?		
No prescription plan or only partial plan?		
On disability?		
Prisoner?		
Homeless?		
Over 65 years old?		
Under 18 years old?		
Unable to communicate verbally?		
Unable to speak English?		
Unable to read or write?		
Undocumented immigrant?		
Mental illness, including depression?		
Caregiver for someone else?		
Have a primary care physician?		
Does he/she spend time in bed during the waking hours?		
Caregiver	**Yes**	**No**
Does the patient have a caregiver?		
Is the patient's caregiver elderly?		
Does the patient's caregiver work?		
Living conditions	**Yes**	**No**
Does the patient live in an unsafe neighborhood (ie, Is hospice/home health unable to visit during night/day due to safety concerns?)?		
Does the patient live in a nursing facility?		
Stairs to bathroom?		
Running water?		
Electricity?		
Telephone?		
Food stamps?		
Rural location?		
Transportation	**Yes**	**No**
Does the patient have reliable transportation?		
Knowledge, planning	**Yes**	**No**
Does the patient have a living will/advance directive?		
Does the patient know about hospice care?		

Signature of clinician _____ Date_____

SUMMARY

As stated by Elizabeth Prewitt in the 1997 ACP position paper, "Inner-City Health Care," when applied to care of the poor, "the medical model alone is woefully inadequate."[44] It has been suggested, "to adequately serve the needs of the socially marginalized near the end of life, clinical care and education must step 'out of the box,' and connect with the actual life experiences of patients and families."[14,18]

With issues of access and communication at the fore, health care providers must make every effort to understand the specific barriers each individual perceives, because perceived barriers may differ significantly from patient to patient. This article has demonstrated that assuming these perceived barriers can be predicted is clearly wrong. The importance of connecting and listening, then taking appropriate measures to overcome each patient's specific barriers, cannot be overestimated.

REFERENCES

1. Morrison RS, Maroney-Galin C, Kralovec PD, et al. The growth of palliative care programs in United States hospitals. J Palliat Med 2005;8(6):1127–34.
2. Agness C, Murrell E, Nkansah N, et al. Poor health literacy as a barrier to patient care. Consult Pharm 2008;23(5):378–82, 385–6.
3. Crawley LM. Racial, cultural, and ethnic factors influencing end-of-life care. J Palliat Med 2005;8(Suppl 1):S58–69.
4. Freeman HP, Chu KC. Determinants of cancer disparities: barriers to cancer screening, diagnosis, and treatment. Surg Oncol Clin N Am 2005;14(4):655–69, v.
5. Hughes A. Poverty and palliative care in the US: issues facing the urban poor. Int J Palliat Nurs 2005;11:6.
6. Winston CA, Leshner P, Kramer J, et al. Overcoming barriers to access and utilization of hospice and palliative care services in African-American communities. Omega (Westport) 2004;50(2):151–63.
7. Albano JD, Ward E, Jemal A, et al. Cancer mortality in the united states by education level and race. J Natl Cancer Inst 2007;99(18):1384–94.
8. Betancourt JR, King RK. Unequal treatment: the institute of medicine report and its public health implications. Public Health Rep 2003;118(4):287–92.
9. Ward E, Jemal A, Cokkinides V, et al. Cancer disparities by race/ethnicity and socioeconomic status. CA Cancer J Clin 2004;54(2):78–93.
10. Born W, Greiner KA, Sylvia E, et al. Knowledge, attitudes, and beliefs about end-of-life care among inner-city African Americans and latinos. J Palliat Med 2004; 7(2):247–56.
11. Francoeur RB, Payne R, Raveis VH, et al. Palliative care in the inner city. Patient religious affiliation, underinsurance, and symptom attitude. Cancer 2007; 109(Suppl 2):425–34.
12. Jenkins C, Lapelle N, Zapka JG, et al. End-of-life care and African Americans: voices from the community. J Palliat Med 2005;8(3):585–92.
13. Kramer BJ, Auer C. Challenges to providing end-of-life care to low-income elders with advanced chronic disease: lessons learned from a model program. Gerontologist 2005;45(5):651–60.
14. Moller DW. None left behind: urban poverty, social experience, and rethinking palliative care. J Palliat Med 2005;8(1):17–9.
15. Tarzian AJ, Neal MT, O'Neil JA. Attitudes, experiences, and beliefs affecting end-of-life decision-making among homeless individuals. J Palliat Med 2005;8(1): 36–48.
16. Williams BR. Dying young, dying poor: a sociological examination of existential suffering among low-socioeconomic status patients. J Palliat Med 2004;7(1): 27–37.
17. Gross DJ, Alecxih L, Gibson MJ, et al. Out-of-pocket health spending by poor and near-poor elderly medicare beneficiaries. Health Serv Res 1999;34(1 Pt 2): 241–54.

18. Bach PB, Pham HH, Schrag D, et al. Primary care physicians who treat blacks and whites. N Engl J Med 2004;351(6):575–84.
19. Green CR, Ndao-Brumblay SK, West B, et al. Differences in prescription opioid analgesic availability: comparing minority and white pharmacies across michigan. J Pain 2005;6(10):689–99.
20. Morrison RS, Wallenstein S, Natale DK, et al. "We don't carry that"—failure of pharmacies in predominantly nonwhite neighborhoods to stock opioid analgesics. N Engl J Med 2000;342(14):1023–6.
21. Apfelbaum JL, Chen C, Mehta SS, et al. Postoperative pain experience: results from a national survey suggest postoperative pain continues to be undermanaged. Anesth Analg 2003;97(2):534–40 [table of contents].
22. Cleeland CS, Gonin R, Baez L, et al. Pain and treatment of pain in minority patients with cancer the eastern cooperative oncology group minority outpatient pain study. Ann Intern Med 1997;127(9):813–6.
23. Cleeland CS. Barriers to the management of cancer pain. Oncology (Williston Park) 1987;1(Suppl 2):19–26.
24. Anderson KO, Richman SP, Hurley J, et al. Cancer pain management among underserved minority outpatients: perceived needs and barriers to optimal control. Cancer 2002;94(8):2295–304.
25. Anderson KO, Mendoza TR, Valero V, et al. Minority cancer patients and their providers: pain management attitudes and practice. Cancer 2000;88(8):1929–38.
26. National Hospice and Palliative Care Organization. Available at: http://www.nhpco.org/files/public/Statistics_Research/NHPCO_facts-and-figures_2008.pdf. Accessed September 1, 2009.
27. Christakis NA, Escarce JJ. Survival of medicare patients after enrollment in hospice programs. N Engl J Med 1996;335(3):172–8.
28. Gordon AK. Hospice and minorities: a national study of organizational access and practice. Hosp J 1996;11(1):49–70.
29. Smith TJ. Health service studies in the terminally ill cancer patient. In: Bennett CL, Pajeau, Tammy S, editors. Cancer policy. Boston: Kluwer Academic Publishers; 1998.
30. Smith TJ. End of life care: preserving quality and quantity of life in managed care. In: Perry M, editor. American society of clinical oncology educational book. Alexandria (VA): American Society of Clinical Oncology; 1997. p. 303–7.
31. O'Mahony S, McHenry J, Snow D, et al. A review of barriers to utilization of the medicare hospice benefits in urban populations and strategies for enhanced access. J Urban Health 2008;85(2):281–90.
32. Hogan C, Lunney J, Gabel J, et al. Medicare beneficiaries' costs of care in the last year of life. Health Aff (Millwood) 2001;20(4):188–95.
33. Blackhall LJ, Frank G, Murphy ST, et al. Ethnicity and attitudes towards life sustaining technology. Soc Sci Med 1999;48(12):1779–89.
34. Lorenz KA, Rosenfeld KE, Asch SM, et al. Charity for the dying: who receives unreimbursed hospice care? J Palliat Med 2003;6(4):585–91.
35. National Network of Libraries of Medicine. Available at: http://nnlm.gov/outreach/consumer/hlthlit.html#A1. Accessed September 2, 2009.
36. Paasche-Orlow MK, Schillinger D, Greene SM, et al. How health care systems can begin to address the challenge of limited literacy. J Gen Intern Med 2006; 21(8):884–7.
37. Schillinger D, Bindman A, Wang F, et al. Functional health literacy and the quality of physician-patient communication among diabetes patients. Patient Educ Couns 2004;52(3):315–23.

38. Reisfield GM, Wilson GR. Health literacy in palliative medicine #153. J Palliat Med 2008;11(1):105–6.
39. Rosenfeld P, Dennis J, Hanen S, et al. Are there racial differences in attitudes toward hospice care? A study of hospice-eligible patients at the visiting nurse service of New York. Am J Hosp Palliat Care 2007;24(5):408–16.
40. Crawley LM. Palliative care in African American communities. J Palliat Med 2002; 5(5):775–9.
41. Cassel JB, Lyckholm LJ. Rethinking our M.O. J Palliat Med 2007;10(3):649–50.
42. Anderson KO, Mendoza TR, Payne R, et al. Pain education for underserved minority cancer patients: a randomized controlled trial. J Clin Oncol 2004; 22(24):4918–25.
43. Hilfiker D. Unconscious on a corner. JAMA 1987;258(21):3155–6.
44. Inner-city health care. American college of physicians. Ann Intern Med 1997; 126(6):485–90.

End-Stage Liver Disease: Challenges and Practice Implications

Lissi Hansen, PhD, RN[a]*, Anna Sasaki, MD, PhD[b,c],
Betsy Zucker, MSN, FNP[d]

KEYWORDS

- End-stage liver disease • End of life • Palliative care • Pain

An estimated 5.5 million Americans have chronic liver disease. It is the twelfth leading cause of death in the United States, accounting for more than 27,000 deaths annually.[1] As the seventh leading cause of death among people aged 25 to 64 years, end-stage liver disease (ESLD) affects many Americans in the most productive years of their lives.[2] Because of a large and growing disparity between the availability of donor livers and the number of patients waiting for a transplant, increasing numbers of patients die before receiving a transplant,[3–5] or may not be candidates for liver transplant because of comorbidities.[6] In fact, the vast majority of individuals with ESLD are not liver transplant candidates. Despite the increasing number of individuals who are dying of ESLD, little is documented about their end-of-life challenges as the disease progresses. The purpose of this article is to highlight specific challenges for people with ESLD, their families, and their implications for health care providers: ascites, spontaneous bacterial peritonitis, hepatic encephalopathy, malnutrition, altered drug metabolism, renal insufficiency and hyponatremia, hepatocellular carcinoma, and pain. The authors also present a case study to illustrate disease progression and difficulties facing patients, family members, and providers.

END-STAGE LIVER DISEASE

Although the average layperson associates liver disease with alcohol abuse, alcohol itself causes only a small percentage of chronic liver disease in the world. Currently,

---

[a] School of Nursing, Oregon Health & Science University, SN 6S, 3455 South West US Veterans Hospital Road, Portland, OR 97239, USA
[b] Portland Veterans Affairs Medical Center, Mail code P3 GI, Box 1034, 3710 South West US Veterans Hospital Road, Portland, OR 97239, USA
[c] Oregon Health & Science University, Portland, OR, USA
[d] Liver Clinic/DHSM, Portland Veterans Affairs Medical Center, Mail code P3 GI, 3710 South West US Veterans Hospital Road, Portland, OR 97239, USA
* Corresponding author.
E-mail address: hansenli@ohsu.edu

Nurs Clin N Am 45 (2010) 411–426
doi:10.1016/j.cnur.2010.03.005
0029-6465/10/$ – see front matter © 2010 Elsevier Inc. All rights reserved.

hepatitis B is the leading cause of liver disease worldwide, although hepatitis C is becoming an increasing problem.[7] Cryptogenic cirrhosis, which has been associated with nonalcoholic steatohepatitis (NASH) and the metabolic syndrome, is the fastest growing cause of cirrhosis and liver failure. The metabolic syndrome is a constellation of conditions consisting of Type II diabetes, hyperlipidemia, hypertension, and obesity.[8] People with this syndrome are at high risk for cardiovascular events. How alcohol and the metabolic syndrome affect liver damage and fibrosis are still largely unknown. Other etiologies include inborn errors of metabolism, such as hemochromatosis (iron overload); Wilson's disease (copper overload); and alpha-1 antitrypsin deficiency.

Most commonly, cirrhosis is a process of injury and repair that occurs over decades. One exception is hepatitis C infection, which can result in cirrhosis in less than 2 years, especially with recurrent hepatitis C following liver transplant.[9] The progression to cirrhosis is frequently asymptomatic; the affected individual is not aware of the liver disease until a complication of cirrhosis occurs. Cirrhosis can be compensated or decompensated. Compensated cirrhosis occurs when the liver continues to function normally despite the development of progressive damage; it can continue for years. Approximately 80% of patients who are diagnosed with cirrhosis remain compensated for the next 10 years.

Decompensated cirrhosis (ie, a decline in liver function values) is associated with increased mortality from different causes, such as liver failure, renal failure, and infections. The first attempt to predict prognosis for people with declining liver function was the Child classification, which took into account laboratory values (lowered serum albumin and clotting factors) and clinical assessment (degree of encephalopathy, presence of malnutrition, and amount of ascites). This classification has been modified several times and is now known as the Child-Pugh-Turcotte (CPT) score.[10] Based on the sum of the scores for each of the five variables (ascites, encephalopathy, bilirubin, albumin, and prothrombin time) patients are grouped into three classes: A, B, and C. Patients scoring 5 to 6 have "Class A" liver failure. Patients scoring 7 to 9 have "Class B" liver failure. Patients scoring 10 to 15 have "Class C" and far greater mortality (1-year median survival is 45% and 2-year is 38%) than the other two classes.

A more recent scoring system to predict the probability of 3-month mortality is the Model for End-Stage Liver Disease, or MELD.[11] This is a weighted formula using bilirubin, international normalized ratio (INR), and creatinine levels.[12] Currently, patients on the liver transplant waiting list are ranked by their MELD scores. The higher the score (6 to 40) the more severe the disease.[10]

Pathophysiology

End-stage liver disease is a term that is over used and should be reserved for those individuals who have abnormalities of renal function and hyponatremia caused by liver disease. Decompensated cirrhosis with abnormalities of liver synthetic and excretory function (eg, serum albumin and other serum proteins, INR, bilirubin) is more common and occurs when less than 10% of liver-cell mass remains. Death usually results from one of the complications of decompensated cirrhosis, rather than from the additional loss of liver cells.

Cirrhosis is therefore a diffuse process of injury and repair, resulting in a significant increase in fibrous tissue, the loss of normal hepatic architecture, and distortion of vascular and bile flow. Nodules of liver cells form and they are surrounded by fibrous tissue. These nodules have lost their normal blood supply and are nourished through a dense capillary network that envelops the nodules. The normal liver receives up to 85% of nutrition and oxygen through the portal vein, whereas the cirrhotic liver is much more dependent on hepatic arterial flow. Low flow states, such as those that occur with bleeding, render the nodules vulnerable to ischemia and liver cell death. Complications of cirrhosis can be categorized as: (1) those resulting from distortion of blood flow leading to high pressure in the portal vein; (2) those resulting from loss of liver cell mass (eg, hepatotoxins); and (3) those resulting from the incessant injury/repair process (eg, hepatocellular carcinoma).

Distortion of the normal blood flow through the liver results in two major abnormalities: (1) portal hypertension (back pressure into the portal vein and to virtually all the venous structures within the abdomen); and (2) shunting of blood around rather than through the liver, bypassing the liver cells. In fact, abnormalities in normal blood flow through the liver are responsible for most of the complications of cirrhosis. Shunting through the smaller veins of the stomach or duodenum, called portal hypertensive gastropathy/duodenopathy, can lead to upper gastrointestinal (GI) bleeding. Shunting in large veins causes increased pressure in the surrounding vasculature and results in esophageal and gastric varices, which can rupture and bleed dramatically. In the past, there was a 30% 45-day mortality associated with variceal bleeding. Modern techniques of screening and eradication (with sclerosis or banding), however, have reduced mortality rates significantly.[13]

COMPLICATIONS OF END-STAGE LIVER DISEASE
Ascites and Spontaneous Bacterial Peritonitis

As the pressure in the portal vein increases as a result of increasing fibrosis in the liver, there is back pressure into all the veins and venules that drain the GI tract. As a result of this increase in hydrostatic pressure, protein-poor fluid leaks into the peritoneal cavity. The lymph vessels reabsorb this fluid, but when the capacity of lymph flow is exceeded, ascites results. Abdominal pain, back pain, and the development of umbilical hernia are direct consequences of the ascites. Patients with ascites may also experience early satiety and shortness of breath. Their ability to move around is restricted and they may require help to turn, get out of bed, or stand from sitting in a chair. Early in decompensation, diuretics can adequately manage the ascites. Patients are usually prescribed a combination of diuretics. First-line treatment is commonly spironolactone (Aldactone) and furosemide (Lasix). As the disease progresses, ascites becomes refractory to diuretic treatment, and other modalities are employed to reduce the accumulation of fluid (large-volume paracentesis -4 to 16 liters)[14] or to decrease the portal pressure (radiological or surgical-placed shunts).[15,16]

Nurses should provide teaching to patients and their family members related to the progression of the disease, expected effects of prescribed medications, and any side effects. It is important for nurses to emphasize to patients and families that side effects should be reported immediately to patients' providers for further evaluation. Also nurses should reinforce for patients the importance of adhering to a sodium-restricted diet. Family members should be included in teaching because they are often the ones buying food, cooking meals, and assisting with medications.

A potentially fatal complication of ascites is the spontaneous infection of ascites fluid.[15] Because of decreased cellular immunity in patients with decompensated cirrhosis, bacteria can traverse the intestinal wall and grow in the rich culture medium that the ascites presents. Antibacterial proteins present in normal peritoneal fluid are diluted by the quantity of ascites and are ineffective in preventing infection. This condition, known as spontaneous bacterial peritonitis (SBP) is treated with antibiotic therapy.[17] SBP is associated with a high mortality because of the possible progression to sepsis, but more importantly because it can present with minimal symptoms and is diagnosed only late in its course. When patients with cirrhosis and ascites have a rapid increase in the amount of ascites, or if encephalopathy develops without an obvious reason, there should be a high index of suspicion for SBP.

Hepatic Encephalopathy

Hepatic encephalopathy is a complication of cirrhosis that is clinically indistinguishable from other forms of metabolic encephalopathy. Classically there are four stages, with drowsiness, a diminished level of consciousness, and progressive confusion occurring as patients deteriorates into a coma.[18,19] The causes of hepatic encephalopathy are unknown. Originally, ammonia was thought to be the etiologic agent, but the levels did not correlate with the degree of encephalopathy. Many other agents have been proposed over the years, though one single agent has not been proven to cause the condition.[18,20,21]

Although the causal agent is not known, the triggers for encephalopathy are well defined. These triggers can be categorized as gut-related, infectious, or metabolic.[18] Gut-related triggers include intestinal blood and constipation, the latter being the most common in the outpatient setting. Infectious triggers include pneumonia, urinary tract infections, SBP, and any other serious systemic infection. Metabolic triggers include sedatives, dehydration, hypokalemia, alkalosis, and hyperglycemia. In addition, an acute hepatitis caused by medications or virus in the setting of underlying cirrhotic liver disease can result in such a loss of liver cells that coma results. Protein ingestion, however, does not trigger encephalopathy, as was once thought.[22,23] Management of encephalopathy consists of discerning and treating the triggering cause or causes and supporting patients until the encephalopathy resolves.[18] Pharmacologic support includes treatment with lactulose or rifaximin. Lactulose is a nonabsorbable sugar that acts to clean the colon of bacterial neurotoxins; rifaximin is a nonabsorbable antibiotic that eradicates the bacteria that produce these toxins.

Patients developing encephalopathy may undergo obvious personality, cognitive, and behavior changes. These changes may cause anxiety and fear for patients and family members and result in frequent and difficult trips to the emergency department. During encephalopathic periods, patients act in ways that are difficult for family members to understand, such as cursing, being agitated, or being belligerent. Patients with encephalopathy have impaired decision-making capacity, which makes advance-care planning very important early on in the disease process. Although important, this planning often does not happen until late in the process because of various reasons, such as the younger age of patients experiencing ESLD, the hope for a liver transplant, or difficulty with prognostication. During the encephalopathic periods and as patients are getting closer to the end of life, the way the family functions may change adding challenges to each member of the family. Patients loses their independence and family members may take on the role of caregivers for which they may be little prepared and have few skills.[24] Roles may include assisting patients with washing and toileting, monitoring symptoms, and managing medication administration. Nurses play an important role in assessing the support system available to patients and their family members and the unique characteristics of each family. Some questions nurses need to answer include: Who is available to provide physical, emotional, and spiritual support; do patients and their family members have extended family, friends, and neighbors; who is available to help; and who can stay with patients so family members have an opportunity to leave the house and get relief from providing care? Unique characteristics of each family may be related to past experiences with the health care system and their trust in the system. Families who have had negative experiences may be less trusting and therefore less open to interventions, whereas more trusting families may be more open to resource referrals. A social worker or case manager may become involved to facilitate interventions, such as home health agencies, meals on wheels, and hospice.

Malnutrition

Malnutrition is common in patients with decompensated cirrhosis and is multifactorial.[25–28] As the disease progresses, there are metabolic shifts caused by the shunting of hormones away from the liver. Patients become insulin resistant, more ingested protein is oxidized and used for energy rather than protein synthesis, and the use of protein and lipid for fuel (ie, starvation) can occur after 12 to 14 hours of fasting.[29] As decompensation progresses, muscle wasting is common. Weakness of the temporalis muscles results in fatigue even with chewing. Salt restriction for management of ascites results in a decreased desire to eat. Inappropriate protein restriction furthers muscle wasting as muscle protein is used to maintain core proteins. Patients with decompensated cirrhosis often complain that food does not taste good; this is caused by pulmonary excretion of sulfur compounds or taste buds affected by the neurotoxin that causes encephalopathy. Some people develop a craving for lemons or limes.

Patients experience muscle weakness and profound fatigue because of malnutrition and muscle wasting. They have an increased risk for infection. Some patients have a thinning of their skin, allowing it to tear easily. Patients should have no protein restriction.[30] Nurses should teach patients and family members to read food labels and choose foods that are high in protein. At the end of life, patients' lack of appetite should be addressed with sensitivity and compassion. The focus should be on comfort. Patients should be allowed to eat and drink whatever they desire. This diet may be very minimal or include nothing at all because patients often feel full because of the pressure of the ascites on the intestines. Family members should be taught to provide sips of water, ice ships, and mouth care to alleviate patients' experience of dry mouth or oral discomfort.

Altered Drug Metabolism

Another complication of cirrhosis that can affect quality of life, comfort, and safety for patients is that of altered drug metabolism, particularly drugs that are taken up and metabolized rapidly by a normal liver (first-pass clearance). Virtually every aspect of drug metabolism is affected by shunting around the liver. First the drug is distributed more quickly into the systemic circulation, which results in higher concentrations at the receptors level. In addition, there are lower serum levels of albumin and other binding proteins, so higher concentrations of the unbound drug may have a greater effect on the target tissue. Finally, because fluid overload is common in these patients (peripheral edema and ascites), drugs dissolved in this fluid will not be cleared as rapidly, but may have a prolonged half-life in the body.[31] This prolonged metabolism may leave providers reluctant to prescribe or administer necessary medications, such as opioids.

In addition to prolonged metabolism in patients with ESLD, accumulation is more likely to occur.[32] Therefore a reduction in dose and a decrease in frequency in administration may be necessary.[33] Nurses should understand how decreased liver function and altered drug metabolism in patients they care for will affect the response to the prescribed medications. When administering medications, knowing the pharmacologic half-life of medications and their clinical effects in patients will allow nurses to administer medications more safely.[33]

Renal Insufficiency and Hyponatremia

The most severe complication of decompensated cirrhosis, and an indication of impending death, is the onset of renal insufficiency and hyponatremia. There have been significant advances in our understanding of these processes, which are known as Type I and Type II hepatorenal syndromes (HRS).[34] HRS is defined as uremia, oliguria, and dilutional hyponatremia with no other cause of kidney dysfunction. Other causes of kidney injury that must be ruled out include dehydration; intrinsic renal damage caused by diabetes; hypertension; drugs (eg, erythromycin or nonsteroidal antiinflammatory drugs [NSAIDs]); immune complex nephritis; and postrenal causes, such as urinary retention or cancer. Type II HRS tends to be chronic, characterized by fluid overload and progressive resistance to diuretics. Management of Type II HRS consists of optimizing diuretics, salt restriction and occasionally, shunt placement.[35] In contrast, Type I HRS is an acute decline in renal function and often develops in the setting of infection or hypotension. If the underlying cause cannot be corrected, the prognosis of Type I HRS is grim, with mortality in 1 to 2 weeks. Type II HRS also has a significant mortality of 50% within 3 months. Hyponatremia can occur in either Type I or II HRS and signifies an additional mortality risk.[36,37] Causes of low serum sodium are complex and not yet completely understood. There is evidence that revising the MELD score by including a measurement of the sodium level may more accurately predict prognosis in these patients.[36,37]

The onset of renal insufficiency, hyponatremia, and decreasing effectiveness of diuretics are clear indicators of how ill, frail, and close to death patients are. Explaining the meaning of these indicators to patients and their family members as they become evident may be helpful for them in preparing for the death and the loss of a relative, addressing unfinished business, and resolving conflicts. Supporting patients and family members during this time is an important nursing role. Nurses should communicate with family members regarding what they can expect the dying process to be like and what signs and symptoms they may see during this period. Death is a process that cannot be rushed. During this process all physical systems stop functioning. Signs and symptoms may not occur in a particular sequence. Emotionally and spiritually patients are letting go.

Hepatocellular Carcinoma

An additional complication of cirrhosis is hepatocellular carcinoma (HCC).[38] Cirrhosis, irrespective of etiology, is associated with a higher risk for development of HCC; certain hepatic diseases have such a high risk that screening for HCC is advocated. These screenings include hepatitis B, hepatitis C, hemochromatosis, and the cryptogenic cirrhosis associated with NASH. Of patients who acquired hepatitis C 30 to 40 years ago, approximately 10% progressed to cirrhosis. There has been a dismaying upswing in the incidence of HCC due to the number of patients who acquired hepatitis C. Many have compensated cirrhosis and are asymptomatic. HCC grows silently and often is diagnosed late in the course of the cancer. Liver transplant or resection may be an effective cure for some of these patients, but even patients who have received transplants have a significant recurrence rate (around 15%).[39]

The Milan criteria is a staging system for liver transplantation for people with HCC.[40] The system is based on the number and size of liver lesions. To be a transplant candidate patients must be within the following criteria: single HCC lesion less than 5 cm in diameter or three lesions each less than 3 cm in diameter, no extrahepatic metastasis, and no vascular invasion. Recently some liver transplant centers have transplanted patients if therapies have decreased the size of the tumors so they fit the Milan criteria. Other treatment modalities for HCC are palliative and may prolong life. These treatments include percutaneous ethanol injection, transarterial chemoembolization, radio-frequency ablation, cryoablation, Y90, or drug-eluting beads. An oral agent, sorafenib, has been shown to prolong survival in some patients.[41] One of the problems with cirrhosis is that it is inherently a premalignant state and new primary HCCs may form that are resistant to the therapies.

Pain

Health care providers once dismissed cirrhotic patients' right upper quadrant (RUQ) pain complaints, believing that the liver is a silent organ incapable of producing a pain response. When liver transplants became readily available, it was clear that sometimes inflammatory adhesions connected the liver with the anterior abdominal wall causing specific pain. The pain associated with these adhesions is a sharp twinge in the RUQ. The pain can be quite severe, but brief. Counseling patients to avoid sudden twisting movements (or anything else that triggers the pain) is more effective than opioids for this pain. Other pain in this area can be caused by musculoskeletal pain (see later discussion) or intestinal cramping that is usually worse in people who are taking lactulose.

Other physical causes of pain with a decompensated liver include lower extremity pain caused by edema, heartburn caused by ascites compressing the stomach in sensitive patients, and muscular pain. Muscular pain is particularly troubling as the disease progresses and may be the main reason for limited mobility. Muscle wasting is common, as described earlier, and activities of daily living that are trivial to the normal person may cause muscle pain in these patients. Back pain is almost universal in patients with ascites because the weakened muscles, unassisted by the stretched abdominal muscles, are called on to keep patients upright, walking, twisting, and stretching. Painful cramping of hand, leg, and foot muscles can occur as a result of weakened muscles or diuretic therapy. Finally, joints are often painful either from hepatitis C arthritis or degenerative joint disease unrelated to the liver disease.

Pain medications

Acetaminophen therapy is often prohibited in patients with cirrhosis because of providers' fears that therapeutic amounts of acetaminophen may be hepatotoxic. In fact, acetaminophen is a safer analgesic than NSAIDs because the latter are more likely to cause renal toxicity.[42,43] Patients with cirrhosis have an increased risk for interstitial nephritis caused by NSAIDs. Sodium retention moreover is common with this class of antiinflammatory agents, resulting in increased ascites and edema. Because the platelet count is already low, the antiplatelet effect of NSAIDs may exacerbate bleeding from the nose, GI tract, and urinary tract, and may also cause subcutaneous bruising. Finally, NSAIDs can cause hepatotoxicity, albeit rarely.[44,45]

Although acetaminophen may be indicated for pain management in people with ESLD, it is important to consider additional sources of the medication. One important aspect related to acetaminophen is to educate patients and their families about combination medications that include acetaminophen. These medications can be prescribed (eg, hydrocodone/acetaminophen [Vicodin]), or over the counter (eg, acetaminophen/dextromethorphan/pseudoephedrine [Nyquil D Liquid]). Taking acetaminophen alone and included in a combination medication may quickly exceed the maximum amount of acetaminophen (4 g) to be taken over a 24-hour period. This complication may exacerbate the problems by adding further injury to an already damaged liver. Therefore, patients with liver impairment should reduce their acetaminophen intake to half of the recommended dose (1.5–2 g) (Joseph Bubalo, PharmD, personal communication, 2009),[46] and particular in individuals with a significant alcohol use.[47]

Because acetaminophen is often ineffective for moderate to severe pain, opioids are often prescribed. In general, shorter-acting opioids are preferred in patients with cirrhosis because they are less likely to accumulate in the body. There are two competing issues in patients with decompensated cirrhosis. In patients with a history of addiction, there is an induction of metabolic enzymes and brain receptors may be decreased, lowering the effect of the medication; on the other hand, for reasons described earlier, there is frequently a prolonged half-life to these medications.[31] Occasionally the side effects can last longer than the analgesic effect, and patients can develop encephalopathy. It is also prudent to ascertain that patients are not becoming constipated because of the opioids and prophylactic laxatives are frequently given (if patients are not on lactulose already). Cautioning patients and their families about this complication can prevent hospital admissions.

Patients dying of ESLD report pain comparable to the level of pain experienced by patients with advanced lung and colon cancer.[48–50] However, health care providers' lack of belief in patients' pain complaints, concern for triggering drug-seeking behavior in a former addict who has hepatitis C caused by injection drug use, and fear of inducing encephalopathy can all lead to the under treatment of pain and discomfort even in dying patients. If patients have had episodes of encephalopathy in the past (for any reason), they are less likely to be prescribed opioids, but with careful and frequent assessment of level of consciousness, a safe opioid regimen can be developed. In addition, patients with cirrhosis who are in pain, like any other patients, will decrease their physical activity. This immobility will lead to even more muscle weakness, increased risk for infection, and more psychological and spiritual pain (see later discussion). Being strong advocates for adequate pain management is important for all providers, but for nurses in particular, as they care for these patients in clinics and long-term and acute-care settings.

Non-pharmacologic therapies for pain

Non-pharmacologic therapies are best used as an initial approach to pain and as adjuncts to analgesics. These therapies include physical and cognitive-behavioral interventions and are used to enhance relaxation, relieve pain, and improve coping.[51] Physical interventions may include acupuncture, massage, and reflexology.[52–54] Cognitive-behavioral interventions may include guided imagery, meditation, and music therapy.[52,53,55] When recommending therapies to be used by patients with ESLD, nurses need to assess patients before any therapy is recommended or given. The severity of the liver disease and patients' level of cognition should be known. Patients may be suffering from hepatic encephalopathy and have difficulty concentrating and following guidance. Therapies, such as deep tissue massage, may be contraindicated because of the risk for bleeding, whereas gentle, light massage may be appropriate.[56]

Psychosocial Responses

Physical pain in patients with ESLD is often accompanied by emotional and psychological pain, because they can no longer work to support themselves or their families. Income significantly decreases, savings become depleted,[49] and they mourn the loss of lifestyle and former relationships with their family members.[57] As episodes of even mild encephalopathy increase, patients should no longer drive. People they were accustomed to taking care of become their caregivers, and they mourn the loss of independence.[58] Body image suffers as they lose muscle mass and are afflicted with ascites. Finally, patients commonly develop fear and insecurity, because GI bleeding and encephalopathy seem to be entirely out of their control. Because

ESLD develops over time, patients put off getting their affairs in order. They may not be confronted with their own mortality until a major complication develops. At that time, they may not be able to participate in advance-care planning decisions because of weakness and encephalopathy. Therefore, it is important for health care providers to initiate advance-care planning discussions with patients and their family members early on in the patients' disease process.

In this population, forgiveness issues are common. Some (particularly those with hepatitis C or alcoholic cirrhosis) have led addictive lifestyles and have hurt and alienated people along the way. As a result, many patients with ESLD have very little support at a time when they need it the most. Often the hardest for these patients is self-forgiveness. Listening to patients who are dying and their family members may be the most important role for nurses at this time even if they do not feel comfortable providing counseling. This counseling can be provided by social workers, chaplains, and mental health care providers. Open and honest communication is often what patients and family members need. They need to have opportunity and time to ask questions and have questions answered in terms they can comprehend. Nurses may help patients and family members finish unfinished business and facilitate relationship closure for them by attending to what is most important to patients and family members.

CASE STUDY

Mr Green is a 48-year-old man with ESLD caused by hepatitis C and alcohol abuse who is referred for liver transplant workup after several gastrointestinal bleeds. He comes to the clinic complaining of severe fatigue, abdominal pain, and distention. He has a remote history of intravenous drug use and needle sharing in the 1970s, which is likely the source of his hepatitis C virus. He has a lifelong history of alcohol abuse, beginning in his mid-20s, drinking at least a six pack of beer daily until 6 months ago, when he was hospitalized with the first of several variceal bleeds. He smokes cigarettes, one pack per day since age 16. He worked as a mechanic in the past, but has been out of work since his first variceal bleed. He is divorced and lives with his girlfriend, who brings him to the clinic. He has decompensated cirrhosis (Child's Class B) with abnormal liver function tests and a MELD score of 12. He is advised that he is in liver failure and a liver transplant is recommended. To be eligible for a transplant, Mr Green must abstain from alcohol, recreational drugs, and tobacco for 6 months, and he must complete a substance abuse program. He must have solid social support. His girlfriend agrees to support him through the liver transplant process if he will turn his life around. She wants him to get better and is pleased that he is no longer drinking.

He developed ascites during his recent hospitalization and now undergoes large volume-paracentesis as an outpatient. His diuretics are titrated upward, and a low-sodium diet is recommended. Despite these interventions, he continues to require large-volume paracenteses every 2 weeks. He has chronic pain, mostly in his abdomen and back, and is prescribed oxycodone, which has been helpful in the past. He has early satiety because of the ascites, and a poor appetite. He develops protein malnutrition and muscle wasting. Although initially resistant to the idea, he eventually enrolls in a substance abuse program and tries to quit smoking.

His girlfriend quits her job to take care of him, but she is becoming frustrated. He has many medical appointments for his transplant workup, paracentesis, and substance abuse program. Finances are tight and her life is on hold, and he does not seem to be getting better. Mr Green is often too tired to go to his substance abuse class, and she does not know whether to make him go. They argue a lot and he seems depressed. An antidepressant is prescribed, and it seems to help. After 6 months, he still has massive ascites and starts to develop renal insufficiency. He is referred for an intrahepatic shunt for management of the ascites. After the shunt is placed, he develops hepatic encephalopathy and is hospitalized several times with confusion. He needs to take lactulose many times a day and has diarrhea that is difficult to manage. Rifaximin is prescribed to help manage the encephalopathy, and helps reduce the amount of lactulose that he needs to take. He continues to have pain and if he takes too much pain medicine he becomes constipated and confused. He is unable to help out much around the house. He does not complete his substance abuse program and has started smoking again. The transplant workup is cancelled, but he hopes he will be able to qualify in the future. Despite the shunt, he continues to have ascites, and it is unclear why. Is he drinking far too much water? Is he watching his salt intake? Is he taking his diuretics?

Almost 2 years after his variceal bleed, he is hospitalized with confusion for the sixth time. It is clear that he cannot qualify for a liver transplant. His girlfriend is unable to continue taking care of him and he is unable to take care of himself. He has low-level confusion most of the time. He is discharged to a nursing home. He is depressed and lonely. He is not ready to die. Although he knows that he does not qualify for a liver transplant, he continues to hope, until the last weeks before death, that things will turn around. He is hospitalized with severe encephalopathy, and his girlfriend is asked about his wishes for end-of-life care. He has not completed an advance directive, no one else is available as next of kin, and she is left to make painfully difficult decisions for him.

NURSING IMPLICATIONS

This case study describes a typical illness course for patients suffering from ESLD and their family members. Patients with ESLD tend to live in a state of poor health. The progression to death is often a slow process and may not be recognized as a terminal illness. Because patients may look better than they are, projection of death is difficult for health care providers.[59] Because of this, patients with ESLD are referred late to hospice if at all.

Nurses interact with these patients and their families in clinics and long-term and acute-care settings and play a pivotal role in advocating for the care patients and family members need as the disease progresses. Nurses are in a unique position to begin a discussion about goals of care and advance-care planning. The trajectory of the disease gives providers many opportunities to initiate and facilitate an interdisciplinary approach in the care of these patients and families. It is essential that nurses understand the complexity of the disease trajectory and the changing needs of patients and their families, and additional issues that may exist because of a history of substance abuse and resultant strained family relations. Toward the end of life, patients and their families require increasingly complex physical, psychosocial, and spiritual support to maintain or improve their quality of life.[60] Symptoms are often complex and wax and wane frequently. Therefore, medications are often titrated and changed to manage symptoms, such as ascites and encephalopathy. Patients and their families may benefit from a palliative care consult for management of pain, encephalopathic, and gastrointestinal symptoms. Nurses spend more time with patients with ESLD and their family members than any other care provider and may be in a good position to elicit values, preferences, and the patients' understanding of their prognosis. **Box 1** includes examples of questions to ask patients and family

---

Box 1
Examples of questions to ask patients or family members

- What needs and services would you like to talk about?
- If you think about the future, how do you see things going in the next few days, the next few weeks, the next few months? (Use the timeframe that is most appropriate.)
- How are you hoping this will go?
- What are you most concerned or worried about?
- When you think about you or your loved one getting really sick, what fears or worries do you have?
- How does your family like to talk about challenging things?
- Families often find it helpful to talk about end-of-life care. Have you been able to have a conversation about this? May I help you start this conversation?

---

members to begin an advance-care planning discussion. When the time comes, this information will also facilitate end-of-life care. Nurses should continuously be clarifying goals of care with patients and their family members, respecting their decisions about the care and treatments, and supporting them by increased coordination of services. Nurses should collaborate with other care providers in providing continuity of quality care to patients with ESLD and their family members and advocate for timely referral to palliative care and hospice. **Box 2** includes hospice guidelines for determining terminal status for patients with liver disease (life expectancy of 6 months or less).[61]

PALLIATIVE CARE

Patients with ESLD like Mr Green and their family members can benefit from being referred to palliative care early on. Palliative care can be beneficial even to patients who are likely to receive a liver transplant. "Palliative care is an approach that improves quality of life of patients and their families facing the problem associated with life-threatening illness, through prevention and relief of suffering by means of early identification and impeccable assessment and treatment of pain and other problems, physical, psychological and spiritual."[62] Palliative care is an interdisciplinary team approach that is offered simultaneously with all other appropriate medical treatment. The focus of palliative care is to identify patients' and their family members' unique goals related to the care and treatment they are receiving. Palliative care should be provided well before end-of-life care. It emphasizes a focus on living well with the disease and addresses how symptoms, and other issues, affect the goals of care.[60,63,64] Members on the team often include nurses, physicians, chaplains, and social workers. When addressing the needs and challenges of patients with ESLD and their family members, other professionals should also be included in the care, such as dieticians, psychologists, and pharmacists.

In the case of Mr Green, an early referral to palliative care would have been helpful to him and his girlfriend. During Mr Green's illness, the palliative care team would, on a continuum, have been able to clarify the goals he and his girlfriend had for his care. Support would have been provided to both of them. The girlfriend would have benefited from help in the care of Mr Green and in transporting him to the many medical appointments. The team would have been able to manage Mr Green's chronic pain, which was complicated by underlying depression, a long history of substance abuse as a potential coping mechanism, and encephalopathy worsening by the shunt

---

Box 2
Liver disease

Patients will be considered to be in the terminal stage of liver disease (life expectancy of 6 months or less) if they meet the following criteria (1 and 2 should be present, factors from 3 will lend supporting documentation).

1. Patients should show both of the following

   - Prothrombin time prolonged more than 5 seconds over control, or International Normalized Ratio greater than 1.5
   - Serum albumin less than 2.5 gm/dL

2. End-stage liver disease is present and patients show at least one of the following

   - Ascites, refractory to treatment, or patients are noncompliant
   - Spontaneous bacterial peritonitis
   - Hepatorenal syndrome (elevated creatinine and blood urea nitrogen [BUN] with oliguria [<400 mL/d] and urine sodium concentration <10 mEq/L)
   - Hepatic encephalopathy, refractory to treatment, or patients are noncompliant
   - Recurrent variceal bleeding, despite intensive therapy

3. Documentation of the following factors will support eligibility for hospice care

   - Progressive malnutrition
   - Muscle wasting with reduced strength and endurance
   - Continued active alcoholism (>80 gm ethanol/d)
   - Hepatocellular carcinoma
   - HBsAg (Hepatitis B) positivity
   - Hepatitis C refractory to interferon treatment

---

placement. The emotional and spiritual needs of Mr Green and his girlfriend would have been assessed and addressed. As Mr Green became weaker and more dependent, the team would have had a relationship with Mr Green and his girlfriend. In collaboration with them, the team would have been able to deliver appropriate supportive interventions and consultations, limit unnecessary treatments, and facilitate transition from home to an alternative-care setting if needed. It would have also been able to provide bereavement support to the girlfriend.

SUMMARY

Most patients live with ESLD for years, often with uncertainty about their prognosis. Many people struggle with complications of the disease. As the disease progresses and complications become more frequent and difficult to manage, the need for continuity of interdisciplinary care, often including palliative care, increases. Nurses play an essential role in the care of these patients from diagnosis to death. Nurses should facilitate advance-care planning early on, continuously clarify goals of care with patients and their family members. Referrals to other members of the health care team should be timely. The care of patients with ESLD and their family members is complex on many levels, and as the disease progresses it becomes even more complex. The complexity is caused by the disease process, the severity and frequency of complications, and also by possible prior substance abuse, strained family relations, and little social support for patients. Therefore, nurses who care for patients with ESLD across the health care setting need to think broadly about the needs of these patients and their family members. Palliative care considerations must be integrated from the time of diagnosis. The liver team must have the knowledge and skills to address basic palliative care concerns. When additional expertise is needed, referrals to palliative care specialists must be made.

REFERENCES

1. Kochanek KD, Murphy SL, Anderson RN, et al. National vital statistics reports. U.S. Department of Health and Human Services. Centers for Disease Control and Prevention. Atlanta (GA): National Center for Health Statistics; 2004.
2. Hoyert DL, Hsiang-Ching K, Smith BL. In: National vital statistics reports. Deaths: preliminary data for 2003, vol. 53. Atlanta (GA): Centers for Disease Control and Prevention; 2005. 15.
3. Keeffe EB. Liver transplantation: current status and novel approaches to liver replacement [review]. Gastroenterology 2001;120(3):749–62.
4. Gheorghe L, Popescu I, Iacob R, et al. Predictors of death on the waiting list for liver transplantation characterized by a long waiting time. Transpl Int 2005;18(5): 572–6.
5. Armstrong GL, Alter MJ, McQuillan GM, et al. The past incidence of hepatitis C virus infection: Implications for future burden of chronic liver disease in the United States. Hepatology 2000;31(3):777–82.
6. Larson AM, Curtis JR. Integrating palliative care for liver transplant candidates. JAMA 2006;295(18):2168–76.
7. Rustgi VK. The epidemiology of hepatitis C infection in the United States. J Gastroenterol 2007;42:513–21.
8. Byrne CD, Olufadi KD, Cagampang FR, et al. Metabolic disturbances in non-alcoholic fatty liver disease. Clin Sci (Lond) 2009;116(7):539–64.
9. Burra P, Hepatitis C. Semin Liver Dis 2009;29(1):53–65.
10. Dolan B, Arnold R. Fast fact and concept # 189: prognosis in decompensated chronic liver failure. Available at: http://www.eperc.mcw.edu/fastFact/ff_189.htm; 2008. Accessed April 23, 2009.
11. Desai NM, Mange KC, Crawford MD, et al. Predicting outcome after liver transplantation: utility of the model for end-stage liver disease and a newly derived discrimination function. Transplantation 2004;77(1):99–106.
12. Gallegos-Orozco JF, Vargas HE. Liver transplantation: from child to MELD. Med Clin North Am 2009;93(4):931–50.
13. Burroughs AK. The natural history of varices [review]. J Hepatol 1993;17(Suppl 2): S10–3.
14. Gines P, Arroyo V, Quintero E, et al. Comparison of paracentesis and diuretics in the treatment of cirrhotics with tense ascites. Results of a randomized study. Gastroenterology 1987;93(2):234–41.
15. Hou W. Acites: diagnosis and management. Med Clin North Am 2009;93(4): 801–17.
16. Sanchez W, Talwalkar JA. Palliative care for patients with end-stage liver disease ineligible for liver transplantation. Gastroenterol Clin North Am 2006;35:201–19.
17. Fong TL. Polymorphonuclear cell count response and duration of antibiotic therapy in spontaneous bacterial peritonitis. Hepatology 1989;9(3):423–6.
18. Sundaram V, Shaikh OS. Hepatic encephalopathy: pathophysiology and emerging therapies [review]. Med Clin North Am 2009;93(4):819–36, vii.

19. Koffron A, Stein JA. Liver transplantation: indications, pretransplant evaluation, surgery, and posttransplant complications. Med Clin North Am 2008;92:866–88.

20. Baraldi M, Avallone R, Corsi L, et al. Natural endogenous ligands for benzodiazepine receptors in hepatic encephalopathy [review]. Metab Brain Dis 2009;24(1): 81–93.

21. Eroglu Y, Byrne WJ. Hepatic encephalopathy [review]. Emerg Med Clin North Am 2009;27(3):401–14.

22. Sargent S. Management of patients with advanced liver cirrhosis [review]. Nurs Stand 2006;21(11):48–56.

23. Plauth M, Merli M, Kondrup J, et al. ESPEN guidelines for nutrition in liver disease and transplantation. Clin Nutr 1997;16(2):43–55.

24. Bolden L, Wicks MN. The clinical utility of the stress process model in family caregivers of liver transplant candidates. Prog Transplant 2008;18(2):74–9.

25. Cordoba J, Lopez-Hellin J, Planas M, et al. Normal protein diet for episodic hepatic encephalopathy: results of a randomized study. J Hepatol 2004;41: 38–43.

26. Nielsen K, Kondrup J, Martinsen L, et al. Long-term oral feeding of patients with cirrhosis of the liver. Br J Nutr 1995;74:557–67.

27. Sarin SK, Dhingra N, Bansal A, et al. Dietary and nutritional abnormalities in alcoholic liver disease: a comparison with chronic alcoholics without liver disease. Am J Gastroenterol 1997;92(5):777–83.

28. Italian Multicentre Cooperative Project on Nutrition in Liver Cirrhosis. Nutritional status in cirrhosis. J Hepatol 1994;21(3):317–25.

29. Muller MJ, Lautz HU, Plogmann B, et al. Energy expenditure and substrate oxidation in patients with cirrhosis: the impact of cause, clinical staging and nutritional state. Hepatology 1992;15(5):782–94.

30. Blei AT, Cordoba J. The practice parameters committee of the American college of gastroenterology. Practice guidelines: hepatic encephalopathy. Am J Gastroenterol 2001;96:1968–76.

31. Hasselstrom J, Eriksson S, Persson A, et al. The metabolism and bioavailability of morphine in patients with severe liver cirrhosis. Br J Clin Pharmacol 1990;29: 289–97.

32. Tegeder I, Lotsch J, Greisslinger G. Pharmacokinetics of opioids in liver disease. Clin Pharmacokinet 1999;37:17–40.

33. Rhee C, Broadbent A. Palliation and liver failure: palliative medications dosage guidelines. J Palliat Med 2007;10(3):677–85.

34. Angeli P, Merkel C. Pathogenesis and management of hepatorenal syndrome in patients with cirrhosis [review]. J Hepatol 2008;48:S93–S103.

35. Carl DE, Sanyal A. The management of hepatorenal syndrome [review]. Minerva Gastroenterol Dietol 2009;55(2):207–26.

36. Biggins SW, Kim WR, Terrault NA, et al. Evidence-based incorporation of serum sodium concentration into MELD. Gastroenterology 2006;130(6):1652–60.

37. Heuman DM, Abou-Assi SG, Habib A, et al. Persistent ascites and low serum sodium identify patients with cirrhosis and low MELD scores who are at high risk for early death. Hepatology 2004;40(4):802–10.

38. Shariff MI, Cox IJ, Gomaa AL, et al. Hepatocellular carcinoma: current trends in worldwide epidemiology, risk factors, diagnosis and therapeutics [review]. Expert Rev Gastroenterol Hepatol 2009;3(4):353–67.

39. Kornberg A, Kupper B, Tannapfel A, et al. Long-term survival after recurrent hepatocellular carcinoma in liver transplant patients: clinical patterns and outcome variables. Eur J Surg Oncol 2010;36(3):275–80.

40. Freeman RBJ. Transplantation for hepatocellular carcinoma: the Milan criteria and beyond [review]. Liver Transpl 2006;12(11):S8–13.

41. Llovet JM, Ricci S, Mazzaferro V, et al. Sorafenib in advanced hepatocellular carcinoma. N Engl J Med 2008;359(4):378–90.

42. Moreau R, Lebrec D. Hepatorenal syndrome – definitions and diagnosis [review]. Aliment Pharmacol Ther 2004;20(Suppl 3):24–8.

43. Drukker W, Schwarz A, Vanherweghem JL. Analgesic nephropathy: an underestimated cause of end-stage renal disease. Int J Artif Organs 1986;9(4):219–46.

44. Mayoral W, Lewis JH, Zimmerman H. Drug-induced liver disease. Curr Opin Gastroenterol 1999;15(3):208–16.

45. Riley TR 3rd, Smith JP. Ibuprofen-induced hepatotoxicity in patients with chronic hepatitis C: a case series. Gastroenterology 1998;93(9):1563–5.

46. Horowitz D. Organ-specific warnings; internal analgesics, antipyretic, and antirheumatic drug products for over-the-counter human use; final monograph; technical amendment. Federal Register 2009;74(226):61512–6 Wednesday, November 25/Rules and Regulations.

47. Tanaka E, Yamazaki K, Misawa S. Update: the clinical importance of acetaminophen hepatotoxicity in non-alcoholic and alcoholic subjects. J Clin Pharm Ther 2000;25:325–32.

48. Desbiens NA, Wu A. Pain and suffering in seriously ill hospitalized patients. J Am Geriatr Soc 2000;48(5):S183–6.

49. Roth K, Lynn J, Zhong Z, et al. Dying with end stage liver disease with cirrhosis: insight from SUPPORT. J Am Geriatr Soc 2000;48(5):S122–30.

50. Desbiens NA, Wu AW, Broste SK, et al. Pain and satisfaction with pain control in seriously ill hospitalized adults: findings from the SUPPORT research investigators. Crit Care Med 1996;24(12):1953–61.

51. Berenson S. Complementary and alternative therapies in palliative care. In: Ferrell BR, Coyle N, editors. Textbook of palliative care. 2nd edition. New York: Oxford University Press, Inc; 2006. p. 491–509.

52. Magill L, Berenson S. The conjoint use of music therapy and reflexology with hospitalized advanced stage cancer patients and their families. Palliat Support Care 2008;6(3):289–96.

53. Lafferty WE, Downey L, McCarty RL, et al. Evaluating CAM treatment at the end of life: a review of clinical trials for massage and meditation [review]. Complement Ther Med 2006;14(2):100–12.

54. Yang ZC, Yang S-H, Yang S-S, et al. A hospital-based study on the use of alternative medicine in patients with chronic liver and gastrointestinal diseases. Am J Chin Med 2002;30(4):637–43.

55. Toth M, Wolsko PM, Foreman J, et al. A pilot study for a randomized, controlled trial on the effect of guided imagery in hospitalized medical patients. J Altern Complement Med 2007;13(2):194–7.

56. Trotter JF. Hepatic hematoma after deep tissue massage. N Engl J Med 1999;341(26):2019–20.

57. Heyink J, Tymstra T, Sloof MJ, et al. Liver transplantation – the rejected patients. Transplantation 1989;47(6):1069–71.

58. Brown J, Sorrell JH, McClaren J, et al. Waiting for a liver transplant. Qual Health Res 2006;16(1):119–36.

59. Fox E, Landrum-McNiff K, Zhong Z, et al. Evaluation of prognostic criteria for determining hospice eligibility in patients with advanced lung, heart, or liver disease. JAMA 1999;282(17):1638–45.

60. Egan KA, Labyak MJ. Hospice palliative care: a model for quality end-of-life care. In: Ferrell BR, Coyle N, editors. Textbook of palliative nursing. 2nd edition. New York: Oxford University Press, Inc; 2006. p. 13–46.
61. Center for Medicare & Medicaid Services. Hospice care; guidelines for determining terminal status. Available at: http://www.cms.hhs.gov/mcd/viewlcd.asp?lcd_id=25678&lcd_version=27&show=all. 2004. Accessed November 9, 2009.
62. World Health Organization definition of palliative care. Available at: http://www.who.int/cancer/palliative/definition/en/. 2005. Accessed March 27, 2008.
63. American Association of Colleges of Nursing. End-of-Life Nursing Education Consortium (ELNEC) [graduate training program] 2006.
64. NHPCO. Advancing care at the end of life. National Hospice and Palliative Care Organization. Available at: http://www.nhpco.org/. Accessed July 1, 2009.

Is a Good Death Possible After Withdrawal of Life-Sustaining Therapy?

Debra L. Wiegand, RN, PhD, CCRN[a,b,]*, Laura Petri, RN, PhD[c]

KEYWORDS

- Good death • Bad death • End of life
- Withdrawal of life-sustaining treatment
- Withdrawal of life support • Critical care

Although most people hope to live a long life and die quietly in old age, death is unpredictable. Significant variability occurs related to when and how death occurs. For some, death is sudden and unexpected. For others death is violent and traumatic. For most people, dying is prolonged, the expected end of a lengthy illness.

Approximately 2.4 million people died in America in 2000.[1] Historically, deaths occurred at home, whereas today most people die in hospitals.[2–5] Deaths of patients in critical care units represent most hospital deaths, with more than a half million patient deaths in the intensive care unit (ICU) each year.[6] Patients enter the critical care setting in physiologic crisis. Treatment is aggressive, usually with the goal of saving patients' lives. Although interventions are effective in stabilizing most critically ill or injured patients, it is estimated that as many as 1 in 5 patients die in a critical care unit.[6] Most patients who die in hospitals do so under circumstances in which decisions need to be made about how long to pursue life-extending treatments.[7–12] Technologic advances have extended life for many. Technology contributes to the illusion that death can be almost forever forestalled.

This work was supported by NIH-T32-NR08346, A Hospice Care in Critical Care grant from the American Association of Critical-Care Nurses, the Delta Mu Chapter of Sigma Theta Tau Grant, and the Southeastern Pennsylvania Chapter of AACN Research Grant.
This paper was written by Laura Petri in her private capacity. No support or endorsement by AACN is intended or should be inferred.
[a] University of Maryland School of Nursing, Baltimore, MD, USA
[b] 655 West Lombard Street, Baltimore, MD 21201, USA
[c] American Association of Colleges of Nursing One Dupont Circle, NW Suite 530, Washington, DC 20036, USA
* Corresponding author. 655 West Lombard Street, Baltimore, MD 21201.
E-mail address: wiegand@son.umaryland.edu

Ramsey[13(p211)] wrote, "death is a natural fact of life, yet no man dies 'naturally' nor do we have occasions in which to practice doing so in order to learn how." Although one cannot practice dying, before one's own death, most people have experiences with the deaths of family members and friends. These experiences shape our views of dying and influence our opinions of what we might want or would not want at the end of life.

Because the use of technology has become so common, withdrawal of life-sustaining therapy (LST) can add complexity to the dying process. Withdrawal of LST is defined as "the cessation and removal of an ongoing medical therapy with the explicit intent not to substitute an equivalent alternative treatment; it is fully antic-ipated that the patient will die following the change in therapy."[14(p1164)] Families of crit-ically ill patients are almost always involved in the decision-making process regarding withdrawal of LST. In this article, perceptions of family members about deaths after withdrawal of LST are described.

Death is a personal, even sacred[15] event. Most people make specific decisions about how they live with a serious illness and often how that illness will determine their dying. Bresnahan[16(p643)] explained, "we are called to make decisions not only about preserving life and health but also about accepting our dying."

Dignity in dying and death may have different meanings for each of us. People are afraid of lingering and being kept alive after they no longer can enjoy their lives.[17] Quality-of-life concerns fuel this fear; many people specify the fear of living in a coma and the fear of living the end of their lives dependent on technology or on the care of others.[7] As one person described it, "I wouldn't want life support if I'm going to die anyway. There's no dignity in it."[17(p165)]

Individuals often fear that they will lose their dignity as they near the end of life. During the dying process the individual may or may not be able to communicate their final wishes and desires. Death occurs without dignity when treatments that the dying person would not want are continued and when basic comfort needs are not met. Dignity is different for each person and has internal and external compo-nents.[18] The internal component refers to inherent human worth. The external component includes physical comfort and freedom from pain.[18] "It is in this realm of external sources of dignity that healthcare professionals can have the greatest impact."[18(p119)]

Illness or injury may leave the dying person unable to communicate wishes. Before an individual's illness or injury, or at any time during the dying process, the individual may specify another person who can represent the patient's wishes. This may be done formally, with a Power of Attorney for Healthcare or other legal document, or infor-mally, with the patients telling health care providers (orally or in writing) who should represent their wishes. This surrogate represents the patient's preferences if the patient is unable or chooses not to be involved in decision making. If the individual did not identify a surrogate, often the family is aware of the individual's preferences regarding care at the end of life. The surrogate provides substituted judgment, making a decision based on what the patient would decide if he or she were able. If the surro-gate does not know what decision the patient would make or would likely make then the surrogate makes a best interest decision. A best interest decision is determined by the surrogate based on what decision the surrogate believes the patient would want. Key to this process is that the wishes of the dying are represented and respected in the decision-making process.

Ideally, surrogates, family members, and health care providers know what patients' preferences are for end-of-life care. Individuals may want treatments withdrawn if certain conditions exist or may have specific care and treatment preferences (eg, not to have a tracheostomy). The dying may want aggressive treatment with the hope of extending life and delaying death, or they may want to stop aggressive treatments and focus more on comfort measures. Palliative treatments, specifically those that decrease symptom burden, should be provided independent of goals of care or the proximal reality of dying. This is contingent, however, on accurate, complete communication.

Surrogates, family members, and health care providers collaborate together as end-of-life decisions are made in the ICU setting. After a decision is made to change the goals of care, a plan is developed to stop further aggressive treatments, and the surrogate, family, and health care team prepare for the actual withdrawal of specific treatments. Critical care nurses prepare families by telling them what is expected of them before, during, and after the withdrawal of LST. Family members prepare themselves emotionally to the greatest extent possible as they anticipate the death of their ill or injured family member. Families also arrange for extended family and friends to say their final good-byes. A time that is best for the family is arranged for withdrawal of treatments.

Medications are administered to prevent potentially uncomfortable symptoms that may occur when LST is withdrawn. After LST is withdrawn death may occur rapidly or there may be a delay of hours to days. From a family perspective, it is unknown if death is considered good or bad after withdrawal of LST. How families later determine whether a patient died well or not is also unknown. Kendall and colleagues[19] noted that there is a dearth of research on what constitutes a good death. It is important to understand the characteristics or attributes of a good death from patient and family perspectives.

Patients with life-limiting illnesses have included the following as characteristics of a good death: dying while asleep,[20,21] achieving a sense of control,[17] awareness of dying,[22] without knowledge of dying,[21] free from discomfort,[19–21,23] dying peacefully,[20,21] dying quickly,[17,20,21] prepared for death,[22,23] giving up roles,[22] achieving a sense of completion,[23] saying good-bye,[22] relief from burden,[17] and with family around or cared for.[17,20]

Researchers have also described good and bad deaths from health care providers' perspectives.[24,25] Nurses have defined a good death as one in which patients and families are involved with decisions, accepting death, planning ahead, saying good-bye, and dying with integrity, open communication, and adequate symptom control.[24] Nurses interviewed by Costello[25] described good deaths as involving control (nursing control), awareness (patient/family knew the patient would die), dignity, and peacefulness. A bad death included pain or other unrelieved symptoms.[25] Nurses described feeling guilty if they were unable to relieve suffering.[25]

Kehl[26(p281)] conducted a concept analysis of good death and defined a good death as "being in control, being comfortable, sense of closure, affirmation/value of the dying person recognized, trust in care providers, recognition of impending death, beliefs and values honored, burden minimized, relationships optimized, appropriateness of death, and leaving a legacy and family care." Characteristics of a bad death included not being in accord with patient and/or family wishes, prolonged dying, the patient being dependent, a traumatic death, patient suffering, a sense of unpreparedness, having disorganized care, having a knowledge of impending death, the family being burdened, dying alone, and the patient being young.[26] Many of the characteristics of good and bad deaths described by Kehl[26] could never be met by the patients and families of the current study because the serious nature of the patients' illnesses and injuries resulted in a sudden unconscious state.

METHODOLOGY

One of the authors (DW) conducted a study with 56 family members of 19 patients who were hospitalized after an unexpected, life-threatening illness or injury for whom health care providers recommended that LST be withdrawn. Results of this initial investigation have been reported.[27-29] Family members from the original investigation were contacted for a final interview to explore family members' perceptions of the withdrawal of LST. After informed consent was obtained, interviews were conducted with 22 family members 1 to 2 years (mean = 18 months) after the death of a family member who had an unexpected life-threatening illness or injury and who died after LST was withdrawn.

Interviews were conducted at a location selected by each family member. Most of the interviews were conducted in family members' homes. Some of the interviews were conducted together as a family, whereas some were conducted with individual family members. A few of the individual family member interviews were conducted by telephone. Permission was obtained to audiotape each interview. A semi-structured interview guide was used to guide each interview.

The audiotapes were transcribed and carefully reviewed. All interview transcripts and field notes were analyzed. Units of meaning, clusters, and categories were inductively determined. Methodological rigor was established. This analysis focused on whether family members perceived their family member died a good or bad death after withdrawal of LST. Both the authors reached agreement when determining units of meaning, clusters, and categories.

RESULTS

The study included 22 family members of 8 patients. Patient illnesses were unexpected and life limiting. Examples of patient illnesses included subarachnoid hemorrhage, complex injuries sustained in an automobile accident, and severe head injury after a patient fell down a flight of stairs. All of the patients were unconscious before removal of LST. The primary LST withdrawn was ventilatory therapy (n = 8). Among the 8 patients, 5 had the ventilatory therapy removed and were extubated, 2 had the ventilator removed from a tracheostomy, and 1 had ventilation removed by turning down ventilatory settings (oxygen and respiratory rate). Additional LSTs removed along with the ventilator included total parenteral nutrition, intravenous fluids, clamping or removing a ventriculostomy drainage catheter, and discontinuing diuretic and insulin infusions. All of the patients died after LST was withdrawn. Refer to **Table 1** for patient and family demographic data.

Family members were asked, "Did your family member (name of the patient) have a good death or a bad death?" Among the 22 family members, 12 perceived that their family member had a good death, 5 perceived that their family member had a bad death (**Fig. 1**), 4 perceived that the patient's death was both good and bad, and 1 was unable to answer the question. Family members commonly compared their ill or injured family members' death to previous end-of-life experiences that they had with other family members or friends.

Good Deaths

Twelve (55%) family members perceived that their ill or injured family member had a good death. Deaths were perceived as good if the family member was comfortable, thus not in pain, the death was fast, the family member (the patient) was not aware, and death was peaceful.

Table 1
Patient (N = 8) and family member (N = 22) demographic data

Demographic Characteristics	N (%)
Patients	8
Age (y)	69 mean
	70 median
	45–82 range
Gender	
Female	6 (75%)
Male	2 (25%)
Race	
Black, non-Hispanic origin	0 (0%)
White, non-Hispanic origin	8 (100%)
Hispanic	0 (0%)
Primary diagnosis	
New cancer diagnosis (ie, new diagnosis of pancreatic cancer complicated by respiratory and heart failure)	2 (25%)
Neurologic events (ie, cerebral aneurysm rupture leading to subarachnoid hemorrhage)	4 (50%)
Trauma (ie, severe injuries sustained in a motor vehicle accident)	2 (25%)
Family Members	22
Gender	
Female	15 (68%)
Male	7 (32%)
Race	
Black, non-Hispanic origin	0 (0%)
White, non-Hispanic origin	22 (100%)
Hispanic	0 (0%)
Relationship to patient	
Adult child	17 (77%)
Spouse	4 (18%)
Parent	1 (5%)

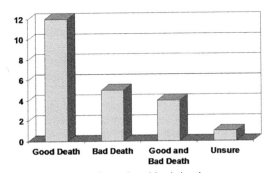

Fig. 1. Family member perceptions of good and bad deaths.

Comfortable

Patient comfort was extremely important to all family members. One patient's husband described, "I don't think she (his wife) suffered once they started the morphine." Another family member stated, "I think she had a good death. I think it was painless." Another patient's family member described.

> There were a couple of occasions when I went out and said, "You know she seems to be a little restless," and a nurse came in and gave her a little bit more (morphine). I didn't think that after the breathing tube came out it was difficult for her because the morphine was being administered. It was being administered at a rate that was certainly enough to ease whatever discomfort she had.

All of the family members who perceived that their family members had a good death perceived that their family members (patients) were comfortable during the dying process after LST was withdrawn.

Death was fast

A good death was described as being a fast death. Fast meant that the family member had been healthy, then suddenly and unexpectedly became extremely ill or injured, and then died after LST was withdrawn. The term fast in this context referred to the length of illness or time from illness or injury to death. A fast death was favorably contrasted to a death that followed a protracted illness, that is, a slow death. One family member described, "I know that it is harder on the family initially, but I think it ends up being easier for the family in the long run." The death was perceived as being easier for the family because the patient who died was ill for a relatively short period of time. The suddenness was perceived as more difficult for the family but thought to be better for the patient. As another family member stated, "A fast death is easier. Because you are forced, it happens, boom. You're forced to take, you have to, deal with it. Whether you deal with it well or not is a different subject altogether, but you're forced to deal with it, and it happens, and it's over with."

Family member (patient) was not aware

None of the patients in this study were conscious after their illness or injury. Although tragic, family members perceived this as good for the patient, considering the circumstances (ie, complex injuries and serious illnesses). One patient's daughter described, "The last I remembered was she was sitting on my deck with no problems. Then at 11:30 PM I get a call, she's in the hospital. She never woke up." Another family member described, "He didn't feel anything, he was in a coma. So he really didn't know anything." Family members perceived that the patients' lack of awareness of the serious nature of their illnesses or injuries contributed to a good death.

Death was peaceful

Family members described the dying process and the actual moments around the time of death as peaceful. Family descriptions of death as peaceful included the peacefulness of the dying environment and the presence of family. One patient's daughter described, "I think that she did have a good death. I think it was painless...she had everybody around her."

Although all of the patients were unconscious, several family members described death as occurring on the patient's terms. One family member described, "She had a peaceful death. She had her family around her, and she certainly knew that had she gone home it would have been harder on everybody, and it certainly would have not been easy on her." Another family member described her family's experience, "My mother was a private person and she waited. I think she waited...she waited until she was alone. Somebody was always with her and at one point we said, OK we're going to go home, we're going to get showers and we're going to come back...and then I got the phone call. There were only a few hours where nobody was with her, and I think she was waiting for that opportunity, just to do it on her own terms."

Bad Deaths

Five (23%) family members perceived that their ill or injured family member had a bad death. Deaths were perceived as bad if the ill or injured family member had a prolonged hospital course with up and down periods, if death was premature, and if signs of discomfort were present.

Prolonged hospital course with up and down periods

It was difficult for family members when the patient's illness course was prolonged (eg, several days to several weeks). Some family members questioned why their family member had to go through the hospital experience. They questioned why their family member survived the initial illness or injury episode, only to die later in the hospital. Other family members questioned why their family member had a day or 2 when it looked like things were going to improve, only to have several additional days during which the family member's condition declined. As one patient's son said, "I hate to see anyone suffer like that. I don't know, it was pretty hard. We always kept thinking he was going to get out of there, but he never made it. He'd get better and he got worse, he got better and he got worse." These family members questioned why they as a family had to go through what they went through in the critical care unit if the end result was not going to be good.

Death was premature

Death was described as premature by 1 family member. The patient's mother described her daughter's death as a bad death. Her mother stated, "I think she had a bad death. Her life wasn't over. She was so young" (patient was 45 years old). For this family member, the perception of a bad death had to do with the fact that the person was dying at a young age rather than the clinical circumstances around the discontinuation of LST.

Discomfort

Signs of discomfort during the dying process were particularly distressing for family members. One patient's daughter stated that her mother was uncomfortable after she was extubated. She described her mother's death as a bad death, "It was really very difficult to watch her under the morphine and slip away and not really herself and gasping for breath. For us [her family], maybe she didn't feel anything, so maybe it was good for her, but I never felt that, until she was so far under the morphine."

Bad and Good Deaths

Four family members (18%) thought that their ill or injured family member's death was both bad and good. One patient's daughter described, "I've been through a fast death of my mother, and I've been through the slow death of my stepmother [patient]. As a family member I think the fast death is easier. It forces you to deal with it, where the slow death you're just waiting and waiting and your emotions are raw. You don't know when it's going to happen. I think my stepmother's death was both [good and bad]. It was very hard ...and then she just kind of slipped into death. It was hard at one point and then it was easy."

Another woman described her mother's death as both good and bad. "It was a good death for mom because she was just so anxious about what it would mean to become debilitated. In other ways it was a bad death, because it was, given her health and who she was, it was premature. I think there were parts of it, in given the trauma that was almost more of what she had wanted; she would want a more sudden death. I just hope it wasn't too painful." Her brother stated, "Under the circumstances, it was as good as it could be. If there is anyway I could have taken those ten days (length of her hospitalization) away from her, I would have. I would have hoped that she didn't make it. But given that she had the ten days, given that it was only ten days, given my hope that she was comfortable through that period. I think, I think it was a good death. I think the actual moment of death was wonderful...Her nurse made those last moments very comfortable for her."

Comparisons to Other Deaths

During the interviews, 10 (46%) family members spontaneously compared their family members' death to other experiences that they had in the past. Among the 10 family members, 3 members who did not perceive the death as good reported that their family member's (patient's) death could have been better. One family member described, "My friend had her husband die a couple months ago. She had played golf with him in the morning. He was down at the desk and she called him for dinner. She went down and he was dead. That's a good death. ...These deaths that go on and on with people suffering and procedures...and all that, I think that's lousy." Again for this family member, the judgment about quality was not about clinical care or the withdrawal of LST but was about the course of the illness or injury before the actual death.

The remaining 7 of the 10 family members reported that their family members' death could have been worse. For example, 1 family member described, "I was glad that it was swift. I didn't want it to be a little mini-stroke here and then another mini-stroke here, and then another. It's kind of weird...at least it just was one." Another family member described, "My father-in-law has Alzheimer's...he is bedridden and he needs to be fed and he has no motor skills any longer and he's not really speaking much...My father [the patient] had a much better death than my father-in-law will have because you know he (my father-in-law) is suffering and my mother-in-law is suffering along with him."

Within Family Differences

In this study, multiple family members participated in 6 of the 8 families. All of the family members in 2 families (8 family members) thought that their family member's death was good. One family (2 family members) thought that their family member's death was both good and bad.

Family members in 3 families (10 family members) varied in their perceptions of good and bad deaths. In the first family, 3 of 4 family members thought their family member's death was bad, whereas the other family member thought the death was good. In the second family, among the 4 family members 2 thought their family member's death was both good and bad, 1 thought the death was bad, and the other thought the death was good. In the third family, 1 family member thought their family member's death was bad, and another family member was unable to answer the question.

DISCUSSION

Cardozo[30] discusses the importance of promoting a good death by not administering aggressive treatments that cannot maintain or improve the patient's quality of life. This is an important fundamental consideration in caring for the critically ill. Sudden critical illnesses and injuries, however, often involve initial uncertainty regarding expected patient outcomes. Because most prognoses are initially unclear, it is clinically appropriate to provide aggressive interventions in an effort to save patients' lives. As the conditions of patients decline, and the possibility of good outcomes fade, it is important that the goals of care transition from curative to comfort so that good deaths can be achieved.

This study offers new understanding of family perceptions of good and bad deaths. Some family members within a family had the same perceptions of their family member's death, whereas other family members within a family had different views of their family member's death. Thus, what may be a good death to one individual may not be to another.[26] What constitutes a good death is a very personal opinion.[26,31] Thus, even individuals within a family may have different perceptions about whether a specific death was good or bad. In addition, if death is viewed as a process, as opposed to an event, the quality of dying may change over time.[26] This may influence family members' perceptions of good and bad deaths.

Engelberg[32] highlighted the importance of using a family-centered approach to determine the quality of dying for seriously ill patients in the ICU. The current study offers new understanding of family perceptions of good and bad deaths in the context of death after withdrawal of LST.

Family members in this study defined a death as good if the family member (patient) was comfortable, the death was fast (from the time of initial illness or injury to death), the family member (patient) was not aware, and death was peaceful. A death was defined as bad if the ill or injured family member (patient) had a prolonged hospital course with up and down periods, if death was premature, and if signs of discomfort were present. Again, the same death could be perceived as good and bad by different members within the same family. Thus, health care providers should intervene to optimize the conditions that can be improved (especially symptom management) but also be aware that even optimal patient care does not preclude perceptions of a death as bad. Families in this study were clear that if a patient experienced pain or died with unrelieved signs or symptoms, it was a bad death. Although the critical care team does not have control of all of the characteristics described by family members, they do have control of promoting comfort and a peaceful environment at the end of life.

Families in this study did not want their family members (patients) to suffer. This finding supports research conducted by other investigators.[17,20,21,23,24,26,33] Family members also perceived that a good death was a fast death (from the time of the initial illness or injury to death). Other studies also support a fast death, but the definition of a fast death, usually refers to the dying process.[17,20,21] Families in this study perceived a death as good if it was peaceful. This supports other researchers who identified the importance of a peaceful environment.[20,21,25] Presence of family members contributes to a peaceful dying environment.[17,20]

A prolonged death and premature death were also considered characteristics of a bad death in a concept analysis conducted by Kehl.[26] Signs of discomfort or unrelieved symptoms are absolute determinants of a bad death.[25,26]

Some of the findings from this study are not consistent with those of other researchers who have studied good and bad deaths. The serious nature of the patients' illnesses and injuries precluded patients and families in this study from achieving traditional characteristics of a good death (eg, being in control, relationships optimized, and so on). Family members in this study perceived their family members' death was good because their family members (the patients) were not aware. This differs from the findings of others who consider the death as bad if patients are not aware of dying.[22,25,26]

THE IMPORTANT ROLE OF HEALTH CARE PROVIDERS IN ACHIEVING GOOD DEATHS

The perceptions from family members in this study make clear that health care providers have multiple opportunities to improve the circumstances of a patient's death. Family members described a bad death as including pain and other symptoms that are not relieved. Family members described death as good if the person dying was comfortable, meaning the absence of burdensome symptoms, and if the dying environment was peaceful. It is important to prevent, to the greatest extent possible, and to intervene quickly to relieve any signs of distress after LST is withdrawn.

Many of the symptoms likely to occur in patients who are dying, including patients for whom LST is being discontinued can be anticipated. Pain, dyspnea, and restlessness were described by family members in this study as concerning symptoms, consistent with the findings of other researchers.[34,35–37] Signs of discomfort after withdrawal of LST may include tachycardia, hypertension, restlessness, and diaphoresis. Respiratory distress may include tachypnea, labored breathing, gasping, and use of accessory muscles. Anticipating these symptoms allows prevention of burdensome symptoms. A low-dose analgesic infusion, usually an opioid, should be administered before withdrawal of LST. This infusion can be rapidly titrated to signs of distress.[38] "As a general rule anytime an increase in an infusion dose is being considered due to reemergence of the signs or symptoms of suffering, intravenous bolus doses should be administered concurrently to achieve a rapid response."[39(p958)] The analgesic infusion (eg, morphine sulfate) physiologically increases pulmonary venodilation and facilitates breathing. Repositioning, oropharyngeal suctioning, reducing intravenous fluids, and administrating anticholinergic medications may decrease pulmonary secretions; bronchodilators and benzodiazepines may also relieve dyspnea.[40,41] Benzodiazepines can also be used to relieve restlessness and possible anxiety. If patients are already receiving continuous infusions of analgesics or anxiolytics, they should be titrated to effect but not higher than that.

Fears of hastening death should not preclude adequate symptom management. Opioid administration to treat pain does not cause respiratory depression when carefully titrated to a patient's distress.[42] Clinical pharmacists, in addition to pain and palliative care specialists, are important resources who can be consulted to assist with managing symptoms.

Palliative care is interdisciplinary care that aims to relieve suffering and improve the quality of life for patients with serious illness and their families.[43] Palliative care can help to promote a peaceful environment for the dying patient and the patient's family. Palliative care can improve communication, build relationships, and control distressing symptoms.[44] "There is...another way of exercising control over the process of death which we might call the palliative care alternatives. Here the control is not exercised over the timing of death but over the symptoms which accompany it."[45(p406)] Palliative care can be integrated into the care of acutely ill or injured patients in the ICU.[41]

Of utmost importance is that comfort is promoted during the dying process after LST is withdrawn. Based on this investigation, if comfort is attained, a good death can be obtained. According to the American Nurses Association, "nurses should not hesitate to use full and effective doses of pain medication for the proper management of pain in the dying patient."[46] As stated by the Hospice and Palliative Nurses Association, "uncontrolled pain should be considered an emergency with all healthcare professionals taking responsibility to provide relief."[47] Other distressing symptoms should also be addressed and managed effectively.

Broader supportive care should also be provided to the dying. In addition to aggressive symptom management, basic comfort measures are invaluable. This includes frequent mouth care, washing, and massage with lotion. Moistening a patient's mouth, a cool moist washcloth to the forehead, lip balm applied to dry lips, administering an antipyretic to reduce a patient's fever, and assisting with turning to one's side supported by pillows promotes comfort. Relief of suffering and promotion of comfort are fundamental to a good dying process.

The critical care nurse should also include interested family members in preparing for a peaceful environment for the dying process. The family may have important ideas that can be incorporated into the care of the patient, which may include special music, a favorite quilt, or a patient's favorite baseball game. In addition, family members should be prepared for what to expect during and after LST is withdrawn. Preparation includes the variability of the dying process, the possibility of noisy breathing, and changes that family will see in the patient's color and skin temperature. Family members should be encouraged to let the critical care nurse know immediately if they perceive that the patient is in any discomfort. This is an opportunity for the nurse to intervene either to alleviate symptoms or to explain why the signs are not of distress.

A well-coordinated interdisciplinary team should be in place to aid in meeting the physical, psychological, social, and spiritual needs of the dying. "Clinicians need to consider dying patients in the context of their families and close relationships and be sensitive to their culture, values, resources, and other characteristics."[48(p22)]

Health care providers are responsible for providing quality end-of-life care and for supporting families through the end-of-life process. Health care providers need to stop, pause, and reflect on the care they provide to the dying: Is the environment peaceful? Is comfort promoted? Is dignity promoted? The provision of quality end-of-life care contributes to dying well and good deaths.

End-of-life care should be directed by the wishes of the dying. Much can be done to promote a peaceful process. As health care providers, "we can relieve suffering, respect personal dignity, and provide opportunities for people to find meaning in life's conclusion."[49(pv)]

LIMITATIONS

There are several study limitations. Family members were not asked if a certain aspect of the dying process was good or bad. For instance, if families had been asked if their loved ones' final moments of dying were good or bad, additional information related to the final moment of death may have been obtained. It would be important to ask this in future research. The original study included a slightly more diverse sample of family members, however, the current study included all White members. Non-White family members were among the family members who did not respond to the investigator's request for a final interview. A more diverse sample of family members may provide different family perceptions of good and bad deaths.

SUMMARY

Is a good death possible after withdrawal of LST? Most family members participating in this study perceived that their loved ones died good deaths. This is especially significant given the context of the deaths: they occurred when LST was withdrawn from critically ill adults after unexpected illnesses or injuries.

This study has implications for clinical practice. Deaths after withdrawal of LST can be recognized even by bereaved families as good deaths. Health care providers need to strive to achieve good patient deaths. It is important that end-of-life care includes effective symptom management. Relief of suffering and promotion of comfort are fundamental to a good dying process. Although the timing and circumstances of a person's death may be bad in many ways, the actual dying and death can be good.

REFERENCES

1. Institute of Medicine. Describing death in America: what we need to know. Washington, DC: National Academies Press; 2003.
2. Gruneir A, Mor V, Weitzen S, et al. Where people die: a multilevel approach to understanding influences on site of death in America. Med Care Res Rev 2007; 64(4):351–78.
3. Lynn J. Introduction. In: Webb M, editor. The good death: the American search to reshape the end of life. New York: Bantam Books; 1997. p. xvii–xix.
4. Robert Wood Johnson Foundation. Chronic care in America: a 21st century challenge. New Jersey: Princeton; 1996.
5. Webb M. The good death: the American search to reshape the end of life. New York: Bantam Books; 1997.
6. Angus DC, Barnato AE, Linde-Zwirble WT, et al. Use of intensive care at the end of life in the United States: an epidemiologic study. Crit Care Med 2004;32(3): 638–43.
7. Cassell J. Life and death in intensive care. Philadelphia (PA): Temple University Press; 2005.
8. Kaufman SR. And a time to die: how American hospitals shape the end of life. New York: Scriber; 2005.
9. Seymour J. Critical moments – death and dying in intensive care. Buckingham: Open University Press; 2001.
10. Smedira NG, Evans BH, Grais LS, et al. Withholding and withdrawal of life support from the critically ill. N Engl J Med 1990;322(5):309–15.
11. Tilden VP, Tolle SW, Nelson CA, et al. Family decision making in foregoing life-extending treatments. J Fam Nurs 1999;5:426–42.
12. Tilden VP, Tolle SW, Garland MJ, et al. Decisions about life sustaining treatment: impact of physicians' behavior on the family. Arch Intern Med 1995;155(6):633–8.
13. Ramsey P. The indignity of "death with dignity". In: Lammers SE, Verhey A, editors. On moral medicine: theological perspectives in medical ethics. Grand Rapids (MI): William B. Eerdmans Publishing Company; 1998. p. 209–22 (originally written in 1974).
14. Prendergast TJ, Claessens MT, Luce JM. A national survey of end-of-life care for critically ill patients. Am J Respir Crit Care Med 1998;158(4):1163–7.
15. May WF. The sacral power of death in contemporary experience. In: Lammers SE, Verhey A, editors. On moral medicine: theological perspectives in medical ethics. Grand Rapids (MI): William B. Eerdmans Publishing Company; 1998. p. 197–209 (originally written in 1972).
16. Bresnahan JF. Catholic spirituality and medical interventions in dying. In: Lammers SE, Verhey A, editors. On moral medicine: theological perspectives in medical ethics. Grand Rapids (MI): William B. Eerdmans Publishing Company; 1998. p. 642–7 (originally published in 1991).
17. Singer PA, Martin DK, Kelner M. Quality end-of-life care: patients' perspectives. JAMA 1999;281(2):163–8.

18. Proulx K, Jacelon C. Dying with dignity: the good patient versus the good death. Am J Hosp Palliat Med 2004;21(2):116–20.
19. Kendall M, Harris F, Boyd K, et al. Key challenges and ways forward in researching the "good death": qualitative in-depth interview and focus group study. BMJ 2007;334(7592):521–6.
20. Hughes T, Schumacher M, Jacobs-Lawson JM, et al. Confronting death: perceptions of a good death in adults with lung cancer. Am J Hosp Palliat Med 2008; 25(1):39–44.
21. Vig EK, Pearlman NA. Good and bad dying from the perspective of terminally ill men. Arch Intern Med 2004;164(9):977–81.
22. Kellehear A. Dying of cancer: the final year of life. Melbourne (Australia): Harwood Academic Publishers; 1990.
23. Steinhauser KE, Clipp EC, McNeilly M, et al. In search of a good death: observations of patients, families, and providers. Ann Intern Med 2000;132(10):825–32.
24. Borbasi S, Wotton K, Redden M, et al. Letting go: a qualitative study of acute care and community nurses' perceptions of a 'good' versus a 'bad' death. Aust Crit Care 2005;18(3):104–13.
25. Costello J. Dying well: nurses' experiences of 'good and bad' deaths in hospital. J Adv Nurs 2006;54(5):594–601.
26. Kehl KA. Moving toward peace: an analysis of the concept of a good death. Am J Hosp Palliat Med 2006;23(4):277–86.
27. Wiegand DL. Withdrawal of life-sustaining therapy after sudden, unexpected life-threatening illness or injury: interactions between patients' families, healthcare providers, and the healthcare system. Am J Crit Care 2006;15(2):178–87.
28. Wiegand DL, Deatrick JA, Knafl K. Family management styles related to withdrawal of life-sustaining therapy from adults who are acutely ill or injured. J Fam Nurs 2008;14(1):16–32.
29. Wiegand DL. In their own time: the family experience during the process of withdrawal of life-sustaining therapy. J Palliat Med 2008;11(8):1115–21.
30. Cardozo M. What is a good death? Issues to examine in critical care. Br J Nurs 2005;14(20):1056–60.
31. Mayer SA, Kossoff SB. Withdrawal of life support in the neurological intensive care unit. Neurology 1999;52(8):1602–9.
32. Engelberg RA. Measuring the quality of dying and death: methodological considerations and recent findings. Curr Opin Crit Care 2006;12(5):381–7.
33. Valentine C. The "moment of death". Omega: Journal of Death & Dying 2007; 55(3):219–36.
34. Beuks BC, Nijhof AC, Meertens JH, et al. A good death. Intensive Care Med 2006;32(5):752–3.
35. Daly BJ, Thomas D, Dyer MA. Procedures used in withdrawal of mechanical ventilation. Am J Crit Care 1996;5(5):331–8.
36. Lynn J, Teno JM, Phillips RS, et al. Perceptions by family members of the dying experience of older and seriously ill patients. Ann Intern Med 1997;126(2): 97–106.
37. Tolle SW, Tilden VP, Rosenfeld AG, et al. Family reports of barriers to optimal care of the dying. Nurs Res 2000;49(6):310–7.
38. Mularsksi RA. Pain management in the intensive care unit. Crit Care Clin 2004; 20(3):381–401.
39. Truog RD, Campbell ML, Curtis JR, et al. Recommendations for end-of-life care in the intensive care unit: a consensus statement by the American College of Critical Care Medicine. Crit Care Med 2008;36(3):953–63.

40. Clark K, Butler M. Noisy respiratory secretions at the end of life. Curr Opin Support Palliat Care 2009;3(2):120–4.
41. Wiegand DJL, Williams LD. End-of-life care. In: Carlson K, editor. AACN advanced critical care nursing. Philadelphia (PA): Elsevier; 2009. p. 1507–25.
42. Campbell ML. Treating distress at the end of life: the principle of double effect. AACN Adv Crit Care 2008;19(3):340–4.
43. National Consensus Project for Quality Palliative Care. Clinical practice guidelines for quality palliative care. 2nd edition. Pittsburgh (PA); 2009.
44. Johnston B, Smith LN. Nurses' and patients' perceptions of expert palliative nursing care. J Adv Nurs 2006;54(6):700–9.
45. Walters G. Is there such a thing as a good death? Palliat Med 2004;18(5):404–8.
46. American Nurses' Association. American Nurses' Association position statement on pain management and control of distressing symptoms in dying patients. Washington, DC: ANA; 2003.
47. Hospice and Palliative Nurses Association. HPNA position statement: pain management. Pittsburgh (PA): HPNA; 2008.
48. Committee on Care at the End of Life. In: Field MJ, Cassel CK, editors. Approaching death: improving care at the end of life. Washington, DC: National Academy Press; 1997.
49. Cassel CK. Preface. In: Field MJ, Cassel CK, editors. Approaching death: improving care at the end of life. Washington, DC: National Academy Press; 1997. p. v–vii.

Recruiting for End of Life Research: Lessons Learned in Family Research

Denice K. Sheehan, PhD, RN

KEYWORDS

• Patient recruitment • End of life • Parental cancer
• Adolescence • Death and dying

There is a growing trend to improve care at the end of life (EOL) based on clinical research. Researchers have expanded the evidence base to guide practice in EOL care,[1–3] but challenges in recruiting participants to EOL research have been reported.[2,4–6] Nevertheless, several researchers suggest that hospice patients and their caregivers are interested in participating in research and deriving benefit from the experience.[6–8] Researchers have highlighted the importance of clinician support in recruiting participants to EOL studies.[2,5,7,9] Hospice staff can identify patients for studies, thereby making the findings applicable to a hospice population.

Studies of patients at their EOL and their families should be designed to answer research questions specific to the population, have realistic entry criteria, and be of short duration.[10] The author's research focused on interactions between parents with advanced cancer and their adolescent children.[11] In addition, the strategies used by families to prepare adolescents for their lives after a parent's death were identified. The author also sought to understand the research experience for these arguably vulnerable families. The author interviewed 26 participants, including parents with advanced cancer, their spouses/partners, and their adolescent children, about their experiences with each other after the parent was diagnosed with cancer.

Recruitment of subjects from a large urban hospice for EOL research began in August 2005. The first participant was referred in January 2006 and referrals continued until June 2006. Following the questions in the interview guide, each participant was asked, "How has this interview been for you?" Most participants responded positively, indicating that it "was a relief" to talk with someone about how they were feeling. Participants said that talking about their experiences during the interview

This work was supported by grants from Sigma Theta Tau International and the Midwest Nursing Research Society, and The Carly Jayne Ensley Award from Akron General Hospital.
Department of Nursing, Kent State University, PO Box 5190, Kent, OH 44242-0001, USA
E-mail address: dsheeha1@kent.edu

made them feel "good," "better," "lighter," or "released." Several adolescents and ill parents also said that it was easier to share their stories with a stranger than with someone they knew; some adolescents believed they could tell the interviewer "everything." A few participants described the interview as uncomfortable or painful, but the majority found them cathartic and "insightful," indicating that it was helpful to reflect on their experiences. These responses provided valuable insights into the benefits and burdens of participating in EOL research.

Recruitment issues in EOL studies have been well documented in the literature.[2,4–6] Strategies for addressing these concerns can help to minimize recruitment challenges.[12] In this article, the perceived benefits, burdens, and barriers to participation in EOL studies are explored and proposed solutions will be addressed.

RECRUITMENT PROCESS

Several strategies are successful in the recruitment of patients and their families for EOL studies. Kirchhoff and Kehl[2] have found that recruiting is most successful when researchers screen patient charts for eligibility. Once prospective participants have been identified, health care providers ask permission from the eligible patients for the researchers to talk with them about their study.[2,13]

In this study with hospice patients and their families, the author included several strategies to increase recruitment of participants. The author presented the study at weekly interdisciplinary team meetings and also met with hospice nurses and social workers individually to describe the study, answer questions, clarify points that were unclear, and elicit their help in identifying patients who met the study criteria. Patients diagnosed with advanced cancer who (a) had children between the ages of 12 and 18 years, (b) were able to speak, write, and understand English, and (c) had the cognitive ability and physical stamina to participate in the study were considered eligible for this study. Exclusion criteria included (a) gross cognitive impairment and (b) lack of physical stamina necessary for the interview. No formal testing was done to ensure that the patients had adequate cognitive function and physical stamina. Rather, the nurse or social worker who referred the patient determined the eligibility of patients, which was later reevaluated by the author at the interview site before conducting an interview. Two parents with advanced cancer were excluded from the study because they lacked the physical stamina to participate in the interview.

Fliers describing the study were given to the hospice nurses and social workers who were primarily responsible for identifying potential participants based on the inclusion and exclusion criteria. The nurses and social workers introduced the study to potential participants, gave them a flier if they were interested in learning more about the study, and asked the participants' permission to give their telephone number to the author. If the patient agreed, the recruiter inquired as to the best time for the author to speak to the participant over the phone. The study recruiter then notified the author about the potential participant.

The author then spoke to the potential participants by telephone to answer their questions; conducted a brief interview to screen out individuals who did not meet inclusion criteria using the screening script; and reviewed the requirements, potential benefits, and risks of participation in the study. A convenient time and place of interview was arranged for the participant. The ill parent was asked if subsequent interviews could be arranged with his or her spouse or partner and adolescent child. Individual interviews were held in a private room at the freestanding hospice, in a skilled nursing facility, or in the participant's home. The time between the interviews and death was short, ranging from 1 to 12 weeks. Six interviews were conducted 3 weeks or less before the parent's death.

A parent's impending death is a time of crisis within families. Regardless of the situation, participants in this study welcomed the opportunity to talk about the interactions between the ill parents and their adolescent children. The well parents and adolescents were also eager to talk, although they had many other priorities in their lives. Every participant answered all questions. As the interviews progressed, the participants became increasingly comfortable with the questions, were more self directed, and elaborated more on their stories. Although several of the participants cried, they all declined offers to end the interviews. None of the participants chose to complete the interview in more than one session.

All participants replied in the affirmative when asked if they were interested in receiving a summary of the research findings, and all the well parents and adolescents agreed to be contacted about participating in future EOL research studies. A summary of the findings was mailed to the adolescents and well parents.

BENEFITS OF PARTICIPATION

Researchers have found that being able to help others at the EOL is important to seriously ill patients[14] and their caregivers.[8] Participating in EOL research provides opportunities to derive meaning from illness and to use one's own suffering to benefit others.[15-18] The parents of young adults with cancer in Grinyer's study[19] believed they had benefited from contributing to the research and perceived the research outcomes as significant. In another study, hospice patients reported that the benefits of participation included opportunities to help the physician or nurse, have a sense of purpose, to be followed more closely by their health care providers, and to improve their symptoms.[6] Thus seriously ill patients have given altruistic reasons for participating in EOL research, describing how one's participation could benefit others. Other participants expressed a wish for personal gain related to the illness; either a hope for more clinical options or merely for the means to feel better.

Ferrell and Grant[20] noted that participants thanked them for studying topics in EOL care that were very important to the participants and their caregivers. Participants have also noted that completing written instruments and participating in interviews serve as a mechanism for communicating needs, thoughts, and feelings not previously voiced by them.[19-21] Murray[22] concluded that providing a trusting participant-researcher relationship for adolescents to tell their stories may be therapeutic. The storytelling also provides the participants with an opportunity to form new perceptions of the self.

In the current study, parents with end-stage cancer, their spouses or partners, and their adolescent children had an opportunity to tell their stories to an interested researcher who documented the ways in which the ill parent and adolescent interacted with each other near the EOL. The participants also had the opportunity to help others with similar experiences by communicating their stories.

The benefits of participating in the interviews were described by 13 participants (5 ill parents, 3 spouses, and 5 adolescents.) The wife of an ill patient expressed how different it was to talk about her husband as he was closer to death:

I've had this conversation before. Now this time the difference is that my husband's going to die real soon so I'm more at peace about my life and the acceptance of what I have to do to move on than I was before. Before it was just a never-ending story of this is going to go on forever. But now things are different.

A 16-year-old girl described the benefits of talking about her experiences rather than holding back her feelings:

It's always helpful talking about it. I like talking about it because it always helps me. Like anybody who's interested in talking about it I'll talk to about because it's just, it's nice to vent about it because like when I would try to hold it in stuff just was worse. When you get it out it's just makes everything a lot better. Just makes you feel like refreshed.

An 18-year-old boy originally agreed to be interviewed when his father asked him to, the night before the scheduled visit. Although the well parent and daughter were interviewed the next day, the young man declined, saying "I hardly know you. I don't know you at all." Two weeks later, however, the social worker called to relay the message that the young man was interested in participating in the study. After he was interviewed, the author asked him why he wanted to do the interview now. He smiled and said, "because you interviewed my dad and sister and they said it helped them a lot." He commented further:

It's been helpful and insightful. It's been helpful because I got to get a lot of my feelings out. And it's been insightful because I got to kinda look into myself and to see what I've done while this has been going on.

The husband of an ill participant also commented on the benefits of reflection and the unique benefits that were derived from the focus of this interview:

It's been good. I've done a lot of talking to people through this whole journey with [ill wife], and every time I talk to somebody, I start reflecting on certain things that she did that were unique and funny about her. So whoever I talk to, it just makes me think of all the things that made me fall in love with her and makes her just a super unique person. So I like talking about it. I kind of internalize…I'm a closet crier, ya know. I don't like to cry in front of other people. I go in the car, go down the basement, or in the bathroom or whatever. But it really helps to talk to people about it. This interview's been very good to kind of verbalize it. You've kind of opened my eyes to the different times that I can remember that were special to [adolescent son] and his mom.

An ill mother said the interview was fine, but lamented that her 14-year-old son did not know her and might never know her. She believed it would be easier if she could write down everything she said in the interview to help him understand her better, and accepted the author's offer of a copy of the transcript.

Some hospice staff believe that the opportunity for research participation improves the hospice's reputation in the community.[13] The hospices that participate in research are more likely to increase their involvement in EOL research. Hospices that participate in EOL research are more likely to be urban, and have an academic affiliation, a larger census, and an inpatient hospice facility.[13] An urban hospice with a daily census of approximately 1300 patients and an inpatient facility was involved in the current study and consistently participated in EOL research.

BARRIERS TO PARTICIPATION

Gatekeepers play a significant role in recruiting patients for research by providing or denying access to potential participants. Hospice staff, family, and caregivers want to protect patients and may be reluctant to invite them to participate in research.[2,5,23] Gatekeeping suggests paternalism and compromises the patient's autonomy.[2] The hospice staff's highest priority is patient care.[6] The researcher's goal is to add to the growing body of knowledge in EOL care by conducting well-designed studies.

Researchers have found discrepancies in perceived burdens of research participation between hospice patients and their caregivers.[6] Patients were less concerned than their caregivers about being too ill, experiencing emotional distress, and pain as potential barriers to participation in research. Patients perceived their participation as a burden for their caregivers; however, the caregivers were less likely to perceive the patient's participation as a burden.

The best recruitment strategy was to participate consistently in weekly hospice interdisciplinary team meetings. Several members had known the author as a hospice clinical supervisor who also presented workshops 10 years earlier, and the inpatient facility staff knew the author as a clinical faculty member who worked with undergraduate nursing students in the facility.

The research plan was initially presented at weekly interdisciplinary team meetings at 5 hospice offices and the inpatient facility. A large number of referrals were expected but when weeks passed with no referrals, a greater involvement in recruiting was found to be necessary. The presentations continued during the interdisciplinary team meetings, and visits were made to every branch office every 2 to 3 weeks. The author listened for potential participants and talked with the team members.

A nurse at the freestanding hospice facility made the first referral. The patient was very interested and agreed to participate in the study. He told the staff that he enjoyed being interviewed. After hearing this feedback, the nurses and social workers referred another patient in the facility several weeks later. This pattern was also evident in the home care offices. The participants were grateful for the opportunity to share their stories with the author. As they talked about their positive experiences with hospice staff, the nurses and social workers referred more patients. Several of the staff who referred families made a joint home visit to introduce the author to the family and left before the interview started. Others just happened to be there for a home visit on the same day as the interview, and heard about the interview first-hand from the families.

Once the interviews began, the families told the hospice team how much it meant to them to "tell their story." In an attempt to close the feedback loop, the author reported back to the team about how well the research was moving along. Once the team members began to trust the author and realize the benefits to the families, the referrals continued nonstop.

The author conducted 26 interviews in 5 months. Over time, the interdisciplinary team members came to trust the value of patients participating in research and also recognized the author's commitment to the process. The author was available at the team meetings and by telephone to discuss eligibility criteria, returned telephone calls to the staff and patients within 48 hours, promptly arrived at the scheduled time for the interviews, and followed up with the referring nurse or social worker regarding the day and time of the interview. The interdisciplinary teams at the home care offices and the freestanding facility were imperative to the study. The teams became more and more interested and invested in the study as it progressed, learning about the process and the findings as well as clinical applications of qualitative research. This approach was a benefit to all.

Of the 10 families approached, 9 agreed to participate in the research and at least 1 member of every family was interviewed. During each screening telephone call, permission to conduct interviews with all eligible family members was given to the author. The interviews were scheduled at a convenient time and place for the families, and were usually conducted within several days of the referral. Flexibility in scheduling the location and time for the interview are very important considerations in EOL research.[2]

On the day of the scheduled interview, 2 of the ill parents did not feel well enough to participate and did not want to reschedule the interview. Both these parents died within a week. In 2 other families, the ill parent initially agreed to the adolescent being interviewed, but then asked to reschedule the adolescent's interview for another day. Although several attempts were made to reschedule, the adolescents were never interviewed. Those parents repeatedly demurred, requesting the author to call back. In both cases, the ill parents died within 2 weeks.

One spouse did not participate because he was too busy at work and felt overwhelmed. He offered to talk with the author at a later date, but several attempts to reschedule were unsuccessful. The ill parent died 12 weeks later. These findings are consistent with findings of other studies in palliative care settings where patients are often too ill to participate[5,10] or wish to defer to a later date, or whose family objects to participation in the study.[10]

A balance between providing opportunities for rescheduling and respecting the family's time for attending to higher priorities and bereavement is essential. The author did not contact any of the families to reschedule interviews after the parent's death.

When asked "How was this interview for you?", 5 participants (1 ill parent, 1 spouse, and 3 adolescents) voiced concerns. A father realized he had been thinking so much about himself while he cared for his ill wife that he may not have been considering what his children were going through. An ill mother found it difficult to discuss death. All participants in a family did not share the same perspectives. For example, in one family the husband said he was uncomfortable, whereas the son and daughter said the interviews were very helpful. In 2 families the adolescents said the interview was difficult, whereas the ill parents and spouses found it to be very helpful. In a third family the spouse was not interviewed, but the ill mother and her daughter thought the interviews were difficult. One husband reflected on his discomfort during the interview:

> Uncomfortable because it made me realize how much I don't know. I mean, when I have to really think of this stuff, and I'm not even sure if I'm thinking, I have the right stuff, I mean. I mean, I should be able to answer it like that and I can't. Like how the kids have changed and I don't know. Maybe I'm selfish. Maybe I've been thinking more about me than them.

A 16-year-old daughter of a woman with cancer expressed concern about the timing of the interview:

> It was hard. But I mean it's better though, because I feel comfortable talking to you about it. But it's just, it's just hard to talk about it now because we have, like when she was in the hospital and sick, we had a prayer service at school. And it was really upsetting and like sad because she was at the hospital and it was just…the whole thing…we didn't know what was going to happen. And then now she comes home and she's doing a lot better and stuff and she's just normal, ya know, going to work and stuff. We had another prayer service and that one wasn't hard because it was like, ya know, you can't be really sad because you come home and you see that she's doing so good. So it's just hard sometimes to talk about it, but then it's like you think about it and it's not because she's doing so well right now and it's…And since she's not in the hospital anymore, she's able to be here with us and go shopping and stuff with us and be able to be at Easter and stuff with us now. So I mean it's just hard when like some people I don't know come up and just talk about it, then it's just hard at first but now I'm fine after.

An ill mother commented that it was always difficult to talk about death, but she would do it again to help other people. Her 17-year-old daughter echoed another teen's comments about the interview becoming easier over time:

Hard at the beginning, easier throughout. Maybe because I haven't thought about that day, the day that she got diagnosed [big sigh]. Uh, I don't know. It's been, it's different because I don't really talk about it with that many people. So...I don't know...it's hard I guess.

One husband's response was very pragmatic:

I never thought about it like that. I never thought about what I feel or nothing like that. Just do what I have to do as a father or as a husband. That's it.

RECOMMENDATIONS FOR RECRUITMENT

The involvement of patients in research requires a clear process of focusing the research questions on the right population. Previous investigators have emphasized the need for researchers to screen charts to determine eligibility, and for clinicians to approach eligible patients about research participation.[2,6,13] Another approach is to screen patients during the hospice admission process for potential participation in research.[7] All of these recommendations advocate clinician support for recruiting participants into EOL studies. Indeed, one of the most consistent recommendations for recruitment into EOL studies is for researchers to partner with clinicians.

The researcher or data collectors trained by the primary investigator are consistently present in the clinical setting or at hospice interdisciplinary team meetings, and have the opportunity to develop collegial relationships with hospice clinicians and gain their trust. Hospice staff expects researchers to be trustworthy,[13] and the research to be justified and useful.[9] Researchers can actively engage hospice clinicians in the planning stages to foster commitment to the study. Consistent updates about process and progress and the findings also help to maintain the clinician's interest in the study.[13]

The researcher must, as soon as possible, contact potential study participants who meet eligibility criteria. Willingness to participate in the study may change over time with respect to the participant's clinical status.[6] Pain, dyspnea, and other symptoms fluctuate, whereas fatigue and unresponsiveness tend to become more common near the EOL. Researchers must be cognizant that when symptoms become more severe and priorities change, research participation may be a burden to patients, families, and hospice staff.

Researchers who are aware of potential recruitment challenges can include appropriate strategies in their research plan. Partnering with clinicians will provide greater access to hospice patients and may potentially inform researchers and hospice care providers about the best ways to improve care at the EOL.

REFERENCES

1. Christ GH, Siegel K, Christ AE. Adolescent grief: "it never really hit me until it actually happened." JAMA 2002;288:1269–78.
2. Kirchhoff K, Kehl K. Recruiting participants in end-of-life research. Am J Hosp Palliat Med 2008;24(6):515–21.
3. Schirm V, Sheehan D, Zeller RA. Preferences for care near the end of life: instrument validation for clinical practice. Crit Care Nurs Q 2008;31(1):24–32.

4. Buss M, Arnold R. Challenges in palliative care research: one experience. J Palliat Med 2004;7(3):405–7.

5. McMillan S, Weitzner M. Methodologic issues in collecting data from debilitated patients with cancer near the end of life [serial online]. Oncol Nurs Forum 2003;30(1):123–9. Available from CINAHL Plus with Full Text. Accessed June 24, 2009.

6. Williams C, Shuster J, Clay O, et al. Interest in research participation among hospice patients, caregivers, and ambulatory senior citizens: practical barriers or ethical constraints? [serial online]. J Palliat Med 2006;9(4):968–74. Available from CINAHL Plus with Full Text. Accessed June 24, 2009.

7. Casarett D, Kassner C, Kutner J. Recruiting for research in hospice: feasibility of a research screening protocol. J Palliat Med 2004;7(6):854–60.

8. Hudson P. The experience of research participation for family caregivers of palliative care cancer patients [serial online]. Int J Palliat Nurs 2003;9(3):120–3. Available from CINAHL Plus with Full Text. Accessed June 24, 2009.

9. Grande G, Todd C. Issues in research. Why are trials in palliative care so difficult? [serial online]. J Palliat Med 2000;14(1):69–74. Available from: CINAHL Plus with Full Text. Accessed June 24, 2009.

10. Ling J, Reese E, Hardy J. What influences participation in clinical trials in palliative care in a cancer centre? Eur J Cancer 2000;36(5):621–6.

11. Sheehan D. Interactions between parents with advanced cancer and their adolescent children [unpublished dissertation]. Ohio: The University of Akron; 2007.

12. Casarett D, Ferrell B, Kirschling J, et al. NHPCO Taskforce statement on the ethics of hospice participation in research. J Palliat Med 2001;4(4):441–9.

13. Casarett D, Karlawish J, Hirschman K. Are hospices ready to participate in palliative care research? Results of a national survey. J Palliat Med 2002;5(3): 397–406. DOI: 10.1089/109662102320135289. Accessed June 24, 2009.

14. Steinhauser KE, Christakis NA, Clipp EC, et al. Factors considered important at the end of life by patients, families, physicians, and other care providers. JAMA 2000;284:2476–82.

15. Agrawal M, Danis M. End-of-life care for terminally ill participants in clinical research. J Palliat Med 2002;5:729–37.

16. Bruera E. Ethical issues in palliative care research. J Palliat Care 1994;10:7–9.

17. Dobratz MC. Issues and dilemmas in conducting research with vulnerable home hospice participants. J Nurs Scholarsh 2003;35:371–6.

18. Wilson-Barnett JW, Richardson A. Nursing research. In: Doyle D, Hanks GW, MacDonald N, editors. Oxford textbook of palliative medicine. 2nd edition. New York: Oxford University Press; 1998. p. 193–200.

19. Grinyer A. The narrative correspondence method: what a follow-up study can tell us about the longer term effect on participants in emotionally demanding research. Qual Health Res 2004;14(10):1326–41.

20. Ferrell BR, Grant M. Nursing research. In: Ferrell BR, Coyle N, editors. Textbook of palliative nursing. 2nd edition. New York: Oxford University Press; 2006. p. 1093–105.

21. Draucker CB. The emotional impact of sexual violence research on participants. Arch Psychiatr Nurs 1999;12:161–9.

22. Murray BL. Qualitative research interviews: therapeutic benefits for participants. J Psychiatr Ment Health Nurs 2003;10:231–8.

23. Ross C, Cornbleet M. Attitudes of patients and staff to research in a specialist palliative care unit. J Palliat Med 2003;17:491–7.

Personal Relationships and Communication Messages at the End of Life

Maryjo Prince-Paul, PhD, APRN, ACHPN[a,b,*], Julie J. Exline, PhD[c]

KEYWORDS

- End of life • Communication • Personal relationships
- Spirituality • Forgiveness

The diagnosis of advanced illness often brings with it an element of limited time. As death draws nearer, time becomes more critical. The end of life is a time-intensive crucible in which patients and family members have important things to express to one another. It may be the last time in a relationship to leave behind words of comfort than expressions of anger or guilt. Embedded in this sacred time are 2 elements of daily functioning: personal relationships and communication. The need to connect through relationships is a fundamental part of being human.[1] Human beings have an innate desire to be in relationships, because relationships connect individuals to the self, families, and God or a higher power.[2] The opportunity to raise awareness, communicate, heal, and reaffirm close personal relationships may improve the quality of life for people who are at life's end. Although close personal relationships and communication seem to be an integral and basic part of human existence, scholars have failed to give adequate attention to their importance at the end of life.

PERSONAL RELATIONSHIPS AND COMMUNICATION AT THE END OF LIFE: THE STATE OF THE SCIENCE

Many groups have identified and established models of scientific evidence regarding a particular phenomenon of interest.[3] Many of these models rank levels of evidence

[a] Frances Payne Bolton School of Nursing, Case Western Reserve University, 10900 Euclid Avenue, Cleveland, OH 44106-4904, USA
[b] The Hospice Institute, Hospice of the Western Reserve, 300 East 185th Street, Cleveland, OH 44119, USA
[c] Department of Psychology, Case Western Reserve University, 10900 Euclid Avenue, Cleveland, OH 44106-4904, USA
* Corresponding author. Frances Payne Bolton School of Nursing, Case Western Reserve University, 10900 Euclid Avenue, Cleveland, OH 44106-4904.
E-mail address: mxp42@case.edu

Nurs Clin N Am 45 (2010) 449–463
doi:10.1016/j.cnur.2010.03.008
0029-6465/10/$ – see front matter © 2010 Elsevier Inc. All rights reserved.

from I to III, with level I indicating the strongest level of evidence.[4] Level I studies are characterized by well-controlled randomized clinical trials with adequate sample sizes, whereas level III evidence usually consists of opinions of expert authorities and case studies. While there has been significant research conducted in the area of patient and provider communication in the context of advanced illness, much less is known about the communication between a dying person and those considered close and important to this dying person. Unfortunately, unlike the areas of pain management and symptom control in patients at the end of life, the state of the science in communication and personal relationships at the end of life is at a low evidence-based level, that is, level III. Supported primarily by case studies, expert opinions, anecdotal evidence, and at a higher level of evidence, descriptive and correlational studies, relational communication science in the context of terminal illness is in its infancy. Because existing studies of relational communication have not focused specifically on the context of end of life, caution is warranted when attempting to generalize these findings to dying patients and their families. Although it is important to keep concerns regarding generalizability in mind, the authors propose that some key concepts and findings on personal relationships and communication are likely to be applicable at the end of life.

PERSONAL RELATIONSHIPS AT THE END OF LIFE

According to Sulmasy,[5] a person is a being in a relationship. Sulmasy suggests that the appropriate care of a dying person requires restoration of all interpersonal and extrapersonal relationships that can still be addressed, even when the person is dying. Although the dying process is highly individualized, dynamic, and ever changing, there is considerable agreement in the literature that personal relationships are a key component of it.[6-8] Furthermore, communication seems to be the catalyst to optimize these relationships.[9-12] Personal relationships are typically embedded in the social well-being domain of most quality-of-life frameworks[13-15] (**Fig. 1**) and are most frequently defined as relationships with self, family, friends, and others, including neighbors and colleagues. Recent published work has begun to uncover an additional understanding of how people who are at the end of life define personal relationships, including the meanings that people assign them, how they function, and how communication occurs within them.[2] Some relationships may go beyond the personal domain to include spiritual relationships, for example, bonds with God or a higher power.

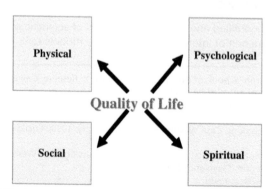

Fig. 1. Quality-of-life framework. (*From* Ferrell B, Grant M, Padilla G, et al. The experience of pain and perceptions of quality of life: validation of a conceptual model. Hosp J 1991;7: 9–24; with permission.)

One of the authors (M.P.P.) has completed several studies in which she has explained different aspects of well-being and communication at the end of life. In the first study, conducted with qualitative interviews of advanced patients with cancer in hospice care, the author identified 6 themes that described the meaning of social well-being at the end of life.[2] These themes include meaning of relationships with family, friends, and coworkers; meaning of relationship with God or a higher power; loss and gains of role function; love; gratitude; and lessons on living. Patients who are terminally ill with advanced cancer often express the importance of close personal relationships at the end of life, and the need to communicate the importance of the relationship through love and gratitude. All participants believed that personal relationships were strengthened by the end-of-life experience, largely through communication of relational messages of love and gratitude.

Building on the results of the previous study, the author conducted a quantitative study[16] of all adult hospice patients aged between 35 and 80 years who were diagnosed with cancer and residing in their private home in a community setting. These patients were recruited from a large, nonprofit hospice program in the midwestern United States. The author explored whether dying patients had communicated expressions of love, gratitude, and forgiveness. In addition, she investigated the extent to which these relational expressions, social well-being, and spiritual well-being predicted the overall quality of life when controlling for physical symptoms in hospice patients at the end of life. There were strong positive correlations among social and spiritual well-being, relational expressions, and quality of life at the end of life (all values of $P<.01$). Spiritual well-being most significantly predicted the quality of life at the end of life, explaining 53.5% of the explained variance. Although the relational expressions variable did make a small contribution to the overall model, it remained statistically nonsignificant.

This study was the first, to date, to begin to measure and test this construct and its expression of "I love you" and "Thank you" in the population with advanced cancer. Despite the increased attention to this construct in the positive psychological literature,[17] there is a lack of empirical support regarding these expressions and their potential effects in the end-of-life domain. These studies provide a strong foundation for the need for future research to understand the specific values of these relationships for people who are dying. Perhaps more importantly, they provide a basis for the importance of attending to these relationships in the clinical care of patients at the end of life.

SPIRITUAL RELATIONSHIPS

Relationships with others may play a pivotal role in spirituality and spiritual well-being. In 2009, a group of 40 national leaders, including physicians, nurses, psychologists, social workers, chaplains and clergy, other spiritual care providers, and health care administrators convened at a National Consensus Conference to define spirituality and to describe how it relates to health care and to patients with life-limiting illness. A further goal of this panel was to make recommendations to advance the delivery of quality spiritual care in palliative care.[18] The 2009 National Consensus Project Guidelines[19] and the National Quality Forum Preferred Practices for Palliative Care[20] served as the foundation for the recommendations of the conference. Spirituality, as defined by the panel and grounded in theological, philosophical, empirical, and clinical literature, is "the aspect of humanity that refers to the way individuals seek and express meaning and purpose and the way they experience their connectedness to the moment, to self, to others, to nature, and to the significant or sacred." This definition reinforces the interrelatedness of the social and spiritual domains of the quality-of-life model (see **Fig. 1**), including God or a higher power as "family" and part of "personal relationship". "Family" may also be viewed as socially and spiritually connected through faith and meaning, whereas relationships with friends and family are sought to be connected through communication.

Spiritual well-being can then be viewed as relational, that is, involving relationships with others and with God (however one sees God), and as action-oriented, involving the interactional part of one's being.[21,22] Spirituality concepts can therefore apply to persons who are religious, nonreligious, or antireligious.[23] A growing body of evidence suggests an association between patients' spiritual lives and their experiences of illness.[6,24–29] Investigators have found that when people are faced with challenging situations, such as a diagnosis of terminal cancer, they draw on approaches that reflect a secure relationship with God or a higher power, a sense of spirituality, and a trustworthy world view.[30–33] Patients with cancer have less psychological distress if they are able to forgive others and if they find strength and comfort from their spiritual beliefs.[34] Patients whose illnesses were not terminal suffered from more depression and poorer quality of life and exhibited anger toward others if they perceived their illness as a punishment from God.[25]

Spiritual well-being is a complex phenomenon that comprises met and unmet spiritual needs as identified by the individual.[35] Some of these needs may be social needs.[2,36–38] Hermann[39] identified the following spiritual needs of dying patient, some of which reflect personal relationships that are typically constituents of a social well-being domain: (1) the need for involvement and control of one's life and care; (2) the desire for companionship with family, friends, and others; (3) the need for religion, including prayers, reading scripture, or attending religious services; (4) the need for life review; (5) the completion of life tasks; (6) the need for positive outlook by taking one day at a time; and (7) the resolution of negative feelings. Hermann then developed the spiritual needs inventory to help nurses recognize the broad perspective of spirituality and to raise an awareness that many of these needs would not be traditionally classified as a part of the spiritual domain. Spiritual needs can only be addressed adequately through an exchange of communication, a dialogue between providers and patients and/or between patients and their significant others. Through careful assessment of these exchanges and the importance that patients assign to them, clinicians can identify the key spiritual needs of patients and attend to them through guided communication.

COMMUNICATION AT THE END OF LIFE

The research conducted by the author (M.P.P.) suggests that interpersonal and spiritual relationships are vital for many patients at the end of life. The opportunity to communicate, raise awareness, and reaffirm close personal relationships may be a conduit that links the social and spiritual domains of quality of life at the end of life. Communication is an important means through which these relationships are formed, maintained, and changed. When patients are aware that they have limited time to spend with others, desires to deepen (and perhaps heal) these relationships may become paramount. Communication is the vehicle that allows such relationships to be acknowledged.

Among the various skills needed in the delivery of clinically competent end-of-life care, the ability to communicate effectively is the most important. Without this skill, little is possible. As George Bernard Shaw stated, "The single biggest problem in communication is the illusion that it has taken place."[40] This assumption can be applied to the clinician who is providing the care and the patient in relationship with self, others, and God or a higher power. Previous research conducted on communication between patient and physician[41–43] provides some understanding of the complexity of the communication dynamics and of the assumption that a clinician's natural abilities are sufficient to guide discussions. For example, Beckman and Frankel[44] analyzed 74 audiotapes of physicians talking to patients in a general family medicine clinic. The study revealed that in only 23% of the cases did physicians give patients a chance to fully disclose and describe their concerns. Perhaps some of these concerns surrounded personal relationships and the communication that was either occurring or not occurring in the time of the illness.

Much can be learned from attending to the factors patients and families have identified as important at the end of life. Clinicians can use their awareness of these key factors to facilitate important end-of-life conversations within personal relationships.' According to Steinhauser and colleagues, as well as other investigators,[6,8,12] attributes of a good death include being in control, being comfortable, being able to help others, saying and sharing important things, being able to be surrounded by family and friends, finding a sense of meaning and peace within oneself, having beliefs and values honored, making a positive difference in the lives of others, being prepared, and having a sense of life completion. By combining the art of communication as a clinician with the knowledge of what patients and families have described as important and necessary at the end of life, clinicians may be better able to facilitate conversations previously left unsaid or to affirm the relationships that have created a "life well-lived."

Communication at the end of life is sensitive, emotionally charged, and requires a skill set beyond most nurses' conception of clinical roles. Communication involves dynamic interactions among individuals with different communication styles based on cultural norms, personal and cultural values, developmental processes, and world views. In cases where death is not sudden, the anticipation of death may allow time for patients and their families to reflect on what needs to be said and how to say it. Communication is the vehicle that allows for such exchange.

Authentic communication at the end of life has the power to enhance people's ability to deal pragmatically with death while enlightening and deepening the meaning of life for dying patients and their loved ones.[45] The dying process often requires the dying patient and loved ones to slow down and pay more attention to the communication that can occu'r between them at the end of life.[46] Studies conducted recently[2,46,47] suggest that the messages most commonly expressed at the end of life involve love, gratitude, and forgiveness.

LOVE AND GRATITUDE

Individuals have a fundamental need for unconditional love, "a love that affirms and supports people just as they are and does not demand that they make themselves different in any way."[48] Love is defined as the integration of 3 biologically based behavioral systems: attachment, caregiving, and sexuality.[49] Love, which is rooted in a fundamental desire to be connected with another, has been linked with happiness and indicators of both psychological and physical health.[50] Expressions of love vary, in part to capture the dimensions of love. Between heterosexual couples, more than 80 different common expressions of love were described in a study, ranging from saying the words "I love you," being understanding and supportive, touching, spending time together, communicating emotion, and giving eye contact.[50] Expressions of love have the potential to positively affect patients' lives. This phenomenon has been examined predominantly in the healthy population and has received only limited investigation in patients with a limited life expectancy.

Gratitude has been defined as an act of appreciation and recognition through the expression of generosity—"Thank you."[51,52] By definition, gratitude is an interpersonal concept, though it can also include spiritual dimension. In internal and emotional terms, gratitude is a positive state that conveys a felt sense of wonder, thankfulness, and appreciation for life.[53] Some of the most profound and reported experiences of gratitude originate from the spiritual or existential domain.[54] For example, praising God for gifts and mercies is a common theme of gratitude in the world's religious traditions.[55] Although most empirical data on gratitude have been collected from undergraduate psychology students and therefore may not be applicable to the end-of-life population, there are some data that may apply to this population, including a seminal study conducted by McCullough and colleagues.[52] In 3 separate studies and with more than 1600 undergraduate psychology students, the investigators developed self-report measures of gratitude and confirmed that gratitude is empirically distinct from constructs such as life satisfaction, vitality, happiness, and optimism and is correlated with emotional well-being, forgiveness, and spirituality. Thus, gratitude and its expression may have a role that benefits the dying patient and loved one.

FORGIVENESS

Most modern scholars and scientists agree on several points about forgiveness.[17] First, they concur with Enright and Coyle[56] that forgiveness should be distinguished from pardon, excusing, and forgetting. Moreover, most scholars stress that the concept of forgiveness is distinct from reconciliation[57,58] and involves a more internal process of reducing bitter, resentful feelings and the desire for revenge, while possibly cultivating positive attitudes toward the offender.[59] In order to forgive, individuals may need to empathize with their offenders, trying to see the situation from the other person's perspective rather than focusing only on their own pain and anger.[60] The process of empathizing and reducing bitter feelings may be a strenuous one, requiring considerable time and effort.[58] When people have experienced severe, ongoing relational hurt, a single expression of "I forgive you" or "I am sorry" from either side may not be sufficient to repair the damage.

Some end-of-life clinicians, having facilitated or witnessed powerful experiences of forgiveness in cases of serious, unresolved conflicts, might assume that forgiveness is a crucial need for all patients at the end of life. However, this assumption has not been demonstrated empirically. Although the forgiveness process has been examined in the general population, further investigation is needed to provide conceptual clarity and valid measurement in the end-of-life population. It may be that just as grief is a process, so is forgiveness,[61] and therefore it may require different measurement strategies and communication guidance in the end-of-life population.

A few studies have begun to examine forgiveness in end-of-life contexts. For example, one recent investigation[62] conducted with 20 terminally ill patients examined the efficacy of a therapeutic intervention designed to facilitate forgiveness. The intervention, which involved 60-minute sessions for 4 weeks, led to improvements in self-reported quality of life. Another 3-arm pilot randomized controlled trial with 82 eligible hospice patients examined whether a forgiveness intervention, among other life completion and preparation activities, would affect physical functioning, emotional functioning, and quality of life at the end of life.[63] Although both studies revealed positive trends toward improved quality of life at the end of life, they also demonstrated the complexity of forgiveness research with dying patients as an intervention in a relationship to the element of time.

The aforementioned studies on forgiveness at the end of life provide a good foundation for future research and clinical efforts. More research is needed, however, to clarify the prevalence and significance of forgiveness at the end of life. Conducting forgiveness research with patients who have a limited life expectancy makes longitudinal research difficult. The complex and highly emotional nature of forgiveness work, coupled with a vulnerable population facing the end of their lives, not only increases the difficulty of facilitating these types of conversations but also complicates the rigorous conduct of research. Few people are qualified to facilitate this precarious work.

Psychotherapy literature in the recent past has reflected the growing interest among clinicians in using forgiveness interventions to help families and individuals seek resolution in damaged relationships, resolve long-standing relational problems, and let go of anger and bitterness.[64,65] Many of these studies have focused specifically on close relationships involving marriage and family; closeness and commitment in relationships can actually be a large part of what motivates people to forgive.[66] Teaching people how to empathize with their offenders is an important element in most forgiveness interventions.[67,68] Training in empathy may be particularly helpful for men, given that men are typically not able to empathize to the degree that women can.[69] In addition, many studies show that genuine, heartfelt apologies are robust facilitators of forgiveness and relational healing,[70] although caution is needed to ensure that apologies are not forced or premature.[71]

Self-forgiveness has become another major area of research.[72] Fisher and Exline[73] demonstrated that when people have harmed others seriously, feelings of remorse (which focus on the specific offense and the harm it caused) can bring some benefits by motivating people to apologize and to attempt relational repair. In contrast, feelings of self-condemnation (which involve seeing one's whole self as bad) are linked with depression and other indicators of poor mental health. An important task for clinicians then may be to convey support, affirmation, and acceptance to patients so that they can face their responsibility for interpersonal hurts without feeling condemned. Where appropriate and possible, qualified clinicians might also help to facilitate apologies as part of a process of self-forgiveness.

Unresolved conflicts with God (or a higher power) constitute another potentially important area for intervention. In the recent past, investigators have suggested that many people have a relationship with God much as they would with another person,[74] and some of them experience feelings of abandonment, anger, and disappointment in their perceived relationship with God. Situations involving death and illness are among the most common causes of such anger.[75] Investigators have shown that prolonged, frequent, or intense anger toward God is associated with mental health problems such as depression, anxiety, anger, and low levels of self-esteem and well-being.[76] Furthermore, anger toward God is associated with other sources of spiritual struggle, including doubts about God's existence, feeling punished by God, and religious conflicts with other individuals or institutions.[77] Spiritual struggles, including anger toward God, might then be an important facet of intervention designed to enhance spiritual well-being (and thus, quality of life) at the end of life. Because many nurses may not feel prepared to address these types of spiritual issues, collaboration with chaplains or spiritual care professionals may often be helpful.

These findings may have practical implications in end-of-life contexts. In **Box 1**, the authors present a list of 'suggestions that may help patients and family members navigate the process of interpersonal forgiveness, apology, self-forgiveness, and resolution of anger toward God.

Box 1
Forgiveness and apology: a brief summary of research findings

Anger and forgiveness

Anger is a natural response to injustice and can be an important signal of what is important to us. Chronic anger can lead to emotional and physical problems, so it is important not to ignore our anger but to learn from it.

Before trying to let go of angry feelings, it may be important to protect oneself from future harm. This might mean setting limits with the person who hurt you. If you do this, it is important to avoid name-calling and hostile criticism. Try saying, "When you did X, I felt hurt." or "It was hard for me when you did X."

People have many different understandings of the word forgiveness. Most scholars agree that forgiving does not mean excusing, forgetting, or pretending that an offense never occurred. Instead, forgiveness means letting go of bitter, grudging, or vengeful feelings. You might forgive someone while not completely trusting him or her.

People often experience forgiveness as a source of emotional relief. Bitter feelings and grudges use up emotional and psychological energy and can become heavy burdens.

Forgiveness can be difficult, especially for severe offenses in which the doer of harm has not apologized or accepted responsibility. The process could be a long one.

People often believe that they should forgive, perhaps because of religious beliefs or social pressure; however, they sometimes find that they cannot totally get rid of their feelings of anger. Writing in a journal or talking to another trusted person can help people resolve anger and find meaning in difficult situations.

Being able to empathize or putting yourself in the other person's shoes can make forgiveness easier. Can you try to see the situation from the other person's perspective?

Apology and self-forgiveness

If and when you apologize, be clear about what you did that was wrong. If you need a better understanding of what exactly you did that was wrong, respectfully ask the other person for clarification.

If the other person does not know about the offense at all, it will sometimes be more painful for him or her to learn about it than to not know. When it seems unwise to apologize directly, some people might find relief from their guilty feelings by confessing the wrongdoing to another close friend, a religious professional, or God. Keeping a journal may also help. You might also be able to take other steps to improve your relationship with the person you hurt; steps that do not involve revealing the offense.

Some people apologize too often and blame themselves for things that were not actually their fault (or that were not really wrong). If you really do believe that you did not do anything wrong, you might still benefit from talking to the other person about the problem and trying to understand why he or she felt hurt or offended. But it is usually best not to apologize unless you really see yourself as responsible for at least part of the problem.

Once you have done what you can to make things right, you might benefit from actively trying to forgive yourself for what you have done, thus releasing yourself from unnecessary guilt and pain.

Anger toward God

People are often reluctant to admit feelings of anger toward God because they see such feelings as morally wrong or taboo. It may be important to give yourself permission to examine these potentially frightening feelings.

People often see God in the same way that they see their parents. It may be useful to think about whether issues with your parents are affecting the way you see God.

Anger and disappointment with God cause some people to doubt God's existence. Sometimes the issue is intellectual; people cannot comprehend how a loving God could act in a way to cause them anger or disappointment. At other times, there is a sense of revenge in the disbelief or by thinking, "I will show you. I just won't believe in you anymore."

At present, there are no instruments or tested interventions that target patients who are coping with relational hurt and forgiveness issues at the end of life. A potentially important future goal for end-of-life care may be to help patients identify important hurts and, where applicable, to consider the possibility of forgiveness or apology. Clinicians have the potential to play a vital role by facilitating such conversations between dying patients and their families. The interdisciplinary team may play an important role in such a situation. Although such conversations may be difficult to navigate, successful attempts to facilitate resolution of interpersonal problems may help to promote good outcomes for the dying patients and their families.

A NOTE ON THE EXPRESSION OF "GOOD-BYE" OR "FAREWELL"

Proposed initially by Callahan and Kelley[78]and Byock[79] as "final opportunities" and "developmental landmarks," the concept of farewell and the related expression of "good-bye" seems to have different meanings to the patient when compared with that to the loved one or significant others. Several investigators[29,80] have researched factors considered important at the end of life by patients, family members, physicians, and other care providers. The relational expression of good-bye has not emerged as an important factor or been identified in other studies conducted with terminally ill patients. In 2 earlier studies, the notion of farewell was introduced within the structure of the interview as a probe question and did not emerge spontaneously within the context of the interview or the study instruments. Therefore, no conclusion can be made about the relevance or importance of saying good-bye in reference to patients' perspectives, and further investigation is needed. However, issues related to farewell may have major importance for loved ones who are bereaved.[47]

FINAL CONVERSATIONS WITH BEREAVED LOVED ONES

Until now, the focus of this article has been on personal relationships and communication at the end of life from the perspective of the dying patient. Recent research with bereaved loved ones suggests that important close relationships and communication messages extend beyond the time of death. In their ethnographic study, "Final conversations," Keeley and Yingling[81] reported on an in-depth exploration from the perspective of the bereaved and of the occurrence and meaning of conversations among dying persons and those close to them. Keeley[47] interviewed 82 bereaved loved ones on an average of 5 years after the death (range: 3 months to 27 years). Respondents described end-of-life communication as an important relational phenomenon. Keeley concluded that these final conversations had the ability, in many cases, to allow sharing of important memories, saying a meaningful good-bye, and to complete relationships by expressing love. For the bereaved, final conversations allowed an opportunity to talk about difficulties with the dying person in a way that enabled them to reach out to the latter, express gratitude, and engage in some reconciliation. The act of conversation and the exchange of dialogue that took place led to the comfort and validation of the beliefs of the bereaved.[46] In addition, bereaved family members who shared a final conversation about religion or spirituality and/or who shared a spiritual experience with their dying loved one experienced a validation of their beliefs.[47]

Although Keeley's research focused on conversations from the perspective of the bereaved family members, it lends support to the importance of end-of-life communication between patients and those considered close and important to them. The universality of the need for conversation and relationship at the end of life rapidly became apparent. In particular, the expression of love was central to final conversations. Dying patients and their families are often willing to engage in conversation and are eager to tell their stories, which has important implications for facilitating end-of-life research. Clinically, end-of-life communication has allowed patients and families to prepare emotionally for their impending loss and empowered the families to let go of their loved ones in ways that were perceived as easier than they had originally believed they would be.

WHAT CAN NURSES DO?

Communication is a skill that is improved with increased awareness and training. At the end of life, most communication is held behind closed doors or in hospital rooms, which may not be conducive to such intimate conversations. Most patients and families do not have effective models to draw from as they try to have satisfying and effective communication at the end of life. For nurses whose practice includes patients who are seriously ill or dying and their families, the facilitation of these discussions rarely comes naturally. Some clinicians might have an innate ability or a natural instinct to carry on such complex conversations; however, like most medical and nursing procedures, the specific skills for facilitating end-of-life conversations must be learned. Nurses may fear, often appropriately, that these discussions lie outside the purview of their role or expertise. Ultimately, nurses alone cannot resolve the issues that surround the relationship and facilitate its healing. Nurses may, however, initiate a conversation with patients and families about the opportunity for communication at the end of life. In addition, they are well placed to make the appropriate referrals to other team members who could work with the patients and family and other health care team members.

Nurses are central in the care of patients and their families at the end of life and are usually the professionals most intimately involved in their day-to-day care. As a result, nurses have a unique opportunity to make a difference in how patients live their final days. The support, guidance, and identification of personal relationships and communication messages by nurses have the potential to make a significant difference in the extent to which terminally ill patients die well and at peace. Furthermore, empirically based findings can help to provide a solid foundation for successful interventions.

WHERE DO WE GO FROM HERE, AND HOW CAN RESEARCH HELP?

The ultimate goal of end-of-life care is to improve the way people die. To improve the quality of nursing care at the end of life, careful application of relevant research findings is crucial. Unfortunately, several major challenges surround the study of communication at the end-of-life. First, valid and reliable instruments need to be developed to measure the phenomenon of close personal relationships and communication at the end of life, including how the relational expressions of love, gratitude, and forgiveness work, and their prevalence and importance (which might shift as death becomes imminent). Second, once adequate confirmation of this phenomenon has been established, specific communication interventions need to be empirically evaluated before being applied to the clinical setting. Increased understanding of how to identify patients and families with relationship issues is key to effective end-of-life clinical practice. In addition, nurses need adequate and proper tools to facilitate conversation and communication among the patient, family, and significant others.

The seminal health communication research by Buckman[42] may be a useful tool (**Box 2**). Although representative of many studies conducted in the context of patient and provider communication, these communication "pearls" may act as a starting point and reference for a clinician to encourage conversation between the terminally

---

Box 2
Communication pearls

- Communication is not one-way.
- Communication includes verbal and nonverbal messages.

Clinicians can

- Create an environment conductive for conversation, which would include quiet space, adequate lighting, and a private area.
- Encourage family members or loved ones not to anticipate what might be said next but listen.
- Provide permission to use silence in the conversation, which may help one feel better about not having the right words to say.
- Facilitate dialogue with no interruption.
- Encourage the use of the phrases "I see..."; "Tell me more..."; "So you mean..."; or "What you are saying is...."
- Encourage family members or loved ones not to change the subject even if it is uncomfortable.
- Encourage touching.

Data from Buckman R. Communication skills in palliative care: a practical guide. Neurol Clin 2001;19(4):989–1004; and ELNEC-Supercore Curriculum 2007; with permission.

---

ill patient and others considered close and important in the dying process. The relational messages expressed could be intrapersonal and interpersonal in nature.

SUMMARY

Avoidance of talk about death and the realization that death is a normal part of the life cycle are prevalent components of United States culture, which is in part because death, as viewed in the United States, is infused with fear and is often beyond the control of patients, families, and even health care providers. Being diagnosed with a life-limiting illness and facing death can evoke many painful emotions including anxiety, sadness, and uncertainty; however, it can also create the potential for profound growth and transformation. Embedded in this experience, and perhaps at the core of its meaning, are close personal relationships. Knowing that a loved one is dying usually elicits pain and suffering for those close to the dying person. Relational partners must also face the reality of the loss of the relationship and the accompanying social loss of the roles they once performed. Thus, despite this anguish of the unknown, having conversations about the relationship and communicating love, gratitude, and/or forgiveness may have potential benefits for the dying person and those considered close and important.

REFERENCES

1. Baumeister RF, Leary MR. The need to belong: desire for interpersonal attachments as a fundamental human motivation. Psychol Bull 1995;117(3):497–529.
2. Prince-Paul M. Understanding the meaning of social well-being at the end of life. Oncol Nurs Forum 2008;35(3):365–71.

3. Guyatt G, Rennie D, Attia J, et al. Users' guides to the medical literature: a manual for evidence-based clinical practice. Chicago (IL): Ama Press; 2002.

4. Ropka ME, Spencer-Cisek P. PRISM: priority symptom management project phase I: assessment. Oncology Nursing Forum 2001;28(10):1585–94.

5. Sulmasy DP. A biopsychosocial-spiritual model for the care of patients at the end of life. Gerontologist 2002;42(90003):24–33.

6. Emanuel EJ, Emanuel LL. The promise of a good death. Lancet 1998;351(Suppl 2):SII21–9.

7. Singer PA, Martin DK, Kelner M. Quality end-of-life care: patients' perspectives. JAMA 1999;281(2):163–8.

8. Steinhauser KE, Clipp EC, McNeilly M, et al. In search of a good death: observations of patients, families, and providers. Ann Intern Med 2000;132(10):825–32.

9. Kristjanson LJ, McPhee I, Pickstock S, et al. Palliative care nurses' perceptions of good and bad deaths and care expectations: a qualitative analysis. Int J Palliat Nurs 2001;7(3):129.

10. Schwartz CE, Mazor K, Rogers J, et al. Validation of a new measure of concept of a good death. J Palliat Med 2003;6(4):575–84.

11. Tong E, McGraw SA, Dobihal E, et al. What is a good death? Minority and non-minority perspectives. J Palliat Care 2003;19(3):168.

12. Kehl KA. Moving toward peace: an analysis of the concept of a good death. Am J Hosp Palliat Care 2006;23(4):277–86.

13. Cohen SR, Leis A. What determines the quality of life of terminally ill cancer patients from their own perspective? J Palliat Care 2002;18(1):48–58.

14. Ferrell BR, Grant M, Funk B, et al. Quality of life in breast cancer. Part I: physical and social well-being. Cancer Nurs 1997;20(6):398–408.

15. Ferrell BR, Grant M, Funk B, et al. Quality of life in breast cancer. Part II: psychological and spiritual well-being. Cancer Nurs 1998;21(1):1–9.

16. Prince-Paul M. Relationships among communicative acts, social well-being, and spiritual well-being on the quality of life at the end of life in patients with cancer enrolled in hospice. J Palliat Med 2008;11(1):20–5.

17. Peterson C, Seligman M. Character strengths and virtues: a handbook and classification. New York: American Psychological Association and Oxford Press; 2004.

18. Pulchalski C, Ferrell B, Virani R, et al. Improving the quality of spiritual care as a dimension of palliative care: the report of the consensus conference. J Palliat Med 2009;12(10):885–904.

19. National Consensus Project. Quality palliative care guidelines. Available at: http://www.nationalconsensusproject.org. Accessed September 15, 2009.

20. National Quality Forum. A national framework and preferred practices for palliative and hospice care: a consensus report. Available at: http://www.qualityforum.org/publications/reports/palliative.asp. Accessed September 15, 2009.

21. Kaut K. Religion, spirituality, and existentialism near the end of life. Am Behav Sci 2002;46(2):220–34.

22. Oldnall A. A critical analysis of nursing: meeting the spiritual needs of patients. J Adv Nurs 1996;23(1):138–44.

23. Dyson J, Cobb M, Forman D. The meaning of spirituality: a literature review. J Adv Nurs 1997;26(6):1183–8.

24. Puchalski CM. Spirituality and end-of-life care: a time for listening and caring. J Palliat Med 2002;5(2):289–94.

25. Pargament K, Smith B, Koenig HG, et al. Patterns of positive and negative religious coping with major life stressors. J Sci Study Relig 1998;37:717–24.
26. Cherny NI, Coyle N, Foley KM. Suffering in the advanced cancer patient: a definition and taxonomy. J Palliat Care 1994;10(2):57–70.
27. Moadel A, Morgan C, Fatone A, et al. Seeking meaning and hope: self-reported spiritual and existential needs among an ethnically-diverse cancer patient population. Psychooncology 1999;8(5):378–85.
28. Kearney M, Mount BM. Spiritual care of the dying patient. In: Chochinov H, Breitbart W, editors. Handbook of psychiatry in palliative care. Oxford (UK): Oxford University Press; 2000. p. 357–73.
29. Steinhauser KE, Christakis NA, Clipp EC, et al. Factors considered important at the end of life by patients, family, physicians, and other care providers. JAMA 2000;284(19):2476–82.
30. Yates JW, Chalmer BJ, St James P, et al. Religion in patients with advanced cancer. Med Pediatr Oncol 1981;9(2):121–8.
31. Hills J, Paice JA, Cameron JR, et al. Spirituality and distress in palliative care consultation. J Palliat Med 2005;8(4):782–8.
32. Pargament K, Ensing D, Falgout K. God help me: I. Religious coping efforts as predictors of the outcomes to significant negative life events. Am J Community Psychol 1990;18:793–824.
33. Pargament K, Hahn J. God and the just world: causal and coping attributions to god in health situations. J Sci Study Relig 1986;25(2):193–207.
34. Breitbart W, Rosenfeld B, Pessin H, et al. Depression, hopelessness, and desire for hastened death in terminally ill patients with cancer. JAMA 2000;284(22):2907–11.
35. Hermann CP. The degree to which spiritual needs of patients near the end of life are met. Oncol Nurs Forum 2007;34(1):70–8.
36. Hermann CP. Spiritual needs of dying patients: a qualitative study. Oncol Nurs Forum 2001;28(1):67–72.
37. Hampton DM, Hollis DE, Lloyd DA, et al. Spiritual needs of persons with advanced cancer. Am J Hosp Palliat Care 2007;24(1):42–8.
38. McMillan SC. The quality of life of patients with cancer receiving hospice care. Oncol Nurs Forum 1996;23(8):1221–8.
39. Hermann C. Development and testing of the spiritual needs inventory for patients near the end of life. Oncol Nurs Forum 2006;33(4):737–44.
40. Shaw GB. The doctor's dilemma. Int J Epidemiol 2003;32:910–5.
41. Back A. Patient-physician communication in oncology: what does the evidence show? Oncology (Williston Park) 2006;20(1):67–74 [discussion: 77–8, 83].
42. Buckman R. Communication skills in palliative care: a practical guide. Neurol Clin 2001;19(4):989–1004.
43. Back AL, Arnold RM, Tulsky JA, et al. Teaching communication skills to medical oncology fellows. J Clin Oncol 2003;21(12):2433.
44. Beckman HB, Frankel RM. The effect of physician behavior on the collection of data. Ann Intern Med 1984;101(5):692.
45. McQuellon RP, Cowan MA. Turning toward death together: conversation in mortal time. Am J Hosp Palliat Med 2000;17(5):312.
46. Keeley M. "Turning toward death together": the functions of messages during final conversations in close relationships. J Soc Pers Relat 2007;24(2):225–53.
47. Keeley MP. Final conversations: survivors' memorable messages concerning religious faith and spirituality. Health Commun 2004;16(1):87–104.

48. Keeley MP. Final conversations: messages of love. Qual Res Rep 2004;5(1): 34–40.

49. Shaver P, Collins N, Clark C. Attachment styles and internal working models of self and relationship partners. In: Fletcher G, Fitness J, editors. Knowledge structures in close relationships: a social psychological approach. New York: Springer-Verlag; 1996. p. 163–84.

50. Hendrick S, Hendrick C. Love. In: Snyder C, Lopez S, editors. Handbook of positive psychology. Oxford (UK): Oxford University Press; 2002. p. 472–85.

51. McCullough ME, Kilpatrick SD, Emmons RA, et al. Is gratitude a moral affect? Psychol Bull 2001;127(2):249–66.

52. McCullough ME, Emmons RA, Tsang JA. The grateful disposition: a conceptual and empirical topography. J Pers Soc Psychol 2002;82(1):112–27.

53. Emmons RA, Shelton C. Gratitude and the science of positive psychology. In: Snyder C, Lopez S, editors. Handbook of positive psychology. New York: Oxford University Press; 2005. p. 459–71.

54. Goodenough U. The sacred depths of nature. New York: Oxford University Press; 1998.

55. Emmons RA, Crumpler C. Gratitude as a human strength: appraising the evidence. J Soc Clin Psychol 2000;19(1):56–69.

56. Enright R, Coyle C. Researching the process model of forgiveness within psychological interventions. In: Worthington E, editor. Dimensions of forgiveness: psychological research and theological perspectives. Philadelphia: Templeton Foundation Press; 1998. p. 139–61.

57. Enright R, Gassin L, Wu C. Forgiveness: a developmental view. J Moral Educ 1992;21:99–114.

58. McCullough ME, Pargament K, Thoresen C, editors. Forgiveness: theory, research, and practice. New York: Guilford Press; 2000. p. 1–14.

59. Worthington EL. Handbook of forgiveness. New York: Routledge; 2005.

60. Hargrave TD. Forgiveness: a review of the theoretical and empirical literature. J Fam Ther 1994;20(1):21–36.

61. Ashby HU Jr. Being forgiven: toward a thicker description of forgiveness. J Pastoral Care Counsel 2003;57(2):143–52.

62. Hansen MJ, Enright RD, Baskin TW, et al. A palliative care intervention in forgiveness therapy for elderly terminally ill cancer patients. J Palliat Care 2009;25(1):51.

63. Steinhauser KE, Alexander SC, Byock IR, et al. Do preparation and life completion discussions improve functioning and quality of life in seriously ill patients? Pilot randomized control trial. J Palliat Med 2008;11(9):1234–40.

64. Butler MH, Dahlin SK, Fife ST. "Languaging" factors affecting clients' acceptance of forgiveness intervention in marital therapy. J Marital Fam Ther 2002;28(3): 285–98.

65. Ingersoll-Dayton B, Krause N. Self-forgiveness: a component of mental health in later life. Res Aging 2005;27(3):267–89.

66. Finkel EJ, Rusbult CE, Kumashiro M, et al. Dealing with betrayal in close relationships: does commitment promote forgiveness? J Pers Soc Psychol 2002;82(6): 956–74.

67. Enright RD, Fitzgibbons RP, Fitzgibbons RP. Helping clients forgive: an empirical guide for resolving anger and restoring hope: American Psychological Association Washington, DC; 2000.

68. Worthington EL. Dimensions of forgiveness: psychological research & theological perspectives. Philadelphia: Templeton Foundation Press; 1998.

69. Exline JJ, Baumeister RF, Zell AL, et al. Not so innocent: does seeing one's own capability for wrongdoing predict forgiveness? J Pers Soc Psychol 2008;94(3): 495.
70. Exline JJ, Worthington EL Jr, Hill P, et al. Forgiveness and justice: a research agenda for social and personality psychology. Pers Soc Psychol Rev 2003; 7(4):337.
71. Exline JJ, Deshea L, Holeman VT. Is apology worth the risk? Predictors, outcomes, and ways to avoid regret. J Soc Clin Psychol 2007;26(4):479–504.
72. Tangney JP, Boone AL, Dearing R. Forgiving the self: conceptual issues and empirical findings. Worthington EL Jr, editor. Handbook of forgiveness. New York: Routledge; 2005. p.143–58.
73. Fisher ML, Exline JJ. Self-forgiveness versus excusing: the roles of remorse, effort, and acceptance of responsibility. Self Ident 2006;5(2):127–46.
74. Kirkpatrick LA. Attachment, evolution, and the psychology of religion. New York: The Guilford Press; 2004.
75. Exline JJ, Park CL, Smyth JM, et al. Anger toward god: five foundational studies emphasizing predictors, doubts about god's existence, and adjustment to bereavement and cancer, 2009. [Epub ahead of print].
76. Exline JJ, Martin A. Anger toward God: a new frontier in forgiveness research. Worthington EL Jr, editor. Handbook of forgiveness. New York: Routledge; 2005. p. 73–88.
77. Exline JJ, Rose E. Religious and spiritual struggles. In: Paloutzian RF, Park CL, editors. Handbook of the psychology of religion. New York: Guilford; 2005. p. 315–30.
78. Callahan M, Kelley P. Final gifts. New York: Poseidon Press; 1992.
79. Byock IR. Dying well: the prospect for growth at the end of life. New York: Riverhead Books; 1997.
80. Greisinger AJ, Lorimor RJ, Aday LA, et al. Terminally ill cancer patients. Their most important concerns. Cancer Pract 1997;5(3):147–54.
81. Keeley M, Yingling J. Final conversations. Acton (MA): VanderWyk and Burnham; 2007.

Helping Parents Make and Survive End of Life Decisions for Their Seriously Ill Child

Pamela S. Hinds, PhD, RN*, Katherine Patterson Kelly, PhD, RN

KEYWORDS

- Pediatric end-of-life decision making
- Parent decision making • Decision-making guidelines

Nearly 25,000 children between the ages of 1 and 19 years die each year in the United States (http://www.cdc.gov/nchs/fastats/adolescent_health.htm,[1] http://www.childstats.gov/americaschildren/tables/phy7b.asp).[2] In a certain though unknown number of these deaths, parents are asked by health care professionals to discuss their child's serious clinical situation, including their child's diminished likelihood of survival and their preferences for end-of-life care for their child. This discussion cannot occur in clinical situations in which the child's death occurs quickly or unexpectedly such as in a life-ending trauma, and it is not likely to occur in certain countries or cultures where decision making is considered to be the domain of the physician only.[3] In several chronic illnesses, however, it is possible and likely that parents in the United States would participate in end-of-life decision making on behalf of their seriously ill child. In general, parents of chronically ill children report that they prefer to be involved in decision making about their ill child's end-of-life care, although they find this to be the most difficult of all treatment decisions that they have made.[4,5] Some, though not all parents, include their ill child in decision making. Whether the child is included or not, parent participation can be an opportunity for clinicians to enact care that may serve as a source of comfort to the parents in the immediate circumstance and in the longer term after the child's death.

Funding source: Portions of the work reported here were funded by the Oncology Nursing Foundation, the Project on Death in America, and the National Institute of Nursing Research (R21 NR008634).

Department of Nursing Research and Quality Outcomes, Children's National Medical Center, The George Washington University, 111 Michigan Avenue NW, Washington, DC 20010, USA
* Corresponding author.
E-mail address: pshinds@cnmc.org

Nurs Clin N Am 45 (2010) 465–474
doi:10.1016/j.cnur.2010.03.006
0029-6465/10/$ – see front matter © 2010 Elsevier Inc. All rights reserved.

nursing.theclinics.com

The authors' purpose here is to describe factors considered by parents who participate in end-of-life decision making on behalf of their seriously ill child, and strategies that nurses and other clinicians can implement to help parents emotionally survive the decision-making experience. The authors also describe a relationship-based model (Relational model of end-of-life treatment decision making) that depicts how clinicians may help facilitate end-of-life treatment decision making by parents on behalf of their ill child. Lastly, the authors offer an updated set of evidence-based practice guidelines that clinicians may find useful from the point of diagnosis of a life-threatening illness when helping parents make and survive end-of-life decision making for their seriously ill child. Although the vast majority of research on parental end-of-life decision making cited here, from which the model and the guidelines were derived, was completed in pediatric oncology or pediatric intensive care settings, there are important points of generalization across diseases and clinical settings.

BACKGROUND

Most of the end-of-life treatment decision making (care discussions that focus on the ill child's quality of life and focus on the child's family as the priority of care when survival is no longer believed possible) occurs in hospital settings. In the United States, 90% of children from ages 1 to 19 years receive hospital-based care during the final week to several months of their lives. Although an increasing number of families are choosing to take their ill child home to die after participating in end-of-life discussions and decision making, most of these ill children die in hospital settings.[6] Palliative and end-of-life discussions between parents, clinicians, and when possible the ill child, primarily take place during these inpatient interactions.

Some parents who prefer to take their child home to die are unable to do so because of the shortage of available home-based services (http://www.nhpco.org/files/public/Statistics_Research/NHPCO_facts_and_figures.pdf).[7] In addition, parents may not have professional bereavement services available to them after they leave the hospital setting. Thus, this final hospitalization may be the last opportunity for clinicians to interact in a supportive manner with parents. Hospital-based clinicians need to implement care strategies that meet parents' immediate support needs and need to have the potential of providing sustaining effects for the parents after the child dies.

CLINICAL CONTEXTUAL FEATURES INFLUENCING PARENTAL END-OF-LIFE DECISION MAKING

Seriously ill children who have experienced a life-threatening or life-limiting chronic illness tend to have a period of palliative care that includes a strong focus on symptom management and reduction of suffering secondary to the illness or its treatment. During this time period, parents and the ill child begin to ponder the chances of the child not recovering from the illness. Parents of chronically and acutely ill children rely on several different factors to assist them in their decision making.[8–10] Most of these factors are readily apparent to the parents, while others, although directly influencing their decision making, are difficult for parents to identify, define, or explain. It is important that health care professionals involved in the care of the seriously ill child and involved with the child's family help parents to explicate fully the factors they consider most relevant to their decision making. This involvement requires careful listening and thoughtful questioning by clinicians to help parents realize and reveal all the factors considered in their decision making. Research completed to date indicates that no single factor predicts or explains the parental decision making; some parents identify between 3 and 8 influencing factors.[11–13] The factors vary, but have in common a relationship element in that each factor reflects a caring concern for someone else, most commonly the ill child, or reflects valued information provided by trusted others.

Parents of seriously ill children are most commonly unable to tolerate a prolonged discussion of end-of-life treatment decision making or discussions about the grave status of their child. Parents report that although they privately consider the possibility that their child may not survive, this realization is too overwhelming to consider for more than a few intense moments at a time. Some parents have also reported thinking that it is too risky to speak aloud of their child's possible death, because this may make it more likely that the child would die.[14,15] The overwhelming realization of the child's grave situation can result in parents briefly acknowledging the situation and then immediately shifting the discussion to focus on a future desired event for the child, such as a family vacation.

Clinicians often fear that this conversation shift indicates that parents do not understand the gravity of the clinical situation; clinicians then shift the conversation back to the clinical situation in an effort to reinforce parental understanding. Parents, however, report that this clinician strategy is not helpful to them; they explain that they are well aware of the seriousness of their child's condition. Instead, parents have acknowledged at the time and subsequent to this behavior that they needed to maintain hope that their child would survive in the face of overwhelming horror related to the realization that their child could not survive. Without this kind of hope, parents fear they would not be able to function at this time and thus would risk not being able to take care of their ill child.[14,16]

Parents report desiring information about their child's clinical status, but more than a third describe this information as upsetting and unsettling.[17] There are also times when parents have reported not being able to consider or speak of their child's situation[18] and are thus not able to actively participate in end-of-life decision making during such times. Despite these human responses to information about their ill child, parents in the United States prefer to be involved in their child's treatment decision making, including at the end of life.[19]

FACTORS INFLUENCING PARENTAL END-OF-LIFE TREATMENT DECISION MAKING

The following factors have been reported in 2 or more studies of parental decision making and represent categories of influencing factors that are the most frequently reported by parents. The factors listed later are thus not the complete list of factors considered, and the order that the factors are presented does not signify the importance or frequency of occurrence.

Parental Trust of Clinicians

Parents acknowledge that trusting their child's clinicians, especially the child's physician, helps them to participate in treatment decision making.[4,20,21] Parents trust the clinicians to make reasoned judgments on behalf of the ill child and to consistently look out for the child's best interests. Involving parents in treatment and quality-of-life goal setting early in the child's course of illness and throughout the child's care continuum, including end-of-life, helps parents to trust that clinicians are indeed looking out for their child's best interests.[22] Parental trust of physicians and physician judgment making were reported to be associated with parental peace of mind related to treatment decision making in a study that relied on parent response to a questionnaire.[20]

Having Information About the Child's Status

Parents report that having access to understandable information about their child's health status influences their ability to participate in end-of-life decisions. This information includes the certainty that all reasonable attempts to save the child have been done and to the best possible ways.[4,23–25] In addition, parents appreciated information from experienced clinicians about how their child's status compares to other children in similar situations. Parents prefer that this kind of sobering information be couched in terms of what is unique and special about their ill child. Some parents prefer having direct recommendations from clinicians about treatment decision making and are apt to ask clinicians: "what would you do if this were your child?"[4,26]

Time to Understand the Serious Prognosis and Approaching Death

Parents have reported the benefit of having advanced knowledge of the child's serious and worsening condition and awareness of the child's impending death.[27,28] In one study, parents indicated a preference for at least a 24-hour awareness preceding the child's actual death.[29] In this same study, participating parents indicated that they had thoughts at times that death was preferable for their very ill and suffering child. It may be important to note that the above information was gathered from bereaved parents and thus was retrospectively solicited.

Feeling Supported by the Child's Clinicians

Parents' perceptions of being respected and trusted by their child's clinicians to make good decisions on behalf of their ill child in turn helps them to participate in their child's end-of-life treatment decision making.[11,24,30,31] Parents also report feeling supported by clinicians who allow them to speak of hope while participating in end-of-life decision making. More recent findings indicate that one way for clinicians to convey respect and support to parents of seriously ill children is to inquire about and honor the parents' internal definition of being a good parent to their seriously ill child.[30,32]

Although parents' definitions of being a good parent varied somewhat, core elements included being well informed about their child's situation, making informed and unselfish decisions in their child's best interest, being at their child's side even when doing so was difficult, showing the child how well loved the child is, advocating for the child with the clinical staff, promoting the child's health in all possible ways, and helping the child to make good life decisions.[30] Of importance, parents report that their ability to achieve their definition of being a good parent to their ill or dying child provides important emotional relief and meaning to them at the time the child's death and following the child's death. This immediate and later benefit to parents gives added importance to the clinician's role in supporting parents' efforts to achieve their personal definitions.

Parental Valuing of Their Ill Child's Preferences

Parents have indicated that they consider their child's stated or perceived preferences when contributing to end-of-life decision making. Parents report that they do not necessarily need to speak to their ill child directly at the time of such decision making about the child's preferences, because they tend to know these preferences from previous conversations or from sensing what their child would prefer.[4,33] Chronically ill children who have lived with a life-threatening or life-ending illness have had repeated opportunities to observe the changes in other ill children, and tend to ask about these children or tend to comment on their impressions of the status of these children to their parents. Chronically ill children are thought to have a more mature understanding of death than their healthy peers,[34] as conveyed in conversations with their parents or clinicians.

Faith

Across studies, a high number of parents have indicated that their religious faith sustains them during their treatment decision making. Thoughts that help parents to participate in end-of-life decision making include a certainty that the child would be in a better place after death and not be alone.[4,13] Some parents have reported that helping their child to believe in a greater being is part of being a good parent to a seriously ill child.[30]

Observing the Ill Child's Physical Changes

Parents have reported being persuaded by changes in their child's body that their child could not survive the illness. Similarly, parents have reported appreciating when clinicians share images of their ill child's internal body changes, because this helps them to conclude that their child's condition is serious. In contrast, parents have described not having such clues when their ill child was on a ventilator that seemed to modulate the child's physical responses.[35,36]

Monitoring Scientific Advances

Parents have described making contacts with others through various methods or using electronic searching of scientific literature to determine if any new treatments that might be relevant for their ill child are becoming available. Such parents have been quick to add that they are not doubting the capabilities of their child's clinicians,

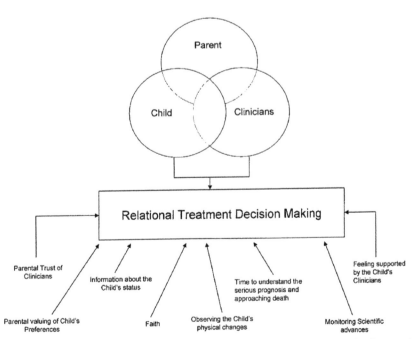

Fig. 1. Relational model of end-of-life treatment decision making: depicting the factors that influence parental decision making.

Box 1

Evidence-based guidelines for the health care team to facilitate parental end-of-life decision making

From diagnosis forward

1. At the time of diagnosis and throughout treatment, actively seek opportunities to provide honest and complete information to parents about treatment and their child's response to treatment.[37]

2. At the time of diagnosis and throughout treatment, involve parents in treatment and care-related discussions and decision making. Be available to discuss and rediscuss decisions and related concerns with parents.
   - At the time of diagnosis and at junctures in care, consistently ask parents to participate in goal setting for their child's medical care and quality of life.[13,38]

3. Verbally and nonverbally reassure parents that they are "good" parents whose knowledge of their child's preferences and their commitment to the child is unquestioned.[30]
   - Offer to assist parents in sharing information with their child.[39]

4. Give assurances that all that can be done to help the ill child is being done and being done well.
   - Expect and understand that parents are likely to seek other expert opinions about treatment and care.

From deterioration of the child's condition/situation forward

5. As the child's disease progresses or condition worsens, provide clear verbal, written, and visual explanations of the child's status.

6. Inform the parents of treatment (disease directed) and care (nondisease directed) options as they become available in the treatment setting or elsewhere.

From initiation of end-of-life discussions forward

7. Include interdisciplinary team members in end-of-life discussions with parents.
   - Share interdisciplinary assessments with parents.[38]
   - Document end-of-life discussions and make these discussions readily accessible to all members of the interdisciplinary team.

8. When discussing end-of-life care options:
   - Strongly emphasize the interdisciplinary team's commitment to the ill child and to providing expert care at all times.
   - Offer professional recommendations if parents so request.
   - Offer to describe how the ill child would likely respond to each care option (ie, the child's likely physical appearance, ability to communicate, and so forth).
   - Offer to describe the behaviors and symptoms that the ill child is most likely to have during the end of life.[27]
   - Inquire about parents' preference to discuss their faith and its influence on care decision making.[13]
   - Invite parents to share what they think are their ill child's preferences regarding end-of-life care.[30]

9. When discussing end-of-life options with parents, anticipate:
   - Parental vacillation between certainty and uncertainty about the decision.
   - Parents' need for clarification and additional information or repeated review of information to address their uncertainties.[37]

- Parental need for practical information about ways to explain the end-of-life decision to other family members.
- Being asked to offer personal advice (ie, "if this was your child, what would you do?").

10. Allow the parents time to consider the care options.
  - Anticipate that some parents would ask for estimates of how long their ill child would live.[28]
  - Anticipate that the parents would appreciate expressions of feelings and support by the team members.[30,37]

Providing ongoing support:

11. Maintain sensitivity to any specific ethnic, cultural, or religious preferences during the terminal stage.

12. Convey respect for the parents' right to change decisions when it is clinically feasible.

13. Demonstrate commitment to maintaining the child's comfort and dignity and to affirming parents' role.

14. Do not question the parents' decision after it has been made (ie, "are you sure that this is what you want?").

but that they are making certain they have done all that they can do as parents to save their child.[35,36]

RELATIONAL MODEL OF END-OF-LIFE TREATMENT DECISION MAKING

The factors discussed earlier identified as influencing parental participation in end-of-life decision making on behalf of their seriously ill child share a common element: they are all relationship-based. The relational nature of the factors reflects the influence of effective communication with clinicians, maintains trust relationships with clinicians, and allows parents to express their emotions. The factors also reflect the parents' caring and protective relationship with their ill child. Relational decision making involves the parents, ill child, and clinicians as depicted in **Fig. 1**. Their combined efforts are influenced by the factors mentioned earlier, with the combined outcomes being an increased focus on symptom management and reduction of suffering, on child and family quality of life, and on agreement regarding treatment options and choices.

REVISED EVIDENCE-BASED PRACTICE GUIDELINES FOR FACILITATING PARENTAL END-OF-LIFE TREATMENT DECISION MAKING

In 2001, 2 sources of evidence (completed studies on parental end-of-life treatment decision making, published recommendations from diverse professional associations) were analyzed by an interdisciplinary team of health care professionals to provide a base for evidence-based practice guidelines for use by clinicians when working with parents of children who had incurable cancer.[24] Although this set of guidelines was specific to one type of pediatric life-threatening disease, the evidence-based recommendations that comprise the guidelines may have broader applicability. The authors offer here an updated set of guidelines to assist parents in making and surviving end-of-life decision making from the point of diagnosis forward (**Box 1**). Each guideline reflects the relationship basis of end-of-life decision making in pediatrics and, most particularly, involving members of the interdisciplinary care team and the parents. This relationship begins at diagnosis and continues consistently throughout treatment, and includes offering medical information in various forms regarding the ill child's clinical status and providing personal advice as well as expressions of emotions and support. The relationship basis also involves members of the interdisciplinary team with each other, and includes providing information about the status of the child and the parental decision making as well as providing support for each other on the caregiving team. The blend of professional and personal involvement in end-of-life decision making on behalf of seriously ill children and their parents demands continuous clinician effort, availability, sincerity, and as a result, self-care.

SUMMARY

In the United States, parents of seriously ill children whose survival is no longer viewed by expert clinicians as medically possible are likely to be invited to participate in end-of-life discussions and decision making on behalf of their child. These parents want to protect and save their child's life even while they are participating in the discussions and decision making. Clinicians can directly help parents through the discussions and end-of-life decision making using a relationship-based approach that conveys clinician competence, compassion, sincerity, availability, and respect for parents' abilities to make reasoned decisions on behalf of their ill child. In this helping role, clinicians need to be mindful of the multiple factors that influenced the parents' decision making, and be attentive to the importance of these factors at the time of and following decision making. Most particularly, clinicians need to attend to how the parents define being a good parent to their very ill child. Being mindful of these aspects of care at this point in a child's life helps the clinicians to help the parents in the immediate circumstances and into the future in ways that continue to offer the parents comfort after their child has died.

ACKNOWLEDGMENTS

The authors acknowledge with sincere gratitude the formatting contributions to this work from Dorienda R. Britton.

REFERENCES

1. Centers for Disease Control and Prevention. Adolescent health. Available at: http://www.cdc.gov/nchs/FASTATS/adolescent_health.htm. Accessed November 2, 2009.
2. Forum on Child and Family Statistics. Adolescent mortality. Available at: http://www.childstats.gov/americaschildren/tables/phy7b.asp. Accessed November 2, 2009.
3. Carnevale FA, Canoui P, Cremer R, et al. Parental involvement in treatment decisions regarding their critically ill child: a comparative study of France and Quebec. Pediatr Crit Care Med 2007;8(4):337–42.
4. Hinds PS, Oakes L, Furman W, et al. Decision making by parents and healthcare professionals when considering continued care for pediatric patients with cancer. Oncol Nurs Forum 1997;24(9):1523–8.
5. Hinds PS, Schum L, Baker JN, et al. Key factors affecting dying children and their families. J Palliat Med 2005;8(Suppl 1):S70–8.
6. Field MJ, Behrman RE. When children die: improving palliative and end-of-life care for children and their families. Washington, DC: The National Academies Press; 2003.

7. National Hospice and Palliative Care Organization. NHPCO facts and figures: hospice care in America. 2009. Available at: http://www.nhpco.org/files/public/Statistics_Research/NHPCO_facts_and_figures.pdf. Accessed December 3, 2009.

8. Davies B, Deveau E, Veber BD, et al. Experiences of mothers in five countries whose child died of cancer. Cancer Nurs 1998;21(5):301–11.

9. Michelson KN, Koogler T, Sullivan C, et al. Parental views on withdrawal life-sustaining therapies in critically ill children. Arch Pediatr Adolesc Med 2009;163(11):986–92.

10. Sharman M, Meert KL, Sarnaik AP. What influences parents' decisions to limit or withdraw life support. Pediatr Crit Care Med 2005;6(5):513–8.

11. Hinds PS, Oakes L, Quargnenti A, et al. An international feasibility study of parental decision making in pediatric oncology. Oncol Nurs Forum 2000;27(8):1233–43.

12. Kirschbaum MS. Life support decisions for children: what do parents value? ANS Adv Nurs Sci 1996;19(1):51–71.

13. Meyer EC, Burns JP, Griffith JL, et al. Parental perspectives on end-of-life care in the pediatric intensive care unit. Crit Care Med 2002;30(1):226–31.

14. Hinds PS, Birenbaum LK, Clarke-Steffen L, et al. Coming to terms: parents' response to a first cancer recurrence in their child. Nurs Res 1996;45(3):148–53.

15. Hinds PS, Birenbaum L, Pedrosa AM, et al. Guidelines for the recurrence of pediatric cancer. Semin Oncol Nurs 2002;18(1):50–9.

16. Monterosso L, Kristjanson LJ. Supportive and palliative needs of families of children who die from cancer: an Australian study. Palliat Med 2008;22(1):59–69.

17. Mack JW, Wolfe J, Grier HE, et al. Communication about prognosis between parents and physicians of children with cancer: parent preferences and the impact of prognostic information. J Clin Oncol 2006;24(33):5265–70.

18. Oppenheim D, Valteau-Couanet D, Vasselon S, et al. How do parents perceive high-dose chemotherapy and autologous stem cell transplantation for their children. Bone Marrow Transplant 2002;30(1):35–9.

19. Contro N, Larson J, Scofield S, et al. Family perspectives on the quality of pediatric palliative care. Arch Pediatr Adolesc Med 2002;156(1):14–9.

20. Mack JW, Wolfe J, Cook EF, et al. Peace of mind and sense of purpose as core existential issues among parents of children with cancer. Arch Pediatr Adolesc Med 2009;163(6):519–24.

21. Nuss SL, Hinds PS, LaFond DA. Collaborative clinical research on end-of-life care in pediatric oncology. Semin Oncol Nurs 2005;21(2):125–34.

22. Baker JN, Hinds PS, Spunt SL, et al. Integration of palliative care practices into the ongoing care of children with cancer: individualized care planning and coordination. Pediatr Clin North Am 2008;55(1):223–50, xii.

23. Brinchmann BS, Forde R, Nortredt P. What matters to parents? A qualitative study of parents' experiences with life-and-death decisions concerning their premature infants. Nurs Ethics 2002;122(21):388–404.

24. Hinds PS, Oakes L, Furman W, et al. End-of-life decision making by adolescents, parents, and healthcare providers in pediatric oncology. Cancer Nurs 2001;24(2):122–36.

25. Hunt K, France E, Ziebland S, et al. 'My brain couldn't move from planning a birth to planning a funeral': a qualitative study of parents' experiences of decisions after ending a pregnancy for fetal abnormality. Int J Nurs Stud 2009;46(8):1111–21.

26. Truog RD. "Doctor, if this were your child, what would you do?". Pediatrics 1999;103(1):153–4.

27. Pritchard M, Burghen E, Srivastava DK, et al. Cancer-related symptoms most concerning to parents during the last week and last day of their child's life. Pediatrics 2008;121(5):e1301–9.
28. Pritchard M, Srivastava DK, Okuma JO, et al. Bereaved parents' perceptions about when their child's cancer-related death would occur. J Pain Symptom Manage 2009;38(4):561–7.
29. Hunt H, Valdimarsdottir U, Mucci L, et al. When death appears best for the child with severe malignancy: a nationwide parental follow-up. Palliat Med 2006;20(6):567–77.
30. Hinds PS, Oakes LL, Hicks J, et al. "Trying to be a good parent" as defined by interviews with parents who made end-of-life decisions for their children. J Clin Oncol 2009;27(35):5979–85.
31. Meert KL, Thurston CS, Sarnaik AP. End-of-life decision-making and satisfaction with care: parental perspectives. Pediatr Crit Care Med 2000;1(2):179–85.
32. Woodgate RL. Living in a world without closure: reality for parents who have experienced the death of a child. J Palliat Care 2006;22(2):75–82.
33. Hinds PS, Drew D, Oakes LL, et al. End-of-life care preferences of pediatric patients with cancer. J Clin Oncol 2005;23(36):9146–54.
34. Hurwitz CA, Duncan J, Wolfe J. Caring for the child with cancer at the close of life: "there are people who make it, and I'm hoping I'm one of them". JAMA 2004; 292(17):2141–9.
35. Hinds P, Haase J. Quality of life in children and adolescents with cancer. In: King C, Hinds P, editors. Quality of life from nursing and patient perspectives. Boston (MA): Jones and Bartlett; 2003. p. 143–68.
36. Hinds PS, Oakes LL, Hicks J, et al. End-of-life care for children and adolescents. Semin Oncol Nurs 2005;21(1):53–62.
37. Truog RD, Meyer EC, Burns JP. Toward interventions to improve end-of-life care in the pediatric intensive care unit. Crit Care Med 2006;34(11):S373–9.
38. Baker JN, Barfield R, Hinds PS, et al. A process to facilitate decision making in pediatric stem cell transplantation: the individualized care planning and coordination model. Biol Blood Marrow Transplant 2007;13(3):245–54.
39. Beal EA, Baile WF, Aaron J. Silence is not golden: communicating with children dying from cancer. J Clin Oncol 2005;23(15):3629–31.

Living with Cancer: Perspectives on a Five Year Journey

Neville E. Strumpf, PhD, RN[a],*, Karen Buhler-Wilkerson, PhD, RN[b,†]

KEYWORDS

- Ovarian cancer • Living with cancer
- Caregivers • Palliative care

"There is a land of the living and a land of the dead and the bridge is love, the only survival, the only meaning."
—Thornton Wilder, The Bridge of San Luis Rey

THE BEGINNING

For a month prior to diagnosis (in 2004), there were vague symptoms: bloating, gastrointestinal distress, nausea, and general unease. Oddly enough, we read a newspaper article during that time about ovarian cancer and its insidious presentation, considered the possibility of ovarian cancer, and then rejected it. K.B.W. had recently celebrated her 60th birthday and we were about to leave for a two week vacation in Ireland. But as the date loomed closer, symptoms worsened and could no longer be ignored. A visit to a primary care physician first suggested gastritis, but with no abatement in symptoms, a CT scan was ordered. The day before our scheduled departure, the physician called with news that K.B.W. had ascites.

As nurses, we concluded immediately that the probable diagnosis was ovarian cancer. Our fears were quickly confirmed by an oncologist who treated K.B.W.'s earlier breast cancer (alas, we were not strangers to this multifaceted disease). A rapid, but careful decision was needed to determine where treatment would occur—whether at our employing institution, with its renowned academic medical center, or elsewhere. In the end, we chose "home," where we felt some sense of "control" (if such exists under these circumstances).

Nevertheless, there was still a two week wait for surgery, which corresponded precisely with the time period of our now aborted vacation. Although bags were

[a] Hartford Center of Geriatric Nursing Excellence, University of Pennsylvania School of Nursing, 418 Curie Boulevard, Philadelphia, PA 19106-4217, USA
[b] Barbara Bates Center for the Study of the History of Nursing, University of Pennsylvania School of Nursing, Philadelphia, PA, USA
[†] Deceased.
* Corresponding author.
E-mail address: strumpf@nursing.upenn.edu

Nurs Clin N Am 45 (2010) 475–489
doi:10.1016/j.cnur.2010.04.003
0029-6465/10/$ – see front matter © 2010 Published by Elsevier Inc.

nursing.theclinics.com

packed and calendars cleared, we had nowhere to go. The unknown remained before us. With much time on our hands, we read the literature in carefully limited doses. What, after all, does one do with more than 6,000,000 hits when Googling ovarian cancer?

Distraction was the key to sanity, and we created good moments, which became a trademark survival mechanism. We shopped at K-Mart for Martha Stewart sheets and towels when she was convicted of fraud; went to escapist movies (*Spiderman*) or watched provocative Irish films (not necessarily comforting with their Catholic sense of foreboding); sought solace on week-ends in the country; and gathered with family and friends who were aware of the diagnosis. To the extent possible, we focused on the day, and the fact that we "knew only what we knew at the moment," which was far from everything, including, at this point, the results of surgery or the prospects for treatment later. We did our best to keep at bay the alarming statistics on ovarian cancer, with its frequent recurrence, treatment morbidity, and limited prognosis.

In between diagnosis and surgery, three episodes of severe abdominal swelling and shortness of breath occurred, necessitating trips to the emergency room for paracentesis and drainage of many liters of ascitic fluid. The day before surgery we watched a video provided by the physician's office, although the words "gynecologic cancers" were never used. The film portrayed four women of varying ages, races, and social circumstances, all of whom had undergone both simpler and more complex surgeries. General descriptions were provided of the likely hospital course and postoperative recovery. At the conclusion, we knew little and perhaps just as well.

On the morning of surgery, K.B.W. was accompanied to the doors of the operating room by her two devoted sons and N.E.S., where we said good-bye as cheerfully as possible. She recalls how cold it was, how lonely and terrifying the wait for surgery can be. For family left behind, there remains an equally agonizing and even longer wait, staring at others immersed in their own thoughts, jumping to attention with every announcement, gazing at the wall monitor for progress on a loved one's movements from administration of anesthesia, to actual surgery, and finally to the post-anesthesia care unit. When the surgeon called, perhaps 3 or 4 hours later, he reported a successful "debulking of the tumor" (horrible phrase), and said that a brief visit was possible. Even with support from the peri-operative nurse responsible for the family waiting room, and considerable foreknowledge about the appearance of a post-operative patient, the first sight of a loved one attached to complex technical apparatus and demonstrating the visible manifestations of pain is deeply disturbing and induces near-total helplessness.

HOSPITALIZATION

Within days, we were informed that the stage of ovarian cancer was IIIC, meaning far advanced, but gratefully, not metastatic. For two weeks, N.E.S. was at the hospital daily, but rarely more than 6–8 hours, generally timed to coincide with physician rounds, conversations with nurse specialists, and specific treatment or teaching sessions. Being at once nurses, and a patient and a caregiver too, affords many insights inextricably bound to nursing itself. As knowledgeable professionals now in the caring hands of others, some of whom we had trained and many of whom we knew personally or who knew of us, we were mindful of the demands placed on staff nurses and the practical realities of hospital care. We thus consciously balanced our capabilities in self-sufficiency with our needs for attention.

Despite excellent care by an accomplished baccalaureate and master's prepared nursing staff, and an ever-present team of skilled residents under the supervision of a superb attending physician, N.E.S. understood and accepted the need for vigilance on a busy hospital unit with many complicated obstetric and gynecologic cases. Late on a Saturday evening, after a week in the hospital, K.B.W. became increasingly short of breath, and attributed it to the large number of floral arrangements, which were then removed at once. In a much earlier era of nursing care, flowers were in fact routinely taken from the room at night, in order to protect the patient from the ill effects of miasma or "bad air." Efforts to employ this old-fashioned technique, and to alert the resident on call to the problem, elicited minimal concern, and by Sunday morning, when N.E.S. arrived to assess the situation further, it was worse. The nurse in charge, a colleague, still remembers it as a "day from hell," when a severe thunderstorm caused a flood in the basement that created a power outage throughout much of the hospital, except for a bare minimum of electricity provided by an auxiliary generator. Against this backdrop, several emergencies unfolded on the unit, ours being merely one of them. Despite heparinization, faithful adherence to deep-breathing exercises with a respiratory spirometer, and frequent mobilization, hypercoagulability of the blood caused a pulmonary embolus, diagnosed by N.E.S. hours before its likely detection otherwise.

K.B.W.'s recollections of the event focus mainly on the trauma of an excruciatingly painful transfer from bed to stretcher to table for a lung scan, only for the technician, moments later, to discover that the equipment was disabled by the power failure. A functioning machine, attached to an alternative source of power, had to be found, and another painful transfer had to be made. On that day, N.E.S. could do little to shake still vivid memories of caring, as a young staff nurse almost 40 years before, for a woman dying from ovarian cancer with a desolate husband at her side, her belly swollen, utterly unresponsive to chemotherapy, and in unremitting pain.

From the beginning, K.B.W. confronted her physician with questions about her prognosis. Within days of surgery, she was asking what her chances were of living until her 70th birthday. K.B.W. was just 60, and we were both well aware of the statistics. We respected and appreciated the impossible nature of such questions, especially the difficulty in answering with precision, despite our honest and forthright desire "to know." Our consummate physician, as he probably did hundreds of times before given his clientele of women with gynecologic cancers, chose a balanced path, described by Renee Fox,[1] a noted medical sociologist, as one between "positive tenacity" and "medical uncertainty."[(p157)] Frankly, neither of us remembers his answer exactly, but our recollection is of a response that was assured, practiced, and most importantly, comforting. Throughout our journey, we have remained ever grateful for the wisdom, balance, honesty, and nuance that have characterized every uniquely intimate conversation with K.B.W.'s attending physician and many of his fellows. We appreciate that delivering a precise prognosis, except by inference, is impossible, and to date none has been offered. Furthermore, we probably do not want it anyway. We will know when the end is near.

Based on face-to-face interviews with physicians, Nicholas Christakis[2] writes compellingly, in *Death Foretold*, that doctors associate prognostication with death and believe that formulating negative prognoses and communicating them to patients constitute "self-fulfilling prophecies." Many physicians argue that concrete estimates of survival can cause as much harm as good, and as Christakis discovered, prognoses, when made, are most often incorrect. It is one thing to discuss prognosis with your physician. But it is another to extend that conversation beyond the doctor's office. So many of our nonmedical colleagues frequently asked us, point blank, "What is the prognosis?" Apparently the human desire for a definitive answer, realistic or not, well placed or completely misplaced, is powerful and pervasive.

K.B.W. hated the nights and dreaded sleeplessness. Nothing made time pass, and the slow passage of the clock's long hand easily turned five minutes into a discouraging five hours. Yes, patients, if they ever do finally doze off, are awakened for routine nighttime checks, although we learned, after a little experimentation, that a night light minimized this disruption to a degree (with a night light, the nurses did not flip on those glaring overhead fluorescent bulbs). The appearance of the residents on morning rounds, usually about 6 AM, brought a sigh of relief—a difficult and lingering night was at last over.

Privacy, or the lack of it, had to be dealt with, too. This is a tradeoff, one we readily recognized and accepted with the deliberate decision to remain on "home territory" for treatment. There was no breach, per se, of any details of illness, but communications among colleagues were inescapable. The best strategy was straightforward and honest information, usually in the form of periodic e-mails, neither denying diagnosis nor minimizing the need for further treatment. This tempered most rumors, which only occasionally cropped up, the most lethal being word of terminal cancer and placement on hospice.

Spirituality, our own and that of others, was crucial. We were surprised and touched by an outpouring of religious tokens, including a rosary purchased at the Vatican, images of Our Lady of Guadalupe, Lourdes water, Native American objects of healing, and a small statue of a Hindu God, as well as prayers by friends of all faiths: Jews, Muslims, Christians, and a few persons eschewing any religious affiliation whatsoever. In a highly secular and scientific world, such revelations exposed a deeply personal humanity. The frequency of spiritually-based comments from so many physicians and nurses was striking. Although pure speculation on our part, it may be that physicians and nurses, especially those who care for persons with life threatening and incurable diseases, do rely, as we do, on a deep sense of faith. Many mentioned, in more casual conversations, the impact on healing of faith, prayer, and a strong system of support.

DISCHARGE

The literature is replete with innumerable arguments for thoughtful and early discharge planning, and a sizable body of evidence exists concerning the positive outcomes of such care. Even in a university setting where significant data have been amassed on this topic, notably the work of Mary Naylor on transitional care,[3–5] our discharge seemed rushed and frenetic. In a matter of hours, irrigation of a peripherally inserted central catheter (PICC), injections of Lovenox, and wound inspection and management had to be mastered.

Yes, a home care nurse would visit, but discharge of a fragile person, swollen by 30 pounds of excess fluid and barely able to get in and out of bed or to use the toilet without assistance was no small thing for any caregiver, even a nurse. When supports readily available in the hospital disappeared, particularly the security created by a web of experts, the weight of care suddenly felt immense and frightening. The discharge planner saw to it that equipment and medical supplies arrived in timely fashion, but it was small recompense in comparison with the myriad tasks of daily physical care, meal preparation, attention to medications, and endless efforts to promote comfort.

Added to this were daily internal struggles to metabolize our situation and to make sense of what had happened. Our therapist made a home visit, and her advice was helpful and sensible. In handling the transition from "our beautiful life" to "living with cancer," she urged us to make a concentrated effort to experience something joyful every day and to maintain our deep-seated confidence that we would weather this storm. An unexpected byproduct was far more time together than usual, including the silences, often as deeply understood as words themselves. It was a valuable and serendipitous gift.

TREATMENT AND RECOVERY

Although typically chemotherapy for ovarian cancer begins weeks after surgery, circumstances warranted immediate treatment, which started in the hospital with taxol and carboplatin. Thus, the weeks immediately following discharge from the hospital also required adjustment to the rigors of chemotherapeutic agents and their side effects, most significant among them fatigue, hair loss (in anticipation, K.B.W.'s hair was cut very short prior to surgery), dry mouth and oral changes, muscle aches and pains (especially in response to repeated injections of Neulasta), and loss of appetite (for months, only "white" foods appealed to K.B.W., for example, scrambled eggs, mashed potatoes, chicken, soups, pasta with butter, ice cream). For two "foodies" and enthusiastic cooks, as well as avid followers of the local restaurant scene, this was an enormous change. Not only were worries about neutropenia ever present, but we also attended closely to K.B.W.'s International Normalized Ratio (INR) in response to coumadin. In tandem, this meant worries about any possibility of infection (avoidance of crowds, young grandchildren) and innumerable dietary considerations (no fresh or uncooked food, limited intake of Vitamin K). Preoccupation with illness and its management consumed nearly all psychic space.

K.B.W.'s decidedly uncharacteristic introspection and detachment from her surroundings were initially troubling, and it is difficult to remember exactly when life began to resume a sense of normalcy. When it happened, however, her alertness, energy, and engagement were noticeably different. We interpret this transition as a necessary step in harnessing inward strength, mentally and physically, to heal. With time, and between chemotherapy sessions, which occurred every three weeks, K.B.W. gradually resumed meal preparation (and dining out), took longer and longer daily walks, socialized more, and regained capacity for concentration on other than junk magazines.

Chemotherapy, with the exception of one reaction to taxol, went smoothly, and the CA-125 tumor marker encouragingly returned to normal after two rounds of therapy. We ventured to a meeting of the American Academy of Nursing, where K.B.W. received a media award for her contributions to an exhibit at Philadelphia's Fabric Workshop, "RN: The Past, Present, and Future of the Nurses' Uniform." We began preparations for the Thanksgiving and Christmas holidays, and decided, perhaps foolishly, to get a standard poodle puppy, which was added to a household already dominated by six cats! It looked like the New Year would bring some closure to this chapter of our ordeal.

MAINTENANCE THERAPY

On what we thought was the eighth and last visit for chemotherapy, the surgeon-oncologist recommended an additional year of taxol, despite the fact that remission had been attained. The recommendation was the result of a now well-known study by Markman and colleagues,[6] which reported that prolonged maintenance therapy with paclitaxel or taxol (ie, 12 months vs 3 months) was associated with longer progression-free survival but not with longer overall survival, and this benefit appeared to be limited to patients with the lowest CA-125 levels (and presumably, the lowest tumor burdens) at study entry. We learned later that this study was the focus of hotly debated early stopping rules for clinical trials which show positive results before accrual of subjects has ended, thus suggesting treatment effects that may be overly optimistic.[7,8] Elsewhere, the ethical conflicts in providing informed consent in clinical trials[9] were noted, along with the need, in the absence of a confirmatory clinical trial, for physicians to discuss the possible survival benefits of maintenance therapy with patients.[10] Our physician carefully and objectively discussed these potential benefits with us. We found little reason not to continue treatment, other than its side effects, which were undeniably a hindrance but otherwise were by no means completely debilitating. Reading the literature, discussing it with one's physician, and being the patient bring into clear focus the embedded clinical realities and scientific complexities of reasoned approaches to ongoing treatment. Medicine still remains as much art as science.

With another year of chemotherapy before us, the newly acquired puppy was marvelously therapeutic, becoming a helpful focus as K.B.W. readjusted her sights on a much extended period of recovery. We were committed now, more than ever, to go on living, and during that year traveled to Venice, the Adirondacks, and the Grand Canyon, all of which were carefully scheduled to avoid the nadir following chemotherapy.

Oddly enough, the chemotherapy sessions were emotionally therapeutic, affording the chance to bond with many other women and families experiencing life threatening gynecologic cancers. We congregated in a special suite, with permanently assigned staff who knew each patient well, and in an environment that was both comforting and reassuring. Later, for reasons of their own, hospital administrators eliminated this special unit in favor of a new cancer center in a modern building. Sadly, what might have been gained by spacious and light-filled lobbies, technical efficiencies, and streamlined staffing patterns, came about by sacrificing the caring, communal space that had existed before it.

REMISSION

More than a year and a half after diagnosis, we arrived at what the New York Times journalist, Dana Jennings, treated for an aggressive prostate cancer, called "post-treatment letdown," the loss of the comforting rituals that over many months make treatment "feel as familiar as a job." With an end to the structure of chemotherapy, and its predictable patterns of complete collapse, renewed energy, and collapse again, "one snuggles up against uncertainty and 'what's next?'[11]

Mishel defines uncertainty as the "inability to determine the meaning of illness-related events." She found that the "longer chronically ill persons lived with continual uncertainty, the more positively they evaluated that uncertainty," thus "opening doors to new alternatives in adjusting to the changing nature of illness."[12] Other than inevitable stresses induced by quarterly tumor marker checks and physician visits, the realities of living with cancer no longer consumed every waking moment, unless symptoms became more bothersome or new ones surfaced.

Rarely described in the medical literature or discussed by physicians are the "ambiguous boundaries and the complex interplay between doing good and doing harm."[1(p150)] Surgery, in the words of Atul Gawande,[13] is an act of "calculated violence" performed with a "righteous faith that it [is] somehow good for the patient."[(p16)] Common sense dictates that no one argues against the merits of surgery or chemotherapy, itself a calculated poisoning, in cases of life threatening illness. Assuming one survives, consequences of treatment inevitably occur, although "foretelling precisely which patients will experience adverse effects, and protecting against these eventualities, is not easily accomplished."[1(p156)]

Perhaps worries about self-fulfilling prophecies prevent many health care providers from discussing symptoms in advance of their actual appearance. Among such undisclosed symptoms are "chemo brain," the cognitive fogginess associated with chemotherapy, which is well known to patients and may take many months to subside. Impairment in memory and concentration is unpleasant for anyone, possibly more so for an academic. Thus, when K.B.W. began the necessary research for a policy analysis of American home care, it was a major step. The research required painstaking effort, and the resulting manuscript needed numerous revisions, but when finally accepted by The Milbank Quarterly, it was cause for genuine celebration.[14]

Adhesions and hernias are additional "iatrogenic" and unspoken complications, which can present with often alarming gastrointestinal symptoms. Sudden, severe abdominal pain and projectile vomiting first occurred in the summer of 2006 while traveling in the Adirondacks. The problem turned out to be a partial obstruction, and with a brief hospitalization and decompression, the matter resolved itself. But it was the beginning of many similarly unpredictable episodes, several of which occurred on a later vacation in France. We were increasingly reluctant to travel, but were encouraged to do so both by our surgeon-oncologist and the gastroenterologist, each of whom concluded that we should continue living life as fully as possible.

We eventually grew more adept at managing these situations through dietary discretion, medications, and abdominal rest when symptoms occurred. Despite many advances in symptom management, few could offer much advice concerning adhesions. Early in 2008, there was a total obstruction due to a hernia, which resulted in major surgery, but also provided an accidental opportunity for a "second-look" and showed no evidence of cancer. Four years had now gone by and we were mesmerized by the thought that the cancer was "beaten."

RECURRENCE

The tumor marker and the CT scan were normal, so the symptoms of yet another bowel obstruction in the fall of 2008 were upsetting, but not overly worrisome. It seemed so routine, in fact, that N.E.S. went home to work during the surgery, with plans to return to the hospital later. When the phone rang much too soon, the news was not good: the cancer had returned and a lengthy and extensive surgery was under way.

The jolt brought by this unwelcome intrusion was devastating in its impact. Although we had always known recurrence was highly likely, we had shoved that reality farther and farther from consciousness. K.B.W. had spent months regaining her physical fitness with regular and vigorous bicycling and exercise, we had just returned from several weeks of hiking and canoeing, and we were increasingly looking forward to more years ahead. In an instant, this hope, even if unrealistic, was shattered.

The meaning of recurrence needed to be processed and decoded. Immediately, we both tried to determine if the cancer was terminal. We were repeatedly reassured that it was treatable. Nevertheless, a careless comment by the discharge planner about enrollment in "pre-hospice" set off new fears that physicians were not telling us the truth. A disagreement also arose with a palliative care nurse specialist over the amount of pain medication, which, while needed, was in its current dose and method of delivery (patient controlled analgesia) interfering with the return of bowel sounds (during surgery, half of K.B.W.'s small intestine was removed). These incidents, no doubt unintentional, contained an undercurrent of presumed terminality. A few well-meaning, but poorly articulated comments about the "awfulness of the disease" from friends, whose mothers had died of ovarian cancer, didn't help either.

One might ask whether we sought the truth — or simply preferred to deny it. Actually, we did both. Objectively, we knew the typical trajectory of ovarian cancer, a trajectory with discouraging aggregate statistics. We also had knowledge of women with ovarian cancer who had lived for many, many years, despite recurrences. We were unwilling to surrender, yet remained keenly aware that at some point, as yet unknown, we would need to summon the courage to recognize the end of the war. We once hated military metaphors for cancer, but they grew more and more apt. Appropriately and accurately, Sarah Kagan[15] refers to "blessings and battles" in her recent book, *Cancer in the Lives of Older Americans*.

Following three weeks in the hospital, and recuperation of many months to heal a large, open abdominal wound, chemotherapy resumed, this time with eight rounds of taxol, carboplatin, and avastin. Once more, we had the privilege and the means to fight, and we were well aware that it was a privilege not granted equally to all, including access to drugs like Zofran (for nausea) and Neulasta (for neutropenia), both of which are extraordinarily expensive and not reimbursed by all insurance plans.

PALLIATIVE CARE AND CAREGIVING

Treatment for recurrent ovarian cancer reframes the meaning of illness for patient and caregiver. Meghani[16] rightly notes that palliative care is not necessarily about those who are "dying," but is designed for those for whom "alleviation of suffering and improvement in quality of life remain very relevant goals." Gradually, we recognized movement to another phase with new questions: How should decisions be made, roles negotiated, temperaments and styles readjusted, tolerance and tolerability among partners managed? Nevertheless, we made every effort to continue our lives as we had for more than five years, living with unpredictability, but nevertheless living fully and with meaning.

The ragged edges of illness cannot disappear and are never completely out of consciousness: Is this the last trip to our beloved Adirondacks, the last Christmas? Should we have any scruples about buying the things that please us? How should each of us spend our time, together and separately? Can we get through a day without mentioning ovarian cancer? Symptom obsession is unavoidable, whether the trigger is an upset stomach, a diarrheal episode, tongue mapping, unusual fatigue, or the reappearance of a hernia. We vacillate between discussing it or not, because such conversations can feel tiresome and endless at times, for both of us. We actually talk often about death, although perhaps too comfortably, as if we could "domesticate it, file down its claws," make it normal.[17] The *when* and *how* of death, however, is another matter, one that causes more than a few sleepless nights.

"Caregiver burden" may have gone out of fashion as a term and a topic of research,[18] but the weight of caring is immense, and must be terribly so for those with far fewer resources than we are blessed to have at our disposal. In her article for *The Milbank Quarterly*, "Care of the chronically ill at home: An unresolved dilemma in health policy for the United States," K.B.W. remarks on the cost of unpaid caregiving by family caregivers (mostly women). Despite the gratification felt by many to serve as caregiver for a loved one, "its physical, mental, and economic costs are undeniable," and often require skill in technically sophisticated medical tasks, exquisite attention to care coordination, and extraordinary resilience in the face of constantly shifting health status."[14(p625)]

The cornerstones of palliative care are thoughtful advance directives, stated goals for treatment and symptom management, and identification of essential psychosocial supports. Each of us must consider our preferences and values in these areas and make them known to health care providers, verbally and in writing. Patients and caregivers understand their needs and experience illness as a unique, personal, idiosyncratic event, not just a disease.[19]

In her book, *After Shock*, for which we were interviewed, Jessie Gruman[20] offers advice on navigating this landscape, including the needs for routine, distraction, personal time, as well as time with friends and family; physical and mental relaxation; reading and writing; explorations and affirmations of spirituality; counseling and therapy. Gruman, a survivor of four life-threatening illnesses, says her book is about "taking care of yourself while your heart is breaking" [(pxv)], and we would agree that her argument for informed choices, even difficult ones, is in itself empowering. We have carefully executed legal documents and have discussed funeral plans.

At the time of Ted Kennedy's death, a friend remarked of him and his wife, "They never wasted a day."[21(pA1)] One of the gifts of cancer is simply that: head-on confrontation with the day, not tomorrow or next week, let alone next year. The day could be spent in a thousand possible ways, many of them mundane, but as journalist Dana Jennings[11] observed: "Cancer and surgery ... make [you] look and listen, smell and touch with the eagerness of an explorer entering uncharted territory." We have learned to avoid misery, and more importantly, being miserable. But we practice it over and over again!

SUMMARY

Often we were asked, and asked ourselves, who is the target audience for this article and what is its message? In short, we were invited to write a personal narrative detailing for professionals the impact of cancer on two lives among thousands. As nurses, we also illuminate the experience of two individuals who become a patient and a care giver, and are in turn cared for by those personally close to them or with whom they share a deeply rooted set of common beliefs, values, and expertise.

We had, and continue to have, excellent and advantaged care. Still, we suggest that health professionals continue to explore new ways to prepare patients and families for their journeys, especially anticipation of symptoms and likely illness trajectories. In recent years, many advances have been made in the treatment of pain, nausea, vomiting, and fatigue, but there is much to be learned about less clear cut symptoms like abdominal adhesions and chemo brain. Although rarely a problem for us, most patients and family members are likely to need easy and clear access to the relevant provider for symptom management, especially during and immediately after chemotherapy, following discharge for major surgery, and as end stage disease becomes more apparent. Although patients no doubt do at times "worry themselves into another problem," anticipatory guidance on symptoms that could emerge is much needed and would be welcomed by most patients and families. In addition, more attention must be given to adequate preoperative preparation for cancer surgery. Can we provide better support for patients waiting in the operating room, for example, or take greater pains to ensure a restful night's sleep during hospitalization? For patients and families who will endure months and possibly years of chemotherapy, what is an ideal environment for the administration of these therapies? Based on our experience, we would recommend an environment that affords privacy and communality, silence and conversation, and opportunities for meaningful dialogue with health care professionals. Our story reaffirms the centrality of expert and compassionate care, along with timely and honest communication, as crucial to the preservation of integrity, dignity, control, and hope in the face of serious illness.

EPILOGUE

We hoped our conclusion, completed at the end of August 2009, was the end of our story. Since then K.B.W. was hospitalized five times in eight weeks for severe abdominal pain and vomiting. When her doctor told us that K.B.W. had multiple and inoperable bowel obstructions from adhesions, hernias, and carcinomatosis, it felt as if the last rung had been taken from the ladder of hope upon which we had stood for so long. Gently we were told by K.B.W.'s physician that the likelihood of ever again achieving normal bowel function was slender—bringing to an end all of the special joys associated with cooking, eating, entertaining, and traveling. K.B.W. is adjusting far better than most to this cruel punishment (and definitely better than N.E.S.), bravely attaching herself to total parenteral nutrition (TPN) each evening, enduring the indignity of a draining gastrostomy tube, medicating herself constantly for abdominal pain, and accepting another round of chemotherapy with doxirubicin (Doxil).

In a review of current management strategies for ovarian cancer in *Mayo Clinic Proceedings*, the authors note that palliation is all that remains with inoperable bowel obstruction, adding this sobering comment: "There is little clear cut justification for the use of parenteral nutrition" in these cases.[22(p769)] K.B.W. refers to her TPN as BLD (breakfast, lunch, and dinner) and continues to take daily walks, drive her antique Porsche, get a pedicure, enjoy visits with friends and family, and work on her next scholarly paper (she says this one is not the last). We focus daily on what we can do, rather than on what we can't. K.B.W. is teaching N.E.S. what she never bothered to learn, from operating a DVD player to turning on a gas grill, at the same time demonstrating to everyone around her the true meaning of courage, perseverance, and laughter. Thanksgiving and Christmas are coming and we are grateful for the time still granted to us—we wait and hope as we sit on what we call a "palliative plateau."

> "If I am to stand up, help me to stand bravely. If I am to sit still, help to sit quietly. If I am to lie low, help me to do it patiently. And if I am to do nothing, let me do it gallantly."

Book of Common Prayer,[p461]

[The manuscript to this point was submitted on November 18, 2009.]

(Editor's note: After the authors submitted their manuscript, N.E.S. continued to chronicle their experience on the "palliative plateau" with periodic email bulletins to more than 300 family, friends, and colleagues. What follows is an edited version of these bulletins.)

From: Strumpf, Neville
Sent: Tuesday, November 24, 2009 9:29 AM
Subject: RE: update on Karen Wilkerson–11-24-09

Dearest Friends,

Karen has had another hospitalization (severe abdominal pain due to trapped barium from an earlier upper GI series, now resolving), two Porsche rides, several glasses of Pouilly-Fuisse, and her first taste of Irish whiskey in months. Mostly, however, she sups on hot water with lemon, which is very soothing.

Pain is now in better control, and there are small signs that her bowel obstructions may be easing (for those of you who are nurses and doctors, you will know what those signs are!). Karen began a once per month course of Doxil on the 17th—this is an anti-tumor antibiotic produced by the soil fungus *Streptomyces*; it is encapsulated in a STEALTH liposome which defies detection by the body's immune system, allowing the drug to circulate longer and get closer to tumor cells. Side effects so far have been relatively minor, other than fatigue. Pain is also now in much better control.

Thanksgiving, always a large and festive occasion celebrated over many years with 20 or more people, will be very modest this year, with only my 91-year-old dad, brother, and two friends joining us.

A dear friend has prepared a rich homemade consommé of beef and veal for Karen (from Julia Child's *Mastering the Art of French Cooking*; if you have never done this, it is a monumental feat), and I am making Karen a homemade lemon sorbet with mint and a dash of vodka. For the rest of the guests, I will prepare my first ever turkey, and have over the course of the past week been collecting much advice as well as reviewing the debates (stuffing in or out, high heat and fast vs moderate and longer.) Under Karen's watchful eye, I plan to brine and then follow the instructions in "Cook's Illustrated"—where 60 recipes and techniques were tested before producing a final version.

Karen continues to be grateful for the continued stream of cards, visitors, and dozens and dozens of other acts of kindness and care. She notes with her characteristic good humor, despite her eating challenges and limitations, that one must be grateful for a functioning GI system at this time of year. We send our love for a Happy Thanksgiving, a day under any circumstances that is always worth the effort. Neville (and Karen)

From: Strumpf, Neville
Sent: Saturday, December 19, 2009 6:05 PM
Subject: RE: update on Karen Wilkerson–12-19-09

It is snowing heavily in Philadelphia—most unusual in December, but silent and gorgeous. Karen and I, and our black standard poodle PhePhe, had a lovely walk to nearby Fitler Square this afternoon.

I am happy to report that my Thanksgiving turkey was a success, and that we had a perfect day. Immediately afterward, Karen did unfortunately develop a fungemia, a fungal infection in her bloodstream, and had yet another hospitalization (her fifth since early October). But she responded well to IV therapy, and has reached a solid "palliative plateau."

We continue to tinker with a medication algorithm to control symptoms, and to increase daily activities in an effort to combat fatigue. But overall, things are a bit better. Karen attended a lecture, and two parties, in the last week, was out driving and doing some errands, and she is actively engaged with Christmas preparations. The tree is decorated, with great help from the grandchildren, and we are anticipating a beautiful Christmas day celebration with family. A thousand thanks to all of you for the support that continues to come our way unabated—we wish all of you happiness and peace at this season and always. With Love and Gratitude, Neville and Karen

From: Strumpf, Neville
Sent: Thu 1/7/2010 10:55 PM
Subject: Update on Karen Wilkerson

Karen and I had the best possible Christmas and New Year. Christmas day itself contained the magic that goes with trees, presents, family (especially grandchildren and their electric trains); and for New Year's Day, Karen found the strength to make hoppin' john (black eyed peas, rice, and bacon) and collard greens to share with family for good luck in 2010.

Since then, Karen has become gradually much weaker. Yesterday, despite all of my best efforts, I was unable to get her symptoms of nausea and pain under control, coupled with worsening balance, mental status, and fluid retention. I e-mailed her physician, who agreed that return to the hospital was the best option.

Our eternally vigilant advocates and nurse friends on the special care unit at The Pavilion at the Hospital of the University of Pennsylvania (HUP) made it all happen very quickly…. and Karen is resting there now fairly comfortably. Her symptoms are in better control, and we had a very useful consult today with HUP's in-patient hospice program. We agreed that on Monday, we would re-evaluate and make a decision about next steps.

Karen's sons, Jonathan and David, and their wives, Kerri and Marie, are with us, and we continue to be surrounded by an incredible web of loving support. What appears to an imminent conclusion to an earthly journey is only in God's hands.

I say with confidence, however, that despite Karen's diminishment, she is brave, patient, gallant, and unafraid, still her own person, still in control of her destiny, entirely without bitterness or anger, and teaching all around her how to live, how to love, and how to die.

From: Strumpf, Neville
Sent: Tuesday, January 12, 2010 12:13 PM
Subject: RE: update on Karen Wilkerson–1-12-10

Following my e-mail on Thursday evening, January 7, reporting Karen's declining health, she rallied almost miraculously. In fact, about 5 minutes after I sent the January 7 e-mail, at 10:55 PM, Karen called to say she was "awake." I read her the e-mail that I had just sent, and her reply was, "Good grief!"

Since then, she has been better each day, with pain and nausea in control with a new medication algorithm, fluids in balance, mind clear as a bell, and sense of humor restored. We learned, during the hospice consult, that neither chemotherapy nor TPN are permitted, and therefore that is a non-option for us at this time. Fortunately, we can continue with very strong support from Penn Home Infusion Services (to manage the PCA pump and the TPN) and Penn's Caring Way Program to manage symptoms.

An extraordinary medical and nursing team at HUP remains at our disposal via e-mail and phone. On Saturday evening, with the kindness of nurses and staff on The Pavilion, we had a joyous combined birthday celebration for Karen's son Jonathan, and the grandchildren, Sonya and Billy, who were permitted to visit the hospital. (They came with their favorite "stuffies" to keep Karen company at night).

We had pizza from Toccanelli's, and a chocolate birthday cake with lighted dinosaurs on top, thanks to the kitchen staff and the concierge.

The plan is for Karen to come home tomorrow. We are learning that this is a very unpredictable journey with the following lessons:

1. Continue to live each precious day to the fullest;
2. Understand that the future cannot be controlled; and
3. Expect that events will continue to reveal the awesome adventure of life.

From: Strumpf, Neville
Sent: Sunday, January 31, 2010 10:05 PM
Subject: RE: update on Karen Wilkerson–1-31-10

Karen came home on Jan. 13, and had a wonderful visit with her brother for the weekend immediately following that included a special meal featuring homemade Greek lemon soup prepared by our personal trainer (who is Greek), and a walk down the street for a haircut with Karen's favorite hair guy.

On Sunday, Jan. 24, Karen developed severe symptoms of nausea, vomiting, pain, fever, confusion, and weakness, and was transferred yet again to the hospital (this time, by ambulance).

Over the course of this past week, we made a decision to move to in-patient hospice care at the Hospital of the University of Pennsylvania, on the special unit (The Pavilion) where Karen has been cared for since late September. We are moving in the direction of less "aggressive" care, yet keeping in mind the fluidity of the situation. Although occasionally confused, Karen remains ever herself, and had a pedicure and a massage in recent days, as well as wonderful visits with family and close friends. She longs to come home, and if possible, we will do that.

From: Strumpf, Neville
Sent: Sun 2/14/2010 6:23 PM
Subject: Karen's earthly journey is complete

Dearest Friends,

So many of you have followed our journey lovingly and patiently for a very long time—you can never know what that has meant to us, regardless of the form that concern might have taken—which was considerable and abundant.

Last Sunday, Karen had a remarkably good day following our epic snowstorm, and asked to be wheeled around the hospital to view it, in all its magnificent snowy-white glory. (Karen insisted that a photograph be taken of the two of us in front of the Rhoads Building Courtyard at HUP.)

Later that evening she wanted a glass of wine, very rare for her at this juncture. We toasted to 17 years in life together—the anniversary of our coming together would have been today, Valentine's Day. She said, "How wonderful!" as we clinked some clunky hospital wine glasses. We watched part of the Super Bowl, and most importantly the halftime concert by The Who. And poetically, the Saints won.

After that Karen went to sleep so peacefully. On the day of her death, Saturday, February 13, we were serenaded in the early morning by the night supervisor—and a former student of mine—who so gorgeously sang "Our Father Who Art in Heaven." Karen opened her eyes and said, "Thank you." It was unquestionably one of those unforgettable moments that brings one full circle—a student who becomes a valued colleague, and who in the end takes you home.

Karen's children and their wives spent much of the day with her on Saturday, while I took a short break of several hours. I returned to the hospital about 7 PM and suggested that the children leave. Karen died at 8:30 PM. A wonderful night nurse tenderly left me, and later the children, with lots of time, and much support, at this most intimate of moments.

All of the physicians who were on call from the gynecologic-oncology service came to say good-by to us, and to Karen, as had many of her doctors and nurses throughout the previous few days. We were all touched and blessed by Karen's life—her humor and courage, her grace under duress, and her unyielding will to live until the very end.

Love, Neville

(Editor's note: Word of Karen's death triggered an avalanche of tributes and an outpouring of love. As Neville said, "The magnitude and force of her life, her 'incandescent presence,' as one neighbor put it, have been reflected in hundreds of e-mails, websites, facebook pages, announcements, photo displays, cards, gifts and mementoes, tears, laughter, and an immense circle of love.")

On Thursday, Feb. 18, an overflow gathering of more than 300 of Karen Buhler-Wilkerson's closest friends joined her family in celebration of an extraordinary life at Philadelphia's Trinity Memorial Episcopal Church. Neville Strumpf delivered the eulogy.)

ACKNOWLEDGMENTS

The authors express their gratitude to Renee C. Fox for her wise counsel during the preparation of this paper, Sarah H. Kagan for her ever-present clinical wisdom, Ruth Ouimette for a helpful early read, and the nurses and physicians at the Hospital of the University of Pennsylvania for their exquisite compassion and care throughout our journey. We are particularly indebted to the staff on The Pavilion, where K.B.W. was hospitalized ten times in the final months of her life. Additionally, N.E.S. expresses her gratitude to Jim Gardner for his careful editing of the manuscript and his editorial assistance with e-mail bulletins sent after the manuscript was completed, and which are appended at the end.

REFERENCES

1. Fox RC. Toward an ethics of iatrogenesis. In: La Fleur W, editor. Dark medicine: rationalizing unethical medical research. Bloomington (IN); Indianapolis (IN): Indiana University Press; 2007. p. 149–64.
2. Christakis N. Death foretold: prophecy and prognosis in medical care. Chicago: University of Chicago Press; 1999.
3. Naylor M, Brooten D, Jones R, et al. Comprehensive discharge planning for the hospitalized elderly: a randomized clinical trial. Ann Intern Med 1994;120(12): 999–1006.
4. Naylor M. Comprehensive discharge planning and home follow-up of hospitalized elders: a randomized controlled trial. J Natl Med Assoc 1999;281:613–20.
5. Naylor M, Brooten D, Campbell R, et al. Transitional care of older adults hospitalized with heart failure: a randomized clinical trial. J Am Geriatr Soc 2004;52(5): 675–84.
6. Markman M, Liu PY, Wilczynski S, et al. Phase III randomized trial of 12 versus 3 months of maintenance paclitaxel in patients with advanced ovarian cancer after complete response to platinum and paclitaxel-based chemotherapy: a Southwest Oncology Group and Gynecologic Oncology Group Trial. J Clin Oncol 2003;13: 2460–5.
7. Cannistra S. The ethics of early stopping rules: who is protecting whom? J Clin Oncol 2004;22:1542–5.
8. Korn EL, Freidlin B, Mooney M. Stopping or reporting early for positive results in randomized clinical trials: the National Cancer Institute Cooperative Group experience from 1990–2005. J Clin Oncol 2009;27(10):1712–21.
9. Markman M. Ethical conflict in providing informed consent for clinical trials: a problematic example from the gynecologic cancer research community. Oncologist 2004;9(1):3–7.
10. Thigpen T. Maybe more is better. J Clin Oncol 2003;21(13):2454–6.
11. Jennings D. Losing a comforting ritual: treatment. NY Times. June 30, 2009;D5.
12. Mishel MH. Reconceptualization of the uncertainty in illness theory. Image J Nurs Sch 1990;22:256–64.
13. Gawande A. Complications: a surgeon's notes on an imperfect science. New York: Henry Holt and Company; 2002.

14. Buhler-Wilkerson K. Care of the chronically ill at home: an unresolved dilemma in health policy for the United States. Milbank Q 2007;85:611–39.

15. Kagan SH. Cancer in the lives of older Americans: blessings and battles. Philadelphia: University of Pennsylvania Press; 2009.

16. Meghani SH. A concept analyis of palliative care in the United States. J Adv Nurs 2004;46(2):152–61.

17. Scarboro E. Giving myself consent to let go [review]. NY Times. September 6, 2009;6. Available at: http://www.nytimes.com/2009/09/06/fashion/06love.html?_r=1&pagewanted=print#. Accessed April 23, 2010.

18. Levine C, Murray TH. The cultures of caregiving: conflict and common ground among families, health professionals, and policy makers. Baltimore (MD): The Johns Hopkins Press; 2004.

19. Lowenstein JK. The weight of shared lives: truth telling and family caregiving. In: Levine C, Murray TH, editors. The cultures of caregiving: conflict and common ground among families, health professionals, and policy makers. Baltimore (MD): The Johns Hopkins Press; 2004. p. 47–53.

20. Gruman J. After shock: what to do when the doctor gives you—or someone you love—a devastating diagnosis. New York: Walker & Company; 2007.

21. Rimer S. Kennedy's closest confidante, in politics and life. NY Times. August 29, 2009; A1, A12. Available at: http://www.nytimes.com/2009/08/29/us/politics/29vicki.html. Accessed April 23, 2010.

22. Aletti GD, Gallenberg LC, Cliby WA, et al. Current management strategies for ovarian cancer. Mayo Clin Proc 2007;82(6):751–70.

Index

Note: Page numbers of article titles are in **boldface** type.

A

Abdominal massage, for constipation in palliative and end of life care, 287–288
Adolescents, cancer in parents of, recruiting for end of life research, **441–448**
Advance care planning, in model of care for sickle cell disease, 380–381
Aging, demographics of illness and, 271–273
Ascites, in end-stage liver disease, 413–414
Asphyxial threat, in patients with dyspnea, 365–366
    fear activation by, 365
    fear and pulmonary stress behaviors across cognitive states, 366

B

Bacterial peritonitis, spontaneous, in end-stage liver disease, 413–414
Bad death, after withdrawal of life-sustaining therapy, **427–440**
Barriers. See Disparity, in health care.
Behavioral assessment, of respiratory distress in patients who can not report dyspnea, 365
Bereavement, coping with, in model of care for sickle cell disease, 389–392
    final conversations with loved ones, 457–458
Bisphosphonates, for pain management in palliative and end of life care, 308

C

Cancer, barriers to palliative care for low-income patients in late stages of, **399–409**
    access to hospice, 403
    access to pain control, 402–403
    communication and understanding, 404
    education and health literacy, 404
    overcoming, 404–406
    study of, 400-401
    perspectives on living with, **475–484**
Caregivers, perspectives on living with cancer, **475–484**
Children. See Pediatrics.
Chinese herbal therapies, for pain management in palliative and end of life care, 310
Cognitive behavioral techniques, for pain management in palliative and end of life care, 309
Cognitive impairment, prevalence of dyspnea and, at end of life, 363–364
Communication, barriers to palliative care in low-income patients in late stages
    of cancer, 404
    issues with, in model of care for patients with sickle cell disease, 378
    messages and personal relationships at the end of life, **449–463**
        expressions of good bye or farewell, 457
        final conversations with bereaved loved ones, 457–458

Nurs Clin N Am 45 (2010) 491–500
doi:10.1016/S0029-6465(10)00063-0
0029-6465/10/$ – see front matter © 2010 Elsevier Inc. All rights reserved.

nursing.theclinics.com

Moving?

Make sure your subscription moves with you!

To notify us of your new address, find your **Clinics Account Number** (located on your mailing label above your name), and contact customer service at:

Email: journalscustomerservice-usa@elsevier.com

800-654-2452 (subscribers in the U.S. & Canada)
314-447-8871 (subscribers outside of the U.S. & Canada)

Fax number: 314-447-8029

Elsevier Health Sciences Division
Subscription Customer Service
3251 Riverport Lane
Maryland Heights, MO 63043

*To ensure uninterrupted delivery of your subscription, please notify us at least 4 weeks in advance of move.

Printed and bound by CPI Group (UK) Ltd, Croydon, CR0 4YY

03/10/2024

01040453-0005